Culture, Religion, and Ethnomedicine

The Tibetan Diaspora in India

Igor Pietkiewicz

UNIVERSITY PRESS OF AMERICA,® INC.
Lanham • Boulder • New York • Toronto • Plymouth, UK

4501 Forbes Boulevard
Suite 200
Lanham, Maryland 20706
UPA Acquisitions Department (301) 459-3366

Estover Road
Plymouth PL6 7PY
United Kingdom

Printed in the United States of America
British Library Cataloging in Publication Information Available

Library of Congress Control Number: 2008930727
ISBN-13: 978-0-7618-4134-0 (paperback : alk. paper)
ISBN-10: 0-7618-4134-2 (paperback : alk. paper)
eISBN-13: 978-0-7618-4204-0
eISBN-10: 0-7618-4204-7

A free companion website that includes extensive additional material, including full-color photographs, is available at www.CULTUREandMEDICINE.com

∞™ The paper used in this publication meets the minimum requirements of American National Standard for Information Sciences—Permanence of Paper for Printed Library Materials, ANSI Z39.48—1984

Contents

Preface		v
Acknowledgments		ix
Introduction		xi
1	Tibetan Culture, Religion, and Acculturation	1
2	Health and Illness Behaviors	36
3	Religion and Health	94
4	Tibetan Buddhism in Tibet and in Exile	116
5	The Traditional Tibetan System of Medicine in Tibet and in Exile	142
6	Empirical Research	163
7	Presenting and Analyzing the Qualitative Data	184
8	Discussion and Conclusions	240
Appendixes		253
Bibliography		265
Index		281

Preface

While the idea of doing research on the Tibetan diaspora came up unexpectedly, it dovetailed with my previous interests. As a psychotherapist, I was interested in health issues, and had analyzed the principles behind various paradigms of medicine. Having focused on the idiom of health and disease, I had also investigated the adaptive, informative, and transgressive function of illnesses. Arthur Kleinmann's writings on medical anthropology, in which he described cross-cultural phenomena in clinical contexts, were a source of inspiration.

Following some clinical observation and literature study of patients suffering from cancer, I decided to perform research in that area. The area chosen for study was very broad, however. I identified a great number of variables, and having too little knowledge on qualitative research methodology, I became discouraged. Consequently, I distanced myself from this study and focused on my clinical work in a psychiatric ward. Every day, I spent most of my free time in the company of a Tibetan Buddhist monk-teacher who had come to stay with me for a few months. This gave me the opportunity to practice the Tibetan language, and perform Buddhist rituals. Before the lama returned to his monastery in Northern India, he insisted that I should visit Asia again. Never before had I considered using my own religious background (i.e. Tibetan Buddhism) for academic purposes, but I decided to plan a second trip to Asia to gather material for my investigation.

My general knowledge of the Tibetan healing system stemmed from my previous contact with the Tibetan *amchees* (doctors trained in traditional Tibetan medicine) in India and Nepal, my experience of having a medical check-up done by them and taking Tibetan herbal pills for indigestion. At that point, I suspected that most Tibetans were probably using the traditional

Tibetan system of medicine as their main treatment option. However, these assumptions were soon to be confronted with reality in the course of my study: that more and more Tibetans were turning to Western medicine, especially when faced with serious illness.

Again, there were many subjects for potential research which interested me—individual religious experiences of Buddhist practitioners, the issue of conversion to Buddhism, motivation for undertaking monastic life, and personal image of Buddha. I was also interested in doing some comparative studies between Tibetan Buddhist monks in India and Christian monks in Europe. But because my strongest interests were health issues, I wanted to learn more about the traditional Tibetan system of medicine. Apart from the specific research conducted in the context of the Tibetan diaspora, this book draws upon my personal observation and experience, which stems from my relationship with Tibetan culture and Tibetan Buddhism. It is the final outcome of a long self-experiential and academic process, the results of which are presented as follows.

The Introduction provides a short background for my basic research problem and specific theoretical problems. Chapters One, Two, and Three expand upon the theoretical framework associated with the research questions. In the first three chapters, I elaborate on the interdependencies between culture, religion, and health, the expressions of which are to be found in the qualitative data analysis. I also present the findings of research conducted in other cultural contexts, where similar phenomena have been reported. Chapter One outlines Tibetan culture, religion, and the refugees' process of acculturation in the Indian environment. Chapter Two explores health and illness behaviors, while Chapter Three focuses on religion as it relates to health.

Chapter Four presents the fundamental concepts present in Tibetan Buddhism, which are relevant to the research questions and crucial for a better understanding of the qualitative material. I present these concepts from the *emic* perspective (in accord with the perceptions and understandings deemed appropriate by native informants), and make reference to Buddhist teachings commonly made available to the general public. In this chapter, I attempt to show these teachings not from an academic standpoint but from the practitioner's point of view—that is, as such teachings come to be understood by Tibetans who are exposed to religious socialization and immersed in this symbolic system.

Chapter Five introduces the basic principles of the traditional Tibetan system of medicine. In this chapter, I describe its major concepts, and diagnostic and treatment methods, as well as the relevant idioms of disease. Familiarity with these is essential to understanding the illness behavior and illness pathways analyzed in this study.

In Chapter Six, "Empirical Research," I describe the research design and the presentation of the study sample, as well as the context. I also explain the methodology, detailing the benefits and principles of grounded theory and the gradual process of data analysis.

Chapter Seven, "Presenting and Analyzing the Qualitative Data," presents my findings in a step-by-step analysis of the qualitative data—resulting in a grounded theory of illness behavior among Tibetan diasporic society.

Finally, in Chapter Eight, I discuss the research problems with reference to the theoretical framework described in Chapters One, Two, and Three, along with critical reflections and recommendations for future research. To provide a visual reference for some of the issues explored in the course of my research I designed a companion website that includes extensive additional material including full-color photographs taken in Asia. To access that material visit: www.cultureandmedicine.com

Acknowledgments

A number of people contributed to this study, and I am deeply grateful to them. First of all, I would like to express the utmost gratitude to my beloved teachers: His Eminence Sangye Nyenpa Rinpoche, Venerable Tenga Rinpoche, and Venerable Khandro Rinpoche for their instructions, guidance, and blessings throughout my years of study. Secondly, I would like to thank Professor Halina Grzymala-Moszczynska, the head of the Psychology of Religion Department at the Jagiellonian University in Krakow, Poland. Her support and experience as a mentor were crucial for the creation of this work. I would also like to thank my family and the close friends who supported me emotionally on my chosen path. The comfort and reassurance I received from them were vital to the process, and became a source of courage, strength, and hope.

Introduction

Tibetan culture has been going through a major transformation since the brutal Chinese invasion of 1949. Since that time, it has been exposed to powerful influences both within and outside Tibet. The policy of the Chinese government aimed to suppress and destroy the cultural heritage of Tibetans by introducing "re-education"—so called—and strict laws prohibiting any acts of nationalism, or practice of the spiritual behaviors so essential to the Tibetan people. In 1959, as a way of saving his life and culture, the leader of the Tibetans and the symbol of their traditional customs and values—His Holiness the Dalai Lama—decided to flee from his country to India. Once there, he managed to re-establish a Tibetan government in exile, as well as some educational and spiritual institutions. The present seat of His Holiness the Dalai Lama became know as the "Little Lhasa"—a place where a continuous influx of Tibetan refugees is still reported. Due to the establishment of the Tibetan community in exile, many of the cultural treasures, values, and practices—including symbols, cultural heroes, and rituals—have been saved. The traditional Tibetan national costume (*chupa*), hairstyle, decorations, cuisine, language, and religious behaviors are still commonly used as specific ethnic markers, and sources of ethnic identity.

At the same time, the Tibetan culture became susceptible to changes associated with the acculturation process. Not only do the Tibetans in India experience a clash between their own culture of origin and the host culture, but they are also significantly exposed to Western culture. This is especially true in the densely populated settlements, where the Internet, Hollywood films, and pop music are available. There, Western values as well as lifestyles are transferred via tourists from Europe and America. (For a discussion of this, see Chapter One, Section 1.3.1, "Factors Affecting Acculturation").

As a result of various biological, ecological, and psychological factors, many Tibetans develop a wide variety of health problems. How they respond to illness became the focal point of this research. While a few existing studies elaborate on illness behavior and help-seeking pathways among the Tibetans, there is not much information on how specific variables affect these processes. In the course of my study, I identified several affecting factors, and analyzed the relationships between them to produce a grounded theory of illness behavior among members of the Tibetan diaspora.

PURPOSE OF THE STUDY

The purpose of this study was to examine health and disease in the Tibetan community in exile, along with common reactions to illness. My research subjects function in a specific acculturative context, in which individuals are exposed to both the influence of the host culture (the Indian community, their values, religious beliefs, etc.) and Western culture (people coming from Europe or America). Analysis of the qualitative material will give some insights into how acculturation affects illness behavior, meaning making, help-seeking pathways, and coping strategies.

THEORETICAL PROBLEMS

The key issues of the interdependencies between culture, religion, and health were guided by the following general research questions:

1. What are the interdependencies between culture, religion, and health? It is evident that this problem will include different aspects of culture (e.g., traditional beliefs, values, coping strategies), its salutary, pathogenic and pathoplastic functions, as well as issues associated with emigration and acculturation. Religion, which is a symbolic system present in one's culture, will be analyzed as a way of meaning-making and a source of coping strategies. I will elaborate on my main research question by answering the following sub-questions:
2. How does culture affect health? What are its positive and negative influences?
3. How does culture affect the idiom of health and ill-health? What is the relationship between culture and meaning-making?
4. How does culture affect illness behavior and help-seeking pathways?
5. What are the main areas of interdependence between religion and health?

6. How does religion affect physical and mental health values?
7. How can religion serve as a coping strategy?

RESEARCH PROBLEMS

The general research problem: "What are the most typical patterns of illness behavior?" was further analyzed according to five specific research questions:

1. How do contemporary Tibetans construct the idiom of disease? How do they perceive and interpret their health problems?
2. How do Tibetans perceive and assess potential treatment methods?
3. What are the common help-seeking pathways?
4. What factors affect illness behavior and help-seeking pathways, and how?
5. What is the relationship between religion and illness behavior among Tibetans?

I believe that this study may contribute to the psychology of religion, by illuminating some examples of religious coping in a Tibetan Buddhist context. It will also provide vivid illustrations of how Tibetans approach the philosophical and physical problem of suffering. The dynamics of change in illness behavior, as it is influenced by the acculturation process, will also be discussed, as an area of interest to both sociologists and medical anthropologists. *Culture, Religion and Ethnomedicine: The Tibetan Diaspora in India* presents proof that it is essential to maintain an open mind in a clinical setting, and remain sensitive to cross-cultural issues so as to establish proper rapport with patients and understand their decisions regarding help-seeking and treatment. Unless we can understand the patient's symbolic system, cultural beliefs and values, this goal may be difficult to obtain.

LIMITS OF THE STUDY

Culture, Religion and Ethnomedicine: The Tibetan Diaspora in India does not seek to produce a cross-cultural comparison between India and Tibet or any other countries. For that reason, I did not include comparative analyses with other ethnic groups (e.g., Indians) or between Tibetans living in exile and in their homeland. Most of the research was done in northern India, while Tibetan subjects from southern India were few.

My research was also limited in terms of the time I was able to spend in the East. The duration of the fieldwork done in Asia specifically for this study was four months, not counting my previous travel to India and Nepal. Due to the various constraints on my time, I conducted my research in just a few settlements. Cultural factors imposed an additional limit on the study: There was generally more access to male subjects. Additionally, most of the Tibetans I interviewed were employed in the health sector.

AN EMIC PERSPECTIVE

My decision to approach this study from the *emic*[1] perspective helped those interviewed to feel more relaxed, and encouraged them to share sensitive and intimate information. As a Buddhist practitioner, and having some knowledge of the customs and language of Tibet, I was accepted as being trustworthy, understanding, and closer to them—in other words, a Dharma-brother. On the other hand, because I am of a different ethnic origin, I was sometimes perceived by certain of the younger interviewees as a potential sponsor from the West, which may have affected the elicited data. This aspect was especially evident during subsequent follow-up study via the Internet, when I was frequently asked questions regarding my age, marital status, profession, and so on.

NOTE

1. *Emic* and *etic* are terms used in comparative studies of culture and relate to meaning in ethnographic reporting. An *emic* account is a description of phenomena from the insider's perspective. In other words, the researcher will not only record his or her direct observations, but will also analyze the meaning which is consciously or uncounsciously assigned to the phenomena in that particular cultural context. An *etic* account, on the other hand, will be a description of behaviors or beliefs from a culturally neutral observer's perspective. It involves "classifying and understanding traits as representing cross culturally applicable terms and categories rather than culturally specific meanings" (Schwimmer 2008).

Chapter One

Tibetan Culture, Religion, and Acculturation

1.1 Levels and Dimensions of Culture
 1.1.1 Religion as an Important Component of Culture
1.2 Culture in Transition
 1.2.1 Typologies of Migration
 1.2.2 Refugees as a Distinct Category of Migrants
1.3 Acculturation
 1.3.1 Factors Affecting Acculturation

This chapter will provide a theoretical framework for the issues explored in my study and field work. Following a definition of culture, I will present various levels and dimensions of culture—including religion as an important cultural component. Next, I will elaborate on Tibetan culture in transition, including the issues of migration, exile, the risk factors associated with becoming a refugee, acculturation, and its results. Different models of health and disease versus illness will be explored in the context of Tibetan culture, along with cultural influences on the health variables analyzed. Finally, I will concentrate on the interdependencies between religion and health, highlighting the former as a potential source of coping strategies.

1.1 LEVELS AND DIMENSIONS OF CULTURE

In the present study, I have identified culture as an important variable affecting health and illness behavior. It is essential to open the discussion with a definition of this term. Various analyses of culture usually include the values, beliefs, and practices shared by a group of people. Chanchani and Theivanathampillai (2002, p. 1) cite Taylor's definition of culture as "that complex whole which includes knowledge, belief, art, morals, law, custom and any other capabilities and habits acquired by man as a member of society." Hofstede (1991) describes culture as "mental programming," and points to the fact that from their early childhood, people acquire certain patterns of thinking, feeling. and potential acting. which are culturally dependent and become the "software of the mind."

This type of programming is usually initiated within the family and later carried out within the neighborhood, at school, in peer groups, in the workplace and in the community. It modifies the way people eat, greet each other, and express feelings and emotions. It also determines proximity during a conversation, ways of love-making, and of maintaining body hygiene. Culture is not something that one inherits, but a set of patterns that one needs to learn or acquire. Learning implies that this unique software is modified by the influence of collective programming and unique personal experiences.

Levels of Culture

Hofstede (1991) uses an "onion diagram" to present manifestations of culture at different levels of depth. The two main parts are values and practices. The core of culture is formed by values, which are usually subconsciously acquired in early childhood and remain unconscious to the holders. They shape one's preferences and feelings and thus determine whether a given situation or object is perceived as good or evil, clean or dirty, beautiful or ugly, natural or unnatural, normal or abnormal, rational or irrational.

Values cannot be observed directly. What does remain visible, however, are the practices. This category includes symbols, heroes, and rituals. But although they can be observed, their cultural meaning remains invisible. Symbols carry a particular meaning for people who share the same culture. This sub-category may include words, gestures, pictures, and objects. Some examples might include a traditional costume or hairstyle, a flag, the Coca Cola brand name, or status symbols, such as an expensive stereo or car. Heroes are persons endowed with qualities that are especially prized in a culture. They can be contemporary or historic figures, real or imaginary. Rituals are the collective activities that are considered to be socially essential and thus are carried out for their own sake. They refer to the ways in which people greet and pay respect to each other, or to social and religious ceremonies.

Trompenaars and Hampden-Turner (1997) generated a similar, three-layer model of culture. The outer layer refers to explicit products—the observable reality of the language, food, building, houses, monuments, agriculture, shrines, markets, fashions, and art that characterize a particular culture. The middle layer is formed by norms and values. Whereas norms (as formal writ-

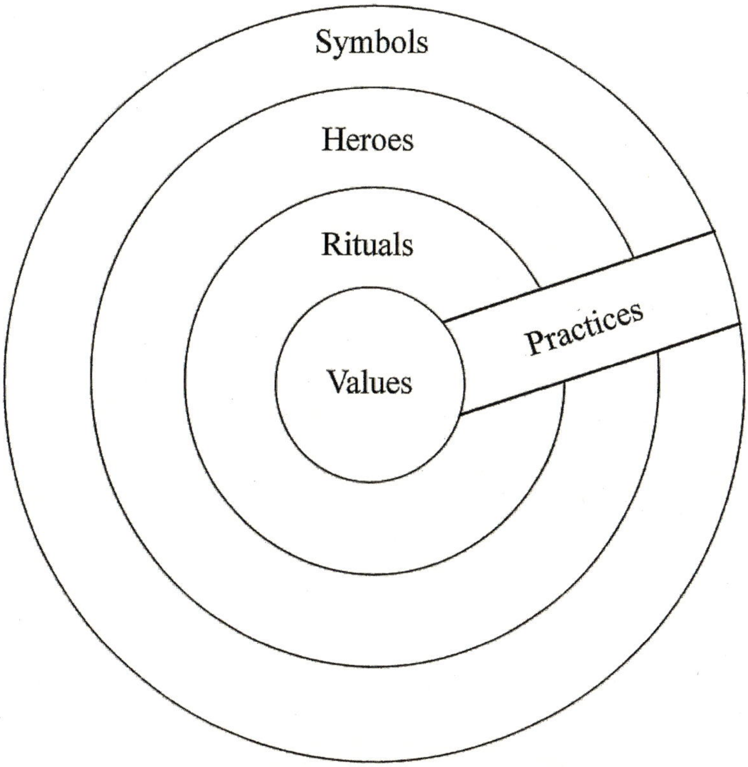

Figure 1.1. Hofstede's "Onion Diagram": Manifestations of Culture at Different Levels of Depth (Hofstede 1991, p.9).

ten laws or informal social control) determine what is assessed as being "right" or "wrong," values relate to the ideals that people share. In other words, norms describe how individuals should behave, and values describe how they aspire or desire to behave.

Finally, there is the core—the assumptions about existence. Faced with everyday life challenges, people often repeat the most effective coping strategies. After some time, they tend to act automatically rather than reflect upon why they do certain things. Questioning basic assumptions may provoke annoyance or confusion. On the other hand, situations in which individuals realize that the old ways of doing have ceased to be effective tend to stimulate cultural change.

According to Hofstede's model, values seem well expressed by the traditional Buddhist principles that are so important for most Tibetans. The things they identify as meaningful, and how they express emotions, are both manifestations of these values. For example, it is highly valued to be kind, pious, and practical, and to perform actions that are defined as virtuous. At the same time, individuals are discouraged from exhibiting anger, jealousy, or pride, or from presenting themselves as weak and dependent on others. Buddhists are also expected to refrain from killing any sentient beings, even the tiniest ones (insects, for example). Even though meat was always an important ingredient in Tibetan cuisine, it would normally be taken from animals that died naturally or by accident. On the level of practices, specific rituals can be identified in the Tibetan community, such as chanting, repeating mantras, circumambulating holy places, and seeking support from lamas. Heroes are represented by the Dalai Lamas or great yogis such as Tilopa, Naropa, or Milarepa. Symbols include mantras (often carved or painted on stones), hand gestures (*mudras*), and various types of offerings, such as butter lamps, or the white scarves known as *kathak*.[1]

Trompenaars and Hampden-Turner (1997) provide a model that lets us view the same culture from a slightly different perspective. According to this model, the explicit products of Tibetan culture include the Tibetan language with its local varieties, traditional Tibetan foods and drinks (e.g., *mo mo*,[2] *thugpa*,[3] *tsampa*,[4] *chang*[5]), garments, decorations, and architecture. Specific ethnic markers include the *chuba*, a traditional Tibetan kimono-like garment, specially designed aprons and head scarves worn by women, and coral necklaces and earrings. Kolas (2004) describes the traditional costume worn by the women of Tibet: "As a minimum, they usually wear their headdress (local Tibetan: *shua*), decorated with bright pink or purple, and their aprons (black at the back, and black, blue or white at the front, depending on their age) over a pair of trousers. Tibetan women from areas outside the county wear other types of headdress, and aprons in different colors, which often makes it possible for local Tibetans to tell where the visitors come from" (p. 184). The ethnic identity and status of women can thus be recognized by their clothes. Buchung (2005) notes that even though chubas are not suitable for the climatic conditions in the Indian subcontinent, the women have managed to adapt them for everyday use.

The manner of dressing up is not only a way of expressing one's ethnic identity, but can be seen as a social strategy in a world where Tibetan culture has been largely commercialized. Penny-Dimri (1994) reports that during popular festivals, local participants would compete for attention by means of their clothing. They would present themselves in traditional dresses (*chubas*) with striped aprons and elaborate hairstyles and ornamentation. According to Penny-Dimri, fashion is a significant factor for those who are trying to reinvent their Tibetan identity. Laymen (usually elderly ones) may also dress up in *chubas*. However, they would prefer to wear them for special occasions, such as celebrations, or for attending religious teaching sessions. *Chubas* are often made of thick cloth and can be uncomfortable in a hot climate. Thus, plain trousers and shirts are usually worn by the men, along with the white scarf (*kathak*) with fine ornaments on it (e.g., dragons, peacocks, or auspicious symbols). Men might wear signet rings with stones or other ornaments, for example, the *gau*—a metal or silver medallion that usually includes some relics. Most people, regardless of age and gender, would also wear a Buddhist rosary called mala on their hands or necks.

Clothes worn by monks and nuns are also specific, explicit products of Tibetan culture. The traditional monastic robes, or, "The three types of Dharma robes"[6] include:

1. "The outer robe" (Tib. *bla gos*) is yellow, and consists of sixty-four pieces. It is only used by the fully-ordained monks[7] during the ordination ceremony, the So-jong Confession Ceremony,[8] or summer retreat.
2. "The lower robe" (Tib. *mthang gos*); and
3. "The monks' shawl" (Tib. *sna'i khams*).

Hofstede (1991) points out that inasmuch as they belong to several different social groups simultaneously, individuals may carry with them different layers of mental programming corresponding to different levels of culture, at the national, regional, gender, generational, social class, or occupational levels. Some of these mental programs may be in conflict, which is the case when religious values clash with generational values, or when gender values clash with the organizational practices of the host culture. This is expressed by the changes occurring in the Tibetan community, which in turn are associated with the acculturation process.

In their daily lives, young people prefer to wear casual Western clothing. Many of them feel attracted to modern fashion trends promoted in the mass media—trends that are not fully accepted by the elderly people. Kolas (2004) notes that even in occupied Tibet, "at school most of the students choose to wear 'modern' dress. However, some Tibetan students still like to demonstrate their ethnic identity, for instance by wearing a red knotted string[9] around their neck (often worn for 'protection'), decorating their jeans with patches of Tibetan apron cloth, or wearing a Lhasa-made 'Stetson' hat" (pp. 187–188). Although many young people still circumambulate holy places, hang prayer flags, or light butter lamps, some question the meaning of such behaviors. This supports the observation of Trompenaars and Hampden-Turner (1997) that some coping strategies may become automatized behaviors. Trying to find one's own Tibetan identity in an acculturative context can be seen as an attempt to cope with such conflicting mental programs.

Dimensions of Culture

Cultures can be described in terms of dimensions in space. Hofstede (1991) presents a four-dimensional model of the differences among national cultures, distinguishing between: 1. large versus small power distance; 2. individualism versus collectivism; 3. masculinity versus femininity; and 4. strong versus weak uncertainty avoidance.

1. *Large versus small power distance:* This dimension refers to how individuals in a specific culture accept the distribution of power. In large power distance societies, people accept a hierarchical order and everyone knows their place. There is no need for justification for power inequalities.
2. *Individualism versus collectivism:* Individualistic cultures promote self-reliance, equality, and individual autonomy. Individuals are expected to take care of themselves and their families. Personal time, personal freedom, and challenge are valued, along with extrinsic motivators (e.g., material rewards at work). Collectivistic cultures value group effort and harmony. They prefer a tightly knit social framework, supported by relatives, the clan, or some other in-group.
3. *Masculinity versus femininity:* This dimension refers to the qualities attributed to gender roles. Masculine cultures affirm assertiveness, competition, toughness, and heroism. Material success, recognition, advancement, and challenge are highly valued. In such cultures, social gender roles will be clearly distinct. In feminine cultures, however, there is an overlap of the social gender roles and both men and women are supposed to exhibit modesty, tenderness, caring, and concern with the quality of life. In the professional area, individuals will aim at establishing good relations with supervisors, peers, and subordinates, with the particular goal of obtaining employment security and stability.
4. *Strong versus weak uncertainty avoidance:* This dimension describes the aspect of ambiguity tolerance—the degree to which individuals feel comfortable with or threatened by that which is new, or seems deviant or weird. It determines to what extent individuals who are faced with ambiguities will maintain a more relaxed atmosphere or exercise rigid codes of belief and behavior to protect conformity.

Trompenaars and Hampden-Turner (1997) elaborate on seven possible dimensions of culture: universalism versus particularism, individualism versus communitarianism, affective versus neutral, specific versus diffuse, achievement versus ascription-oriented, relation to time, and attitude to nature.

1. *Universalism versus particularism:* This dimension defines how people judge others' behavior. There are cultures where people adhere to universally agreed standards and all who fall under these rules are treated equally. Conversely, in particularist cultures, people exercise special obligations to other people; that is, no matter what the rules say, they may feel right in sustaining, protecting, or discounting a person.
2. *Individualism versus communitarianism:* This dimension corresponds to Hoftstede's concept of individualism and collectivism, as described above.
3. *Affective versus neutral cultures:* This refers to the range of expressed feelings and determines whether individuals are more affective (display emotion) or neutral (refrain from expressing emotions). In neutral cultures, feelings and emotions are likely to remain subdued and controlled, whereas in affective cultures people may be more demonstrative.
4. *Specific versus diffuse cultures:* This dimension characterizes to what extent people engage others in specific areas of life and single levels of personality, as opposed to multiple areas at several levels of personality. In a specific culture, when two people meet in different situations (e.g., formal and informal) they will treat these as specific encounters and behave differently in each situation. Conversely, in a diffuse culture, they will adopt different roles or diffuse. For instance, the reputation and authority of a medical professional may leak into another area of his or her life (e.g., private encounters with neighbors).
5. *Achievement versus ascription-oriented cultures:* This refers to how people gain a special, higher status. Whereas in some cultures status is accorded on the basis of achievements, in others it can be ascribed by virtue of age, class, gender, education, etc. Thus, a distinction has been made between achieved and ascribed status, or status based on being versus doing.
6. *Relation to time:* This dimension refers to people's expectations about time, whether they think of time as sequential (a series of events) or synchronic (the past, present, and future interrelated).
7. *Attitude to nature:* This dimension describes whether the members of the culture believe that they are able and should control nature or go along with its laws, direction, and forces. In the former case, they will attempt to impose their will on the environment and change it. In the latter, they will feel that they are part of the environment, and respect it.

In the literature, there is little description of the Tibetan culture from a the dimensional perspective, as presented above. If characteristic features of the traditional Tibetan community are taken into consideration, according to Hofstede's model, they reveal a culture defined by larger power distances, collectivism, and femininity. Specific roles (e.g., of laypeople, monks, nuns, yogis) are well-defined in the society and the hierarchy within specific groups (in a family or a monastery) are well-established. In a traditional Tibetan Buddhist society, group effort and cooperation are highly valued and concentrating on self is more or less discouraged. Modesty, tenderness, piety, loving kindness, and compassion—those qualities attributed to the feminine aspect—are praised most of all. From the perspective of the model presented by Trompenaars and Hampden-Turner, the traditional Tibetan culture discloses qualities defined as particularism and communitarianism. It is also neutral, diffuse, ascription oriented, synchronic in relation to time, and respectful of nature. Many of these qualities are strengthened by the fundamental principles of Buddhist doctrine, which pervades the minds of most Tibetans.

For example, according to the teachings of Dharma all situations one encounters are determined by one's karma. This implies that people and their actions must be considered individually (particularism). There may also be a discrepancy between outer phenomena (actions, situations) and inner phenomena (motivation, emotions). Let's consider a situation in which an adult is beating an adolescent who behaved badly. For an outside observer, it may be difficult to assess whether the behavior of the adult is sustained by anger, or by love and compassion towards the young person. As per the Tibetan perspective, the situation must be judged individually.

In the Tibetan community there are many similar stories that show the relative nature of phenomena. A popular example is a folk story of Drugpa Kunley—a crazy yogi who met a *thanka* painter. The painter was on his way to a lama whom he would ask for consecration[10] of his newly painted picture of a deity. Upon meeting Drugpa Kunley, the painter complained that he had too little golden paint to make the painting as beautiful as he wanted. The yogi asked if he could see the painting and once it was disclosed to him, he urinated on it. The painter was shocked with that apparently outrageous behavior and later complained about it to the lama. When he uncovered his *thanka* before the lama, however, it turned out that the picture was covered with golden paint. The lama explained to the painter that the person he had encountered on the way was a highly realized yogi, and that the painting had already been consecrated.

The teachings on karma also imply that the past, present, and future are interconnected. In simple words, Tibetans maintain that what they experience is a result of their previous actions, and in the present moment they seed the conditions for future experiences and actions. This expresses their synchronic attitude to time. The neutral quality of culture refers to a popular tendency among Tibetans to control emotions, and to resist from crying—which particularly applies to men. The diffuse aspect can be observed in the encounters between high lamas and their students. Whether the situation is formal (e.g., public audience, teaching session) or informal (meeting a *rinpoche*[11] on the street) Tibetans will pay special honors (bow down, never point at the noble person with a finger but with a whole palm, use a special type of honorific language, etc.). Status in Tibetan society is ascribed by virtue of age and class, with special respect given to elderly people in the family and to ordained individuals.

Frequently, certain persons are recognized as special incarnations or emanations. The Dalai Lamas, Karmapas, Panchen Lamas, and many other masters are usually recognized and enthroned from the time they are children, and receive special attention. In Tibetan society, achievement-based status is only conferred upon those who attain spiritual achievements, such as high mastery of the meditation techniques and knowledge of the doctrine. Tibetans also believe that they should live in harmony with their entire surroundings and with other beings, visible or invisible. If they happen to disturb certain beings (e.g., serpent deities) by violating their environment, Tibetans believe that they will need to suffer the consequences of these actions. (This is explained in Chapter Five, "The Traditional Tibetan System of Medicine in Tibet and in Exile.")

In the context of cross-cultural research, it is essential to be aware of cultural characteristics, as they may affect a number of the variables under analysis. Having used some of these cultural dimensions in analyzing and interpreting the qualitative data gathered during the course of my study, I will now focus on the most important aspects of Tibetan culture in exile.

1.1.1 Religion as an Important Component of Culture

To understand religion, it is necessary to know how it is defined and how it functions. The literature on the psychology of religion presents a considerable number of definitions of religion, which concentrate on different aspects of the phenomenon. Pargament (1997) observes that because religion itself is so complex and personal, one is unlikely to produce a single definition which would be adequate and "ultimate." Having analyzed with his students of religion what made religion special, he came up with two types of responses: 1. One of the distinctive characteristics of religion is that it is concerned with the sacred, including God, deities, supernatural beings, transcendent forces, and all that is associated with the higher powers. 2. Religion can be distinguished by its special functions, and is "concerned with how people come to terms with ultimate issues of life" (p. 25).

Similarly, most definitions of religion fall into two categories: substantive definitions and functional definitions. The substantive definitions seek answers to the question: "What is religion?" and are exclusive by nature. Some of them emphasize emotions and experiences, others religious beliefs, practices or rituals, and still others focus on institutions and interactions. However, they all refer to the sacred. The functional definitions, on the other hand, are inclusive and describe what religion does. They involve beliefs, practices, symbols, and experiences, and describe how people deal with the fundamental problems of existence—such as death, suffering, tragedy, evil, pain, and injustice.

How religion operates on the social level is well-presented by Wilson (1988), who describes its latent functions. He points out that in the past religion was important for the maintenance of society and the social order, and provided support for secular authorities. That function was later appropriated and rationalized by agencies outside the religious sphere, and religion became largely privatized. Wilson writes:

> "Religion maintained a certain presidency over all social activities and institutions, but in more advanced societies the process of structural differentiation saw these functions allocated to specialized agencies. Thus it was that, whereas religion was once a primary agency of social control, more technical facilities came to permit much of that task to be embodied in the institutions of law, policing, and public security. Whereas once religion offered a cosmology, an intellectual interpretation of the physical world, in modern times the explanation of the natural order has become the province of scientific enquiry, while the interpretation of the social order has become subject to the increasingly acute awareness of man's own capability to undertake the 'social construction of reality'. Whereas in time past, the legitimation of sovereignty and authority depended on reference to the supernatural, nowadays, the legitimation of authority is typically claimed by virtue of the democratic voice of people" (1988, p. 200).

Subsequently, religion has become less directly involved in areas like economics, politics, social control and education, despite the fact that various churches sometimes retain control over some sections of the system of education. On the other hand, religion has become more of a self-conscious activity, an individual choice in the search for emotional reassurance and intellectual meaning (Wilson 1988).

A good example of a functional definition is presented by Batson, Schoenrade, and Ventis, who define religion as: "whatever we as individuals do to come to grips personally with the questions that confront us because we are aware that we and others like us are alive and that we will die" (1993, p. 8). They point to the fact that out of all species, only humans are significantly aware of their own personal existence, the personal existence of others, the possibility of other worlds, of personal finitude, and that religion is an attempt to deal with existential questions. They articulate existential questions in a straightforward way: "What is the meaning and purpose of my life? How should I relate to others? How do I deal with the fact that I am going to die? What should I do about my shortcomings?" (p. 8).

The authors note, however, that one is often confronted with vital questions that have lasting effects on one's life, but that are not of a religious character—for example, making a decision about marrying someone, taking a specific direction in life, or choosing a career. Nevertheless, Batson et al. explain: "coming to grips with such questions is not religious, for they do not concern matters of existence. By our definition, only when a person is responding to those issues that transcend problems in one's life and concern that nature of life is that individual dealing with religious questions" (1993, p. 10).

Pargament (1997) stresses some of the drawbacks of an approach in which religion viewed functionally becomes a vast phenomenon. He explains that the response to the fundamental problems of existence may also involve things like sports, sex, art, medicine, materialism, nihilism, and so on. Thus, "functional definitions can be unduly broad, violating common conceptions of where religion starts and stops by incorporating any effort to deal with ultimacy beneath the religious rubric" (p. 29). Pargament (1997) defines religion as: "a process, a search for significance in ways related to the sacred" (p. 32). In other words, significance and experiences become religious when the aspirations and responses are connected with the sacred. I have adopted this type of functional definition for the purposes of this study. It will later help characterize the interrelationship between religion and health, which is the essential point of this work.

According to social learning theory, children learn religion just as they learn culture. It happens through modeling the behavior of other people and through social reinforcement. Reinforcement relates to receiving gratification (praise or an encouraging smile) and frustration (punishment or discouragement for wrong behavior). Usually, the most significant figures from whom the child learns how to behave are parents. Batson et al. (1993) stress: "[The] learner is not simply a passive recipient of information and values but one who actively seeks to know and to understand, learning by observing other people's behavior and its consequences, as well as by observing the consequences of his or her own behavior" (p. 54). The concept of social influence can explain the findings of Hoge and Petrillo, who claimed that parents' religious involvement was the most powerful social background predictor of a person's religious involvement (cited in Batson et al. 1993, p. 43).

Classified as part of the category, "Involvement with the culture of origin," this is one of the important cultural variables analyzed in the present study. In discussing the qualitative material gathered and analyzed as part of my field work, I will use a functional definition of religion as a meaning-making system related to the sacred; it will also be viewed as a source of coping strategies. Most of my interview subjects reported that religion was an integral part of their lives. Dharma teachings helped them interpret reality, deal with existential issues, and provided an effective means of overcoming difficulties.

1.2 CULTURE IN TRANSITION

Whereas cultural shifts on the societal level result from changes in the political arena, and due to the process of globalization, transformations on the individual level can be caused by the processes associated with migration. This section defines typologies of migration, presents the concept of "refugees," and describes the characteristics of cultural shifts, such as the acculturation process.

1.2.1 Typologies of Migration

Understanding migration and the phenomena associated with it is crucial to this study, because of the context in which the research was done. The term "migration" refers to a permanent and temporary abandoning of the place inhabited by an individual or larger groups of people (i.e., whole societies) and relocation to a new territory (Kraszewski 2003). There are many typologies of migration, for example, external (which refers to displacement from one place to another, outside a given country or ethnic region); or internal (which refers to displacement within the same region). Another classification is irretrievable versus retrievable, or temporary migration, which may last for a number of months or years. There may be short-term, long-term, or seasonal.

One of the most important distinctions as it relates to this study is the difference between voluntary and enforced migration. Other factors to consider are the number of emigrants (isolated, sporadic, or mass migration; individual, group, or family migration), and their legal status (legal immigrants versus illegal aliens, according to the laws of their homeland and of the host country). Migration can also be classified according to individual motives: for example, it may be political, socio-economic, religious, or cultural. The decision to emigrate can be complex and involves a number of motives. The following sections contain the definition of refugee status, as well as a detailed discussion of the cultural changes connected with forced migration.

1.2.2 Refugees as a Distinct Category of Migrants

Refugees belong to a specific group of people whose exile is triggered by an introduction of certain regulations or a direct activity of various administrative, police, or military authorities. This category includes deportation or displacement during war. Political emigrants may also be termed refugees. They escape from their home country because their life is threatened or they feel that such danger may soon appear (e.g., when a country is conquered by another one or in case of a political coup).

As defined by the United Nations Convention held in Geneva in 1951, the term "refugee" applies to an individual who: "owing to well-founded fear of being persecuted for reasons of race, religion, nationality, membership of a particular social group or political opinion, is outside the country of his nationality and is unable or, owing to such fear, is unwilling to avail himself of the protection of that country; or who, not having a nationality and being outside the country of his former habitual residence as a result of such events, is unable or, owing to such fear, is unwilling to return to it." (The United Nations High Commissioner for Refugees 1996, p. 16).

For the most part, this Convention addressed the problems that emerged in the aftermath of World War II and at the beginning of the Cold War. Therefore, refugee status was initially given to those who had become refugees as a result of events occurring before January 1, 1951. This, however, was ratified in 1967, when the U.N. General Assembly removed the geographical and time limitations written in the original Convention. UNHCR reports: "These schemes had both benefits and drawbacks. They allowed civilians to enter a country speedily with a minimum of red tape, but since there were no binding universal standards that apply to temporary protection, the rights accorded to asylum seekers were often fewer in number and less generous in scope that those provided for under the Convention" (online).[12]

The Convention not only defined the status of refugees, but it also explained the various obligations governments had to undertake, in order to protect asylum seekers. This includes a "non-refoulement" policy (not sending individuals back into a situation of possible persecution), or not penalizing asylum seekers who left behind, or could not obtain, proper documentation and so entered a potential asylum country illegally. The same document also contained an exclusion clause, which defined who was not covered by the Convention (e.g., people who committed war crimes or active soldiers), and cessation clauses—defined circumstances in which individuals ceased to hold refugee status (e.g., they willingly returned home, obtained a passport or residency in another state, or their country of origin returned to a state of democracy after a period of war).

The Convention of 1951 was criticized for a number of reasons. First of all, it did not define the term "persecution." Secondly, some argued that it only applied to individuals, not large groups of people who might seek asylum in a country en masse. It also ignored gender-related issues or burden-sharing. In 1956, the government of India sent a letter to UNHCR that outlined its domestic refugee concerns and expressed a wish not to become a party to the Convention—even though India was a member of UNHCR's Executive Committee, which helped establish global refugee policy.

UNHCR (2006) has reported that the total number of refugees worldwide was about 8.4 million by the end of 2005. (This does not include 4.3 million Palestinian refugees who fall under the responsibility of the United Nations Relief and Works Agency for Palestine Refugees in the Near East.) A decrease in the refugee population was also reported in all regions during 2005. According to UNHCR (2006) statistics, there are 20,198 Tibetans who hold refugee status, 9 asylum-seekers, and 928 individuals who fall into the "various" category, that is, persons of concern to the UNHCR who are not included in other categories. (Data are provisional and subject to change; this status is as of June 2, 2006.)

Most of those interviewed for the present study identified themselves as refugees. Many escaped Tibet after the Chinese occupation and were unable to return without serious consequences (e.g., imprisonment or other forms of punishment). There were also Tibetans who left their country for solely economic reasons. Despite that, they classified themselves as refugees and justified their escape in terms of a search for religious freedom. Much larger numbers are given by the Office of Tibet,[13] which reports that there are about 125,777 Tibetans in exile, and that the approximate distribution of the community is 121,143 in South Asia and 4634 outside South Asia. The office reported almost 70,000 Tibetans living in settlements and the remaining 50,000 in scattered communities in India and Nepal. These differences may be due to the fact that not all Tibetan refugees have been registered by the UNHCR. Table 1.1 shows the distribution of the refugee community in various regions as reported by the Office of Tibet (online).

A continuous influx of refugees was reported in the year following the Dalai Lama's flight, until the introduction of Chinese policies that prohibited people from fleeing Tibet. Beginning in 1980, however, a liberalization of Chinese policy allowed for legal travel to India and made escape from Tibet a realistic possibility. Fifteen thousand Tibetans sought asylum in India between 1986 and 1993, which increased the refugee population by more than 10 percent. Many of them belonged to the young generation (under the age of 25). A large percentage of all refugees were monks and nuns who wanted to escape continuous religious suppression in Tibet and sought shelter in monasteries, which were usually located in the settlements. The growth of the community in exile was also due to the number of births that took place in exile.

The fragility of the settlement economy and infrastructure placed several severe strains on the Tibetan population in exile. Naturally, the amount of land could not increase proportionately to the growth of the community, and

Table 1.1. Population of Tibetan Refugee Community

REGION	*NO.*	*POPULATION*
SOUTH INDIA:		32635
Settlements	5	32572
Scattered Communities	2	63
CENTRAL INDIA:		8436
Settlements	3	6015
Scattered Communities	3	2421
UTTAR PRADESH:		14289
Settlements	6	3581
Scattered Communities	7	10708
HIMACHAL PRADESH:		20307
Settlements	13	6387
Scattered Communities	14	13920
NORTH EAST INDIA:		8622
Settlements	3	5022
Scattered Communities	8	3600
WEST BENGAL AND SIKKIM:		12839
Settlements	4	1750
Scattered Communities	36	11089
LADAKH (Settlements)	3	7558
NEPAL:		15000
Settlements	10	5086
Scattered Communities	15	9914
BHUTAN (settlements):	7	1457
TIBETANS ABROAD:		4634
TOTAL:		125777

there were limited employment opportunities. Housing facilities were also lacking, and the sanitation, health, education, and similar facilities were underdeveloped.

There are three types of Tibetan settlements in India, Nepal, and Bhutan. Tsering Gellek (2001) gives an account of the historical background behind establishment of the settlements: "the Dalai Lama and the Central Administration requested that the Government of India resettle Tibetans in agricultural-based settlements. Land for such settlement had to be requested from various state governments by the Central Government, and as there was not enough land available for agricultural settlements, agro-industrial settlements were also started, most of which are located in the north-west of India in the

State of Himachal Pradesh. Thus with the assistance of the Governments of India and Nepal, and also the Government of Bhutan, the United Nations High Commission for Refugees (UNHCR), foreign donor agencies, and the work, the faith and tenacity of the Tibetan refugees themselves, 54 refugee settlements have been established in India, Nepal, and Bhutan since 1959, comprising 26 agricultural, 17 agro-industrial and 11 handicraft-based settlements" (p. 6).

The largest population of Tibetan refugees can be found in the state of Karnataka, where they are divided into five settlements (established between 1960 and 1974). In each settlement there are from 6 to 22 villages, with populations varying from 3,500 to 11,700 people. All the settlements provide basic education, from nursery to higher secondary school; primary healthcare clinics and hospitals; and access to the traditional Tibetan system of medicine. In three of the settlements in Karnataka, housing for the elderly was also established. I did most of my field work in Dharamsala, the most populous settlement and the seat of His Holiness the Dalai Lama; in Majnu-Ka-Tilla (a Tibetan camp in New Delhi); in Silliguri, and in several other settlements.

Risk Factors Associated with Enforced Migration

Different types of cultural shifts result in specific levels of stress. Because the Tibetan community I studied consisted largely of refugees, I will now describe the risk factors associated with enforced migration. The National Child Traumatic Stress Network (2003) describes different phases of refugee experience and the types of stresses encountered by refugees during these phases. The phases are categorized into Preflight, Flight, and Resettlement.

Preflight is the phase prior to escape from the country of origin, during which refugees anticipate and then cope with all kinds of devastating events. The psychological traumas associated with the war may include: being wounded, raped, tortured, or having one's family or friends killed or wounded. Separation from or loss of a family member or members often results in family disintegration (Tseng 2001). Refugees may witness executions and violence or even be forced to engage in violence. Other traumas involve forced labor in work camps, family separation in age-segregated camps, overcrowding, starvation, poor sanitation, lack of medical services, and lawlessness (Vang and Flores 1999; Chung 2001).

In 2003, NCTSN reported that 300,000 children under the age of 18 had fought in armed conflicts around the world. They explain: "Child soldiers represent a special category of refugees because they both witness and participate in war violence. By their own accounts, front line combat puts child soldiers at risk for rape, torture, war injuries, substance abuse, depression, anxiety, and suicidal ideation. . . . In addition to tangible losses such as home, possessions, friends, and family members, child soldiers may lose trust in authority figures who are unable to provide for their basic needs, or who themselves are perpetrating atrocities. Child soldiers can lose their moral perspective, as they come to believe that looting is not the same as stealing, or that killing for political reasons may, in fact, be justified" (p. 9).

While I have found no reports of Tibetan children acting as soldiers in the Chinese army, such incidents may have been encountered. On the other hand, cases of young Tibetans being forced to participate in the execution of their family members have been reported (Tibetan Center for Human Rights and Democracy 2000b).

During the Flight phase, refugees cope with uncertainty about the future, displacement from their homes, and transport and transitional placement (for example, in refugee camps). Malnutrition, thirst, and lack of medical care are also frequently reported during this phase. Beiser, Simich, and Pandalangat (2003) mention additional indignities and dangers, such as being harassed by the authorities during the immigration process, cheated by agents, and placed deeply in debt for immigration travels by unscrupulous moneylenders. Stress reported by Tibetans during the flight phase is often associated with the long and hazardous escape route through the Himalayas, and the danger of being caught and killed by Chinese troops, as well as hunger, cold, accidents that are likely to occur in high mountains, and being robbed by Indian soldiers (Jacobson 2002; Terheggen, Stroebe, and Kleber 2001; TCHRD 2000b).

The third stage, Resettlement, refers to the period of adjustment to the new environment. It involves a number of challenges associated with the acculturation process, and produces a great deal of stress. Refugees become particularly susceptible to emotional strain resulting from the difficulties they experience in the country offering asylum. Pathak (2004) says: "the inequality of life, uncertainty of job opportunities, financial insecurity, poverty, unemployment, and change in psychosocial environment can be considered as potent cause of strife torn Tibetan society" (p. 88). The traumatic experiences encountered by refugees may seriously increase their risk of mental and physical disorders. Those who have no opportunity for "cultural retreat" or "cultural regression"[14] in particularly difficult moments are more likely to experience emotional strain. NCTSN (2003) reports a number of potential health problems affecting children during the Resettlement phase. These may include anxiety, recurring nightmares, insomnia, secondary enuresis, introversion, anxiety and depressive symptoms, relationship problems, behavioral problems, academic difficulties, anorexia, and somatic problems.

Chung (2001) gives an example of nonorganic or psychosomatic blindness developed by Cambodian women refugees who reported incidents of rape and sexual abuse. Another peculiar symptom became known as the *Ting Moong* (dummy personality): "Ting Moong was a technique employed by Cambodians to survive during the Pol Pot regime, whereby individuals acted as if they were deaf, dumb, foolish, confused, or stupid, and learned to obey orders obediently without asking questions or complaining. Any appearance of intelligence or emotions could quickly lead to torture or execution. Thus continuing to act like a Ting Moong and being afraid to speak up or show feelings is a survival technique to avoid death or punishment and remains with many Cambodians even while in the United States" (Chung 2001, p. 117).

Jacobson (2002) reports association between refugee traumas and the symptoms of anxiety and depression in a Tibetan community. Significant stressors included: leaving the family of origin behind in Tibet to flee to India; theft by Chinese troops; having to sell their homes in Tibet at a severe loss as they fled Chinese incursions during the Border War; fatal illnesses of family members; and the stress of single parenthood. Cases of Post Traumatic Stress Disorder (PTSD) were also reported as a result of traumatic experiences. Sonal Singh (2004) writes: "Around one in five Tibetan refugees in Dharamshala, India, met criteria for post-traumatic stress disorder. Methods of torture reported included electric shocks and suspension in painful positions, beating with iron bars, and setting dogs onto prisoners. On top of this was added the stress of relocation to refugee camps in India, where large numbers of refugees fell ill and died due in no small measure to the unfamiliar diet and much hotter climate. The forty-five years that have passed since the first wave of the Tibetan diaspora have not silenced the psychiatric reverberations of those traumas" (online).[15]

Chung (2001) also points out an important psychological factor affecting refugees' mental health, namely, survivor's guilt. It has been observed that many individuals feel guilty for successfully escaping from the home country and leaving their families behind in a situation that presented potential danger. Communication with the relatives may be impossible, and the refugees experience frustration and obsessive nostalgia. They may also exhibit symptoms of depression or anxiety.

1.3 ACCULTURATION

What happens when two or more cultural groups come together? Such issues are of great interest in understanding the psychology of immigration. Berry (2001) notes that the study of immigrants and immigration is rooted in a number of disciplines, including anthropology, demography, economics, political science, and sociology.

How people adapt in the host country and what attitudes they reveal-in the process is described by the concept of acculturation, which is defined as: "a process that entails contact between two cultural groups, which results in numerous cultural changes in both parties" (Berry 2001, p. 616). In order to function in a new society (even at a minimal level), the immigrants need to gain some knowledge of the host society and adjust to the new situation. This involves acculturation. The host society is the single dominant majority of people sharing a common ancestral language and culture (Bourhis et al. 1997). Berry (2001) highlights the fact that acculturation involves mutual (or reciprocal) change, due to the fact that both immigrants and immigrant-receiving societies and their native-born populations are liable to change.

In their study of the acculturation of Hispanics in the United States, Korzanny and Abravanel (1998) enumerated the following specific indicators of acculturation:

1. Language use: the amount of time a particular language is spoken at home, at work, and with friends.
2. Media behavior: the amount of exposure to television, radio, or other media in one's native language or the language of the host community.
3. Ties to people remaining in the country of origin.
4. Length of residency in the host country. The number of years of residency in the host country were divided by an individual's age. This provided a fraction that indicated the proportion of an individual's life spent in the second culture.
5 Expression of values: this refers to attitude statements that reflect cultural orientations; for example, an individual's most important goals.
6. Composition of interpersonal network: this refers to the proportion of friends who come from the country of origin and those from the host country.

Other indicators may also be included, such as kinship relationships, food customs, marriage and courtship customs, or holidays.

Bourhis et al. (1997) point out that immigrants move along a continuum between trying to maintain their immigrant culture and adopting the host culture, usually at the cost of losing their cultural heritage. Biculturalism is considered to be a midpoint on this continuum. It describes a situation in which immigrants will retain some features of their cultural heritage while adopting key elements of the host culture. According to Berry's Psychological Acculturation Model, they will have to confront two dilemmas:

1. Is maintaining cultural identity and characteristics considered to be of value?
2. Is maintaining relationships with other groups considered to be of value?

Berry (2001) discusses four different acculturation attitudes, namely: assimilation, integration, separation, and marginalization. They explain to what extent people want to have contact with (or avoid) others outside their group versus maintaining (or giving up) their cultural attributes. Assimilation refers to a situation "when immigrants do not wish to maintain their cultural heritage and seek daily interaction with other cultures" (p. 619). Pires and Stanton (2000) explain it as the abandonment of one's first culture in favor of the second one, "the adoption by a minority ethnic group of a host (dominant) culture's beliefs, attitudes, values and behaviors via a linear, progressive learning process or model . . . behavioural patterns will become more like those of the host culture and less like those of the culture of origin. . . . New values and behaviours are acquired additively through increased contact with the new culture and the influence of mass media" (p. 46). Cultural assimilation may precede or happen at the same time as structural assimilation (which involves entry into groups, clubs, and other organizations of the dominant culture).

Separation defines a tendency to place a value on holding on to the culture of origin, and at the same time, avoid interaction with members of the host culture (Berry 2001). Such people refrain from changing their behavioral patterns regarding language, food consumption, or clothing. Integration happens when immigrants aim at both maintaining their culture of origin and engaging in daily interactions with other groups. Finally, marginalization refers to a situation in which individuals reveal little interest in cultural maintenance (e.g., due to enforced cultural loss) or in having relations with members of the host culture (due to exclusion or discrimination).

Similarly, Bourhis et al. (1997) note that some immigrants dissociate themselves from their ethnocultural origin as well as the majority culture of the host country. The authors claim that this may be understood as an attempt at identifying oneself as an individual, one who is not a member of either an immigrant group or the host majority, rather than in terms of marginalization. "Such 'individualists' reject group ascriptions *per se* and prefer to treat others as individual persons rather than as members of group categories. [They] refuse to be bounded by either ingroup or host majority ascriptions" (p. 378–379).

Kosic (2002) explains that the choice of an acculturation attitude may be connected with sociocultural and psychological adaptation: "high adaptation (good job, greater knowledge of host culture) may result in increased social contact and in more positive attitudes toward assimilation; thus the attitudes may be classified as a consequence of adaptation" (p. 197).

Pires and Stanton (2000) present four distinct patterns of acculturation, as identified by Richard Mendoza in his study of Mexican-American adolescents and adults done in 1989. They resemble the acculturation attitudes described by Berry (2001):

1. Cultural Resistance: An attempt to ignore the new culture while maintaining the culture of origin.
2. Cultural Shift: The substitution of new cultural norms in place of native customs.
3. Cultural Incorporation: Adoption of some of the new culture while keeping some of the culture of origin.
4. Cultural Transmutation: Alteration of original and new cultural practices to create a unique subcultural entity.

Presenting some refinements on Berry's characteristics of acculturation, Rudmin (20003) writes that: "integration can only apply to surface aspects of culture, such as choice of languages, cuisine, or music, but not to many aspects of culture for which cultural code switching is not possible. Integration cannot apply to deeper aspects of culture, such as religion, gender roles, or child rearing, because cultural practices in these domains entail enduring commitments that preclude the possibility of code switching. Nor can integration apply to behaviors regulated by law, such as traffic laws, professional standards in medicine, or laws of assault, because choice in these matters is simply forbidden" (online).[16]

Rudmin (2003) describes marginalization as a situation in which individuals want to participate and be acknowledged in the dominant cultural community, the minority community, or both, but fail to do so. He notes that: "Individuals who have no preference to belong to either of these communities cannot be marginalized from them." He goes on to present another type of strategy, namely multiculturalism, which refers to a situation in which "the minority has a preference for cultural practices that are neither from the minority culture nor from the dominant culture, for example, preferences for a sub-culture, or a third culture, or for freedom from cultural constraints and labels."

Smart and Smart (1995) note that adaptation to the new culture may involve several stages: initial joy and relief at having arrived in the new home country, accompanied by hope for a better economic or political future, then post-decisional regret and stress with attendant psychological symptoms; finally, acceptance, adjustment, and reorganization. The authors also describe four possible adaptation responses to the influence of a second culture by Stephen Bochner: "passing," chauvinism, marginalization, and mediation. The first three are marked by passivity, hostility, confusion and isolation. Mediation, on the other hand, involves synthesis of both cultures, a positive integration of both experiences.

Tseng (2001) describes four stages of cultural and psychological adjustment: 1. Premigration Stage, 2. Initial Stage, 3. Middle Stage, and 4. Final Stage. The first stage precedes the actual migration. It is characterized by limited information and actual experience, as well as development of fantasy speculations about life in the host country. These pre-migratory expectations are later confounded by reality. During the Initial Stage (up to 6 months after entry), emigrants need to cope with a number of practical problems, such as learning a new language, and finding employment and housing. While some emigrants may find this stage exciting, others find it confusing and frustrating.

The Middle Stage (between 3 and 5 years) is characterized by a period in which the initial problems have been resolved, and the individuals experience cultural adjustment. During this time they may perceive more cultural differences in relation to value systems, life customs, and interpersonal relationship patterns. Some may try to maintain parts of their culture of origin while adopting new life patterns. The degree of assimilation versus integration will be different among emigrants. The Final Stage occurs 10 or 20 years after migration and defines a balanced stage of adjustment, in which individuals may identify themselves as members of the host society.

Berry (2001) explains the prerequisites for integration to take place: "mutual accommodation is required for integration to be attained, involving the acceptance by both dominant and nondominant groups of the right of all groups to live as culturally different peoples within the same society. This strategy requires immigrants to adopt the basic values of the receiving society, and at the same time the receiving society must be prepared to adapt national institutions (e.g., education, health, justice, labor) to better meet the needs of all groups now living together in the larger plural society" (p. 619).

Berry (2001) also explains that the core phenomenon of acculturation involves "behavioral shifts." This relates to psychological change resulting from cultural contact and new patterns of behavior: "In most cases, there is a rather easy transition involving both 'culture shedding' and 'culture learning': Individuals change the way they dress, what they eat, their greeting procedures, even their values by reducing (suppressing, forgetting) one way of daily living and taking on replacements. The pace and extent of individual change is clearly related to the degree of cultural maintenance in one's own group, which in turn is linked to the relative demographic, economic, and political situation of the groups in contact" (p. 621).

1.3.1 Factors Affecting Acculturation

There are different variables that either foster positive psychological and social adjustment or contribute to acculturative stress. These factors are generally classified into two groups: 1) features of the original and host society (cultural, economic, political, or social); and 2) individual characteristics, for example, demographic variables (age, gender, marital status, education, length of sojourn, etc.), personality characteristics (self-esteem, locus of control), or socio-cognitive and motivational factors, for example, coping strategies, acculturation strategies, social support, and the need for cognitive closure (Kosic 2004). Studies of various groups of migrants reveal how these factors affect life in the host country. Several of these studies, as summarized below, correspond to my observations of Tibetan emigrants in India.

Tseng (2001) found that adjustment presents greater challenges to men than it does to women. Whereas men need to search for new societal roles, women only need to readjust in a domestic setting. But if women lack social interaction they are likely to feel emotionally isolated. Men, on the other hand, may feel frustrated when job opportunities are more available for women. Tseng also mentions the biological burdens of women, such as pregnancy and childbirth, and points out that men are usually the ones who decide to emigrate; females simply follow them.

In terms of matching skills to employment, both highly educated people with professional backgrounds and unskilled, poorly educated workers have the most difficulty in finding an appropriate and satisfactory job. Those with ordinary occupational experience are more privileged in this respect. Adjustment is also easiest for young, single men, who usually experience less responsibility and more freedom in adapting to highly individualistic societies. In contrast, adaptation may be more of a struggle for divorced or widowed females.

Conversely, Yick (2000) found that in Chinese American families, employment is a significant predictor of victimization experiences. In other words, individuals who had employment were more likely to become victims of minor forms of physical violence by a spouse or partner: "Status consistency theory postulates that individuals who are at greater risk of using physical violence are threatened by their lack of resources, and to restore equity in the family, they will employ physical force" (p. 263).

It is significant that many migrant communities make an attempt to recreate and maintain their original sociocultural settings, by forming a "Little Italy," "Little Tokyo," "Chinatown," or "Little Lhasa." Tseng (2001) maintains that such coping strategies can inhibit the process of assimilation into the dominant culture and of learning the language spoken by members of the host society. Many migrants also tend to develop prejudice against the host culture, accompanied by pride in their own cultural heritage. This may result in resistance to acculturation, which is conducive to separatism. Neto's (2002) research on Portuguese youth born in France shows that more social difficulties were reported by those who labeled themselves as Portuguese and intended to live in France only temporarily. On the other hand, those who revealed more assimilative patterns of acculturation had fewer problems.

Neto (2002) also found that fluency in the local language was the strongest predictor of social adaptation. According to Tseng (2001), young people learn the new language and acculturate faster and more easily than older people. Their views and values may more resemble those of the host society than their culture of origin. On the other hand, individuals who interact with family members and members of their own ethnic group are more likely to endorse traditional cultural norms (Yeh et al. 2003). Facility with language acquisition correlates with better adjustment, and is an important factor affecting the formation and maintenance of interpersonal relationships with peers in the host community. Yeh et al. (2003) note that Japanese students in America who had low English proficiency were more likely to socialize with Japanese friends, whereas a higher level of English proficiency was associated with establishing friendships with students from various cultural backgrounds. At the same time, high language competence may involve becoming a translator for family members with limited language abilities.

Differences in speed and level of acculturation between migrant parents and their children may broaden the generation gap and produce additional acculturative strain, by creating or worsening family communication problems and child-parent conflicts (Gil, Vega, and Dimas 1994). This can be exemplified by the Hmong community in America in which children "tend to favor the English language over Hmong and prefer to eat Western foods, such as hamburgers, tacos, or hot dogs, rather than traditional Hmong food. . . . The Hmong parents want to maintain their traditional customs and values, whereas the young Hmong children are quickly learning and adopting American culture and becoming more expressive. However, in the Hmong tradition, children are not expected to express anger, frustration, or contempt toward their parents" (Vang and Flores 1999, pp. 11–12).

Another example is given by Kwak and Berry (2001), who analyzed the adjustment of immigrant Vietnamese, Koreans, and East-Indians in Canada: "Each ethnic group possesses particular core characteristics and values that impact family interactions. When provided with more diverse cross-cultural experiences, adolescents adapt more quickly as compared to their parents, who are more reluctant to accept changes from their originating culture. As a consequence, parents and their children undergo differential rates of acculturation, and this differential process of acculturation accounts for significant sources of intergenerational differences. . . . All three immigrant groups in the present study emphasize filial piety; respect for the elderly and family interests usually take precedence over personal interests. Adolescents are expected to fulfill their responsibilities to family and pay tribute to family lineage. Gender roles are clearly divided. Filial relationships with family members and family harmony are among the highest priorities within their culture" (p. 153).

Although many of the traditional cultural values have been maintained in Asian families, Vietnamese Americans revealed a tendency towards an individualistic over a collective familial approach to achieve familial goals. In Southeast Asian families, the intergenerational conflict appeared due to parents' acculturation resistance. "For Southeast Asian refugee adolescents the root of their intergenerational conflict resides in unrealistic parental expectations since new cultural norms and values obtained by adolescents often contradict those previously learned in Asia. . . . Among value items examined with Southeast Asian refugees in the U.S., differences between parents and their children begin to appear with respect to fulfilling their obligations, seeking fun and excitement, and desiring material possessions, even though education and achievement, harmonious family, and hard work still remain important values" (Kwak and Berry 2001, p. 153).

Changes with reference to parental control were also observed in Korean families. Whereas traditionally strong control was practiced in these families as an expression of warmth and interest, this view of parenting style became problematic for Korean immigrant adolescents, who associated such strict control with hostility and rejection (Kwak and Berry 2001). Furthermore, changes in gender roles were also observed in emigrant East-Indian families: "Greater adherence to traditional gender roles and respect for the elderly and authority persisted, although the tradition of decision making by the eldest male declined as the family structure changed gradually from extended to nuclear" (p. 154). The authors conclude that these generational differences may be understood in terms of parents and children being in different phases of adaptation. In families with a longer sojourn in the host country, parents may have developed more practical and realistic acculturation attitudes. Similar concerns to those described above were reported by Bosnian refugees in America. Adult subjects worried about their children losing touch with their way of life (as a consequence of immersion in the American lifestyle and culture), abandoning their mother tongue (perceived as a threat to Bosnian ethnic and national identity), and becoming Americanized (Weine et al. 2004). It is implied that many of the phenomena associated with acculturation are universal and will be found in different emigrant groups.

Ying and Akutsu (1997) analyzed the sense of coherence[17] and psychological adjustment in five Southeast Asian refugee groups: Vietnamese, Cambodians, Laotians, Hmong, and Chinese-Vietnamese. In expanding upon Antonovsky's theories, Ying and Akutsu report that: "sense of coherence serves as a significant and important predictor of psychological adjustment . . . was found to be a mediator of the significant indirect effects of such key variables as trauma (especially for Cambodians), cultural traditionalism, and English competence on the refugees' experience of happiness and demoralization" (pp. 137–138).

Although there are no studies on the sense of coherence among Tibetans, I believe that those with higher involvement in their culture of origin, and who are accustomed to use religious coping, may reveal a higher sense of coherence. This is because Tibetans who identify themselves as Buddhists are likely to perceive situations as the result of accumulated karma use spiritual methods to make meaning of a given situation, and then manage it more effectively.

To describe the adjustment of Tibetans in exile, Von Somm (1998) refers to the stages of socioeconomic adaptation defined by Thomas Methfessel,[18] namely:

1. Physical survival dominated by a strong "in-group" orientation, separation from the host society's social environment, and dependence on aid programs;
2. A stage of ethnic survival: refugees take part in an active process of adaptation (mostly economic) while trying to maintain their traditional ethnic identity by rejecting certain forms of acculturation;
3. A stage of economic and social integration.

As the new generation grows up in exile, the stage of economic and social integration begins. Knowledge of the homeland among the second generation exiles is based on the stories of their elders or sometimes on more formal learning in institutionalized settings. Von Somm (1988) notes that Tibetans in exile who had been brought up in Tibet tried, for the most part, to perpetuate their way of life in India. But even though the earliest Tibetan refugees in India dreamt of their homeland and wished to return to Tibet one day, many of them still live in India.

According to a study by Goldstein-Kyaga (cited in Misra 2003), Tibetans in India enjoy a better standard of living than in Tibet. Moreover, they have managed to avoid the economic hardships experienced by many of their Indian countrymen. Despite what may be considered a cramped existence by Western standards, they are living in much better conditions than the poverty-stricken Indian farmers or day-laborers just outside their dwellings. In fact, many Tibetans are so well-off that they can invite their families in Tibet to join them in India.

According to Misra (2003), some Tibetans say that voluntary exclusion guarantees the preservation of their identity. They claim that they can pursue their struggle for freedom while living in exile, and can, simultaneously, preserve their religion and tradition. In the eyes of some Tibetans, their exile in India represents a state of permanent pilgrimage in the holy land. Misra refers to a certain resemblance between the physical and religious topography of Tibet and that of Northern India, which lets Tibetans project a false sense of nationhood. "Tibetan religious identity finds an elevated expression in the Indian topography through its places of worship, common gods, goddesses and certain rituals. This symbiosis prevents a Tibetan from feeling completely alienated in India. In other words, a Tibetan in India does not feel entirely displaced, rootless or disoriented as is common with many other diasporic communities" Misra (2003, p. 200). Von Somm (1988) writes: "The new environment has been domesticated by creating a sacred geography marked with classical Tibetan religious objects. The monasteries, mostly built in a traditional style, serve as focal points in the religious landscape. Thus Tibet is to a certain extent recreated in India to guarantee a continuity in space and time" (p. 343).

Tibetans in exile are denied voting rights but are entitled to many of the rights and liberties enjoyed by Indians: their right to protest, and their access to ration cards—two basic but vital features of political and economic equality in India. Many of them are self-employed, engage in business, buy property, and occupy positions in the public sector. Misra (2003) notes how many Tibetans who arrived as desperate refugees have advanced to form a thriving, successful, and self-confident community. Factors supporting this process have included:

1. The establishment of business links in India. (Some Tibetans had managed to transfer their resources to India prior to the 1959 takeover).
2. International aid, in the form of advanced agricultural technology and farm subsidies. This guaranteed a regular and successful yield to those engaged in the farming sector.
3. On the basis of their background experience with a nomadic lifestyle, some Tibetans became good traveling salesmen. This profession brought them a regular and predictable profit.
4. Development of a communal network of contacts and connections, through which advance knowledge of the situation in India could be shared (Misra 2003).

Working in some areas of endeavor, such as the tourist industry or the restaurant business, required some degree of assimilation from Tibetans, since it demanded a greater degree of interaction with the Indians, and attunement with their customs and way of life. But Tsering Gellek (2001) notes that Tibetan settlements were established in exile "with this cautious principle, tempered between establishing amicable relations with locals and maintaining a separate identity. Ironically, the implicit message of not taking jobs away from the local indigent populations, paved the way for the exile's most lucrative industries: carpet weaving and sweater production. These two industries, with special emphasis on the former, created an economic boom for Nepal, and certain areas of India. The carpet industry within a decade of its humble settlement beginnings became Nepal's second largest earner of foreign currency" (p. 7). Handicraft production is one of the chief sources of income for the Tibetan refugee community. Although some Tibetans may be reluctant to work for Indians, in many cases, Tibetans would offer jobs to the locals. Many Indians are employed in the Tibetans' schools, in their craft centers (as carpet weavers), and in their dairies and as farm laborers (Tsering Gellek 2001). Penny-Dimri (1994) reports:

> "Local Indians were employed on a casual labour basis in order to do the farm work for the Tibetan Puruwala residents who were co-operative land share-holders. Indian domestic servants were becoming increasingly popular. Additionally, Indians were engaged on a casual basis by the settlement residents to perform manual work, from climbing a tree to hang the prayer flags, to building a house extension. The general manual labour that would have been performed by themselves or other Tibetan labourers within Tibet, was performed by Indians in the Puruwala settlement. In addition to those Indians who were directly employed by the Tibetans, the latter were in regular daily contact with a number of other local Indians. In the Puruwala settlement, local Indians leased some of the Tibetan property from the administration, which included a carpenter's shop and flour mill. There were Indian customers at the Tibetan settlement general store, Indian patients at the Tibetan health clinic, Indian neighbors, Indians who drove the trishaws, managed the post office and ran various local food stalls, as well as the group of Indian school children who sat under a large tree that was situated between the Tibetan school and Tibetan craft centre. Moreover, there were Indian tradesmen who came on their bicycles every day to sell fresh fruit, vegetables and milk as well as a man who arrived occasionally with a bundle of Western-style skirts, blouses and pants which he sold for 20 rupees each to the women. The general negative attitude of Tibetans toward the Indians did not inhibit the residents of the Puruwala settlement from employing Indian labour or engaging in business with them" (p. 4).

The negative attitudes of Tibetans mentioned by Penny-Dimri (1994) may be connected to their separatist tendencies, or else it may be a defense against prejudice directed towards Tibetans. Whereas Tibetans manage to adapt to a new way of life in exile, they also make strong efforts to remain distinct and protect their cultural identity. Misra (2003) notes that Tibetans refrain from intermarriage with those of other races, and remain committed to their spoken language and food habits, allowing them to remain as a distinct ethnic community. Exceptions to this attitude can also be found. Among representatives of the younger generation (especially men), I have found a few who believed that marrying an American or European would make their journey to the West more possible.

Penny-Dimri (2003) reported that despite maintaining business relationships, there was a considerable social distance between the Tibetans and members of the host community: "A willingness to engage in business does not necessarily imply or lead to other forms of social contact. The Tibetans maintain a social distance, to some degree, in respect to the Indians. In both the Bir and Puruwala settlements the majority of Indians I saw approach Tibetan homes were labourers and tradespeople. Additionally, in Puruwala there were Indian domestic servants and some tribal women from the nearby forest who begged for food. Tibetan women made the observation that the tribal women were suffering from misfortune and that they were not 'professional beggars.' The Puruwala residents were aware that their living conditions were superior to that of the majority of local Indians. In regard to the local Indians, a polite social distance was generally maintained by Puruwala residents. They did not experience the violent Tibetan/Indian conflicts described by the residents of the Bit settlement" (p. 4).

The acculturation of Tibetans in India also involves their exposure to Western culture. There is a significant influx of tourists from all over the world, who visit the Tibetan settlements for various reasons. These Western visitors often become the consumers for the new market of Tibetan goods and services. Misra (2003) notes that "since there exists an ever-growing market for Tibetan artifacts and other products associated with its religions and culture, the exile community is obliged to reproduce these objects" (p. 202). A continuous quest for sponsors has also been reported among Tibetans, who may redefine themselves according to the expectations of their new patrons. Traditional arts (e.g., Tibetan artwork, carpets, performances) are modified according to Western tastes. Von Somm (1998) observes, for instance, that some of the ritual dances and music were shaped and shortened to fit Western standards of entertainment.

Sponsorship is a complex and sometimes difficult issue, one that is deeply intertwined with exposure to Western culture. Many Tibetans in exile have come to rely on it. These sponsorships can be granted to individuals, or may take the form of community funding by welfare organizations. Finding a sponsor may be a highly organized process. Penny-Dimri (1994) reports that individual foreign sponsors are commonly sought to provide a regular income on a one-to-one basis for particular individuals, especially children and monks. There are also welfare organizations that provide money and support for Tibetan community projects, such as building homes and medical centers, or establishing businesses. Visitors from Western countries can be perceived as potential sponsors, and with each influx of tourists, the sponsorship network expands globally. Sponsorships have originated in Australia, Singapore, Hong Kong, Malaysia, Britain, the United States, and Canada. Many of these donations come from Western disciples and devotees of Buddhism, as well as from philanthropists who have an interest in the welfare of the Tibetan people.

Money sent by sponsors can sometimes replace a family income, and so may be equivalent to a breadwinner's wage. Penny-Dimri (1994) gives an example of a family, living in relatively good conditions, yet still receiving a sponsorship: "a family in Dharamsala owned (1) a large two-story home in Dharamsala and recently purchased new carpets from Darjeeling, (2) an allotment of land and a house in an agricultural settlement in South India which they briefly visited during Losar, and (3) a successful business in the sweater trade. Additionally, several siblings lived in Switzerland and provided a variety of goods to them. Nevertheless, their two school-aged children had sponsors."

It is significant that the welfare assistance is often ethnicity-based rather than need-based. This fact often creates tension not only within the Tibetan community but also in the relationships with the hosts. Penny-Dimri (1994) points out that on the one hand, Tibetans proved to be very flexible and adaptable in the new environment, and managed to win a great deal of help from the host government, as well as from foreign non-government organizations and individuals living abroad. On the other hand, Indians seem less resourceful and efficient, and often live in poorer conditions. For example, Tibetan schools have much higher standards and are often supported by various organizations. This contrasts with the Indian schools, in which "children wrote with chalk on small slates and sat on the ground under a tree in one group, while the teacher (a man) sat on a chair in front of them. They apparently had difficulties in following the standard syllabus because of the lack of facilities. The Indian school and students did not receive financial assistance, subsidies or sponsorships and students did not receive free meals or books" (Penny-Dimri 1994, p. 3).

Welfare assistance is still provided to Tibetans, even though their socio-economic well-being surpasses that of the local Indian population. That is why Tibetans may be perceived by the locals as groundlessly privileged. According to Goldstein-Kyaga (cited in Misra 2003), Tibetans lead a far better life in India compared to their standard of living in Tibet. Many Tibetans quoted in this study claimed that their condition had improved "by the grace of the Dalai Lama" and ascribed their success to hard work. They ignored, however, the role of sponsors, welfare agencies, and Indian Government subsidies. Penny-Dimri (1994) also observes that credit would usually go to Tibetan achievements and efforts, but hardly any respondent mentioned the benefits of receiving foreign finance and goods from welfare agencies and sponsors.

(Incidentally: The Tibetans I interviewed for my own research frequently referred to scholarships in a negative light. They claimed that many representatives of the younger generation felt discouraged from studying, obtaining qualifications, and looking for good jobs. Instead, they relied on the idea that they could receive financial help from a foreign donor.)

Computers and the Internet also play a major role in acculturation, especially where young people are concerned. At school, young Tibetans quickly learn how to use computers, and in most settlements there is Internet service. Communication software and chat rooms are vehicles for seeking friends and dates, as well as potential sponsors. Access to Western television, movies, radio, and print media also plays a major role in acculturation.

On the other hand, there are settlements where the level of involvement with the host culture, and exposure to Western culture, are fairly low. This is the case in the more remote settlements I visited, which are mostly inhabited by the older generation. These individuals look as if they were suspended in time. Elderly people were dressed in traditional clothes, wore traditional decorations, and engaged in spiritual practices in the time-honored manner: sitting and repeating mantras with their *malas* in one hand and prayer wheels in the other. When visited by a stranger, they would bow down, holding both hands together,[19] and present the visitor to another person as a sign of salutation and respect. Duff (2003) explains that this was a typical greeting, and sign of homage, in all Buddhist countries until recent times, when Western traditions became dominant.

In the settlements, it is also customary to put out and exhibit one's tongue in greeting. Buchung (2005) says: "The interaction with the outside culture has posed a dilemma for the Tibetans, particularly when there was contradiction between traditional Tibetan beliefs and the modern world view. The Dalai Lama from an early stage asked Tibetans to be pragmatic as they faced such a situation. Tibetans, he said, should differentiate between the essence of their culture and its more superficial ritualistic accouterments. He stressed the importance of preserving the former while being able to forgo some of the latter, particularly in terms of rituals like customary ways of greeting that included sticking one's tongue out, or traditional burial styles which are not feasible at lower altitudes."

An example of such a place is Tezu—a town in the Indian state of Arunachal Pradesh. Cawthron (2003) describes it as one of the poorest and most remote settlements in exile: it was established in 1963 and consists of five camps. In order to survive, Tibetans in the settlement are engaged in farming and they established a small carpet-making center. But importing wool and exporting the finished products is too expensive to make the enterprise financially viable. Trade is also inhibited, because special permits are required for travel in and out of the restricted area of Arunachal Pradesh. Wood and bamboo, available in this area, is used for building houses with thatched roofs. The houses are in poor condition, with their supporting pillars rotting and thatch requiring regular replacement.

Two community health workers, trained at the Delek hospital, run a small health center and provide first aid as well as treatment for minor illnesses. The center is visited by a doctor from the Indian hospital at Tezu, situated 6 km (ca. 3.7 miles) from the settlement. Tuberculosis, malaria, cholera, and dysentery are common complaints. But patients who are suffering from serious conditions must be transported to Tinsukia, a three-hour drive from the settlement, or to Dibrugarh (six hours away).

One social problem facing the settlement is the number of older people who have no family support. While the Tibet Foundation[20] maintains a residence for the elderly that accommodates thirty-eight people, there are many more elderly Tibetans living alone and in poverty. They may be dependent on their neighbors for support, or they may rely on the settlement officer, who distributes charitable funds when they are available. The Tibet Foundation and other organizations may attempt to obtain sponsorships for such settlements. Involvement with the culture of origin is strongly visible in such camps, which present a considerable challenge for those interested in ethnographic study.

Other examples of the effects of acculturation may involve discrimination and prejudice. Penny-Dimri (1994) reports a number of conflicts observed between the Tibetans and Indians of North India, based on ethnic prejudice. These conflicts created tension and served as a trigger for various accusations. They referred to:

1. Gender relationships and sex: "Indian men objected to Tibetan youths 'talking' with their sisters and teasing the young unmarried Indian women. Talking implies familiarity and exposes a crucial cultural difference toward gender relations. The rural Indians (Muslims and caste Hindu) adhere to strict rules in regard to gender relationships and are very concerned about the premarital chastity and purity of the girls. By contrast, Tibetans have a relaxed attitude toward youthful friendships and a pregnancy be-

fore marriage does not present a major social problem" (Penny-Dimri 1994, p. 1).

2. Hygiene practices: Tibetans were accused of being dirty, due to cultural differences related to hygienic behaviors. For example, they only bathed occasionally.
3. Dietary customs: Young, vegetarian Hindu men would make remarks relating to the consumption of meat by monks: "The Hindus condemned the Tibetan monks' practice of eating animals as impure and unspiritual" (Penny-Dimri 1994, p. 1).

Perceived prejudice may also be experienced within one's own ethnic group. Sadutsang (2002) explains: "Tibetans from Tibet and those who had lived in India after 1959 had very different backgrounds. We began to notice subtle differences in their behaviours which were different from those who were already living in India. The group from Tibet were called 'new-comers' and they were much more emotionally labile, even talking to them in a candid way maybe mistaken as being unfriendly, hostile or rude and they may easily feel slighted. They tended to be more suspicious and aggressive. Physical aggression was not uncommon amongst the younger people. Knowledge of Buddhism was limited" (pp. 5-6).

To sum up, there are a number of factors affecting the acculturation of Tibetans in exile. These factors include their political and economic status, job opportunities, cross-cultural differences, such as religious beliefs and practices, prejudice and discrimination, and exposure to Western culture. Difficulties associated with acculturation may include a high level of stress or identity confusion. Having established the different variables affecting acculturation and the effects of the acculturative process itself, in the next chapter I will describe various models of medical treatment in the context of the Tibetan diaspora, as well as the interdependencies between culture and health.

NOTES

1. The Tibetan letters do not even resemble the Latin alphabet. In technical literature, Tibetan terms are often spelled using the Wylie transliteration scheme—a method for transliterating Tibetan script using the Latin letters. For example, a Tibetan word meaning "Buddhist teachings" (Sanskrit: *Dharma*) would be spelled "chos" in Wylie and pronounced, more or less, like "chö". For the reader's convenience, I shall write the Tibetan terms which are popular in the West in italics and as they are pronounced (e.g., *chuba*, *kathak*, *mo mo)*. For some of the Tibetan terms, which are less common in Western countries, I shall provide the Wylie transliteration

in the footnotes. In such cases, the word will be proceeded by "Tib" (e.g., Tib. *chos gos rnam gsum*).

2. *Mo mo* (Tib. *mog mog*) are the traditional Tibetan steamed dumplings.

3. *Thugpa* is a Tibetan noodle soup.

4. *Tsampa*: (Tib. *rtsam pa*) is roasted flour, usually made of barley or sometimes wheat. Tibetans often mix it with their traditional salty butter tea (Tib. *bod cha*).

5. *Chang* is a name for Tibetan beer.

6. Tib. *chos gos rnam gsum*

7. Tib. *dge slong,* Sanskrit *bhikrhu*

8. Tib. *gso sbyong,* Sanskrit *porhadha*: "healing and purifying" or "repairing and purifying." This is a ceremony conducted twice a month (during each full and new moon) in which monks and nuns purify themselves as a result of any broken vows and restore their ordination to purity. Teachings on *gso sbyong* were expounded upon by the Buddha himself, and are presented in the *Vinaya* section of the sutras (Duff 2003).

9. Tibetans often obtain the "blessing stings" from lamas or *rinpoches* during individual or public audiences, or when the lama is giving the *abhisheka* (sometimes translated as empowerment), a tantric ritual. The strings are usually red, yellow, or dark blue in color.

10. Tib. *rab gnas*

11. "Rinpoche" is a term for a very holy person, literally "precious one," but meaning something like, "Holy One Who Is So Valued" (Duff 2003).

12. Source: http://www.unhcr.org/1951convention/new-phase.html

13. The total population figures in South Asia have been compiled from the Internally Displaced People survey, the Office of His Holiness the Dalai Lama in India, and Department of Home records, India. The population figures for Tibetans abroad have been taken from the records of the Department of Information and International Relations, reestablished in 1959 in India as part of the Central Tibetan Administration (CTA). Source: Office of Tibet http://www.tibet.com/Govt/into-tib.html

14. According to Tseng (2001), from a psychological perspective, it is very import ant for immigrants to have a feeling they can return to their homeland and have a "cultural time-out" when the stress becomes too intense.

15. Source: http://www.studentsforafreetibet.org/article.php?id=479

16. Source: http://www.wwu.edu/~culture/rudmin.htm

17. Sense of Coherence (SOC) is a concept developed by Aaron Antonovsky (1990). It defines a "global orientation that expresses the extent to which one has a pervasive, enduring though dynamic feeling of confidence that: (1) the stimuli deriving from one's internal and external environments in the course of living are structured, predictable, and explicable; (2) the resources are available to one to meet the demands posed by these stimuli; and (3) these demands are challenges worthy of investment and engagement" (pp. 7-8). Three of the above components are labeled: comprehensibility, manageability, and meaningfulness. Antonovsky argued that a high level of SOC can be associated with better health and well-being. This became the foundation of salutogenesis—an approach that concentrates on factors sustaining and promoting health, rather that pathogenic.

18. Methfessel, T. (1997). "Socioeconomic Adaptation of Tibetan Refugees in Sough Asia Over 35 Years in Exile." *Tibetan Culture in the Diaspora: Papers Presented at a Panel of the 7th Seminar of the International Association of Tibetan Studies, Graz, 1995*. Korom, J. Frank (ed.). Vienna: Verlag der Osterreichischen Akademie der Wissenschaften, 1997. pp13-24.

19. Tib. *thal mo sbyar*

20. Tibet Foundation is a registered charity established in 1985. The aim of the organization is to develop public awareness of all aspects of Tibetan culture and the needs of the Tibetan people.

Chapter Two

Health and Illness Behaviors

2.1 From Biomedicine to Holism
    2.1.1 Biomedical Model
    2.1.2 Humanistic Model
    2.1.3 Holistic Model
2.2 Interdependence between Culture and Health
    2.2.1 Culture as a Salutary Agent
        2.2.1.1 Healthy Behaviors
        2.2.1.2 Culture and Identity
        2.2.1.3 Culture as a Means of Social Support
2.3 Culture as a Pathogenic Agent
    2.3.1 Unhealthy Lifestyles
    2.3.2 Acculturative Stress
    2.3.3 Identity Confusion
2.4 Culture as a Pathoplastic Agent
    2.4.1 Culture as a Meaning-Making Device
        2.4.4.1 Idiom of Health and Ill-Health
        2.4.4.2 Folk Categories and Explanatory Models
2.5 Illness Behavior
    2.5.1 Help-Seeking Behavior
    2.5.2 Help-Seeking Pathways

2.1 FROM BIOMEDICINE TO HOLISM

As discussed in this study, the effects of culture and religion on health differ according to the model of medicine that is used as a frame of reference. According to Szawarski (1996), there is ambiguity as to the terminology used in the philosophy of medicine: the scientific model is often contrasted with the humanistic. Moreover, the way one views a human being, or health and disease, will be affected by the perspective of a given paradigm. With respect to this study, I will discuss three models of medicine: biomedical, humanistic, and holistic, referring to the division by Davis-Floyd and St. John (1998). The term Western medicine, found later in this book and frequently used by the respondents, does not necessarily imply biomedicine. It may also refer to an approach characterized by the humanistic model.

2.1.1 Biomedical Model

The biomedical model has been the most popular model utilized in the medical sciences. It is associated with the modernistic philosophical tradition that views knowledge as objective and fixed. With this approach, "knower and knowledge are independent, and language is a representation of objective truth and reality. Doctors are authorities as decision-makers and patients are in a deferential position" (Larivaara, Kiuttu, and Taanila 2001, p. 18). Biomedicine is often described as scientific, materialistic, and based on the concept that the role of science is to explain and describe the processes inside the human body, as well as to formulate certain rules. Davis-Floyd and St. John (1998) call this paradigm the "technocratic model." This refers to the technocratic quality of society, which is hierarchical, bureaucratic, and organized around an ideology of technological progress. Medicine practiced according to this model will involve specialized knowledge and technical procedures.

The authors also identify and elaborate on twelve major tenets that characterize this model, namely: 1. Mind-body separation; 2. The body as machine; 3. The patient as object; 4. Alienation of practitioner from patient; 5. Diagnosis and treatment from the outside in (curing disease, repairing dysfunction); 6. Hierarchical organization and standardization of care; 7. Authority and responsibility inherent in the practitioner, not the patient; 8. Supervaluation of science and technology; 9. Aggressive intervention with emphasis on short-term results; 10. Death as defeat; 11. A profit-driven system; and 12. Intolerance of other modalities in the technical hegemony. In short, the model is based on the concept that the mind and the body are two separate substances. Davis-Floyd and St. John (1998, p. 19) explain: "This idea meant that the superior cultural essence of man, his mind—as well as the superior spiritual essence, his soul—could remain unaffected while the body, as a mere part of mechanical nature, could be taken apart, studied, and repaired."

This notion was developed in the time of Descartes, and weakened the European folk view—according to which there was an interaction between humankind and earth as a living organism, infused with a feminine "world soul." In a model in which body and soul remain separate, the former became an object of responsibility and expertise for the medical profession, while the latter became identified as the domain of religion. According to this model, organisms do not much differ from machines. In order to understand this sophisticated bio-mechanism, it can be divided into simpler parts and sub-systems, which are then investigated in detail (*reductionism*). The whole organism is perceived as a sum of organs, functions, and sub-systems, and the specific branches of medicine will specialize in a given area. Health refers to a state in which the biological organism can function properly. Malfunction can be caused by internal factors (viruses, bacteria, genetics) or external ones (impairments of the body, or problems with the environment). The role of the doctor will be to restore or replace a biological function that has been lost.

The concept of the norm is also important, as it determines whether a patient is classified as healthy or sick. Mind and spiritual life are not regarded as being essential for health, and are often ignored. It is also pointed out that mechanizing the human body and perceiving it as a machine can relieve biomedical (or technomedical) practitioners from feeling responsible for the patient's emotional well-being. Healthcare receivers may simply be seen as "interesting cases of x, y, or z." In many instances, objectifying patients may extend to refusal to inform them and discuss details of their health condition, medical procedures, and treatment that is planned.

Medical interviews often include closed questions aimed at eliciting necessary information that confirms the assumptions made by the physician, or that lead to further inquiry. How the patient feels about his or her condition or what it means to the family is not given too much credit. This approach is in opposition to the open-ended, patient-centered type of interview advocated alongside the development of post-modernist thinking. On the other hand, Larivaara, Kiuttu, and Taanila (2001) note that the doctor-centered attitude is suitable and appropriate in acute clinical situation, when the patient's life is threatened and immediate decisions must be made. In such circumstances, the doctor leads the conversation, presenting a sequence of closed questions, and interrupting the patient if they digress from the topic of interest.

What can frequently be observed in clinical contexts governed by biomedicine is an emotional gap between the patient and the practitioner. Doctors themselves often tend to enforce a strict hierarchy. Many of them may be perceived as kind, but also as rigid and officious. During their medical training, they have already learned that they need to protect themselves by avoiding emotional involvement and what is called counter-transference.[1] Diagnosis and treatment "from the outside in" stands in opposition to an approach which assumes that proper healing involves reinforcing the body's innate aptitude for self-healing, which can be done by means of appropriate diet, exercise, cleanliness, and proper lifestyle.

Hierarchy and subordination within technomedicine is expressed in the relationship between individual and institution, in which hospital routines are subject to the convenience of the medical staff, not the patient. Another aspect of hierarchy identifies physicians as being the group positioned over all other healthcare practitioners (including nurses, physician's assistants, and practitioners of other healing modalities, such as naturopathy or ethnomedicine). Furthermore, the emphasis on specialization can be observed in the devaluation of generalists; a primary care practitioner is likely to be allotted a different status and salary than a cardiologist or a neurosurgeon. Whereas specialization enables intense development due to research in a given area, it also makes physicians concentrate on a very narrow scope of human functioning. On the other hand, the more specialized one is, the lesser the expectations that one exercises good interpersonal skills, communication, or empathy. Davis-Floyd and St. John emphasize the disadvantages of such an approach: "Patients have become powerless to assess the relative value of diagnostic and treatment options. Typically, persons with complex or unresponsive conditions are handed around from one specialist to another with little coordination of care until they either give up or succumb to ill effects of the pharmacological disaster that follows" (1998: 31).

Specialization in medicine also leads to standardization. Individuals in a position of power determine the rules for others to follow; for example, which diagnostic procedures, techniques, and treatment methods are appropriate in specific cases. Standards and norms are set up, and often reinforced by the institution's policies, or by the insurance company. In this model, the doctor is presumed to be an expert. His or her authority is emphasized by specific markers, such as a prestigious title, a white coat, or a stethoscope. Using technical jargon not comprehensible to most patients serves a similar function: ensuring distance between the doctor and the patient, and providing the former with a sense of authority and control. Subsequently, the patient feels less responsible for his or her own treatment and becomes a passive receiver of medical actions.

Finally, a characteristic approach to death can be observed in this model. Whereas so much effort is invested in postponing the moment of death, and controlling the laws of nature, when death does occur, doctors often experience it in terms of defeat. In his book, *How We Die,* Sherwin Nuland outlines the problem of biomedical doctors feeling powerless when they are unable to accept the natural order of things, even when the patient is elderly and his or her life energy has come to an end. Davis-Floyd and St. John note: "In a model where death is the enemy and dying tantamount to failure, mortality is a mighty foe. The death of a human being is a defeat for a medical system that strives for ultimate control over nature. Death is a painful reminder that such striving is illusory—no matter how much we dissect life in order to understand it, no matter how many operations we perform or prostheses we insert, we cannot eliminate death" (1998, p. 42).

These are the characteristic features of the model known as biomedicine, which lies at one end of the continuum between the technocratic and holistic approaches to healthcare. We shall now move to the middle part of that spectrum—a model influenced by humanistic thought, known as the humanistic or biopsychosocial model.

2.1.2 Humanistic Model

The humanistic model of medicine stands in the middle of the spectrum, between the technomedical and holistic approaches. Yet the boundaries between the models on this continuum are very much blurred. One can find examples of physicians working in technocratic medical institutions, who use highly sophisticated technologies, yet exercise a special type of attitude towards the suffering person, which is more characteristic of the humanistic model. This will be mediated by the practitioner's individual personality, values, and life philosophy. What is significant about the humanistic approach is an attitude towards the patient marked by kindness and compassion, and by more respect for the patient's autonomy and his or her right to be an active partner in the process of diagnosis and treatment.

The biopsychosocial or humanistic approach takes into account all the aspects of human functioning, that is, the patient's biological and psychological state, emotional and spiritual needs, family and social relationships. All of these things will be considered when the doctor seeks to understand symptoms, determine a diagnosis, and make decisions about how to remedy the patient's suffering. More attention is given to illness narrative: in other words, letting the patient share his or her story. Negotiating the explanatory models for illness held by the patient, the family, and all those involved in the clinical setting becomes one of the aims of treatment. In this model, body and mind are still conceptualized as separate, yet more respect is given to the latter, in comparison with the biomedical model. Proponents of the biopsychosocial model acknowledge the influence of the mind on the body, and vice versa. Subsequently, they advocate that both domains should be addressed during healing. Such an approach has been strengthened by research findings in the field of psychoneuroimmunology.

With this perspective in mind, practitioners should recognize and try to respect the natural tendencies people have: a need to seek privacy and protection when ill, and responding positively to tenderness, a loving touch, and attention, along with an aversion to harsh or punitive contact. Establishing a good rapport between the patient and his or her physician is emphasized as an important factor contributing to recovery. This requires the practitioner to be more mindful and aware of his or her own personality, emotions, difficulties, body language, and verbal expression, all of which play an important role in communication and can be utilized in the context of healing.

A humanistically oriented practitioner is expected to be open to (or at least neutral towards and respectful of) a patient's decision to use complimentary forms of treatment as a way of enhancing physical and emotional well-being. This would not necessarily require the physician to use those complementary or alternative forms of treatment, but at least have a general knowledge of the modalities the patient might refer to. This is necessary so that the physician can assess which of these methods might be beneficial to a particular patient in support of his or her medical treatment. Some treatments may be seen as neutral, while others might present a risk—for example, classical massage is not advised for oncological patients, nor are certain herbs that may interact with pharmacological treatments.

The interaction between the patient and a humanistically-focused doctor should be open and friendly. The patient is seen as a partner in the healing process, not simply as an object of clinical interventions (as is characteristic of biomedicine). Screening interviews are more likely to be patient-centered. As Laarivaara, Kiuttu, and Taanila explain (2001), this type of interviewing is characterized by the doctor encouraging the patients to choose and share the issues that they feel are the most important. This obviously requires more time and effort on the part of the practitioner, who must concentrate on building a good rapport with the patient. While this may be possible for some general practitioners, this type of interviewing is not suitable in an emergency situation—for obvious reasons.

Patient-centered interviewing would result in a shift in the role of the practitioner, who would then be expected to satisfy needs that are usually addressed to a counselor, psychotherapist, or priest. Also, a question arises as to whether this type of interviewing is feasible in a technocratic medical setting, when little time may be allocated to individual patients. Nevertheless, such postulates reflect a longing for attentive and compassionate care, long associated with the ethos of the Hippocratic doctor-healer—a wise and trusted person who cures the body, heals the mind, and comforts the soul of the sufferer.

Within the humanistic model, practitioners acknowledge the need to assist the patient in his or her suffering, even when no further physical recovery can be obtained. In this book, I will discuss the differences between disease (symptoms) and illness (reaction). Both categories are of interest to humanistically oriented physicians, and may produce different treatment objectives. Artur Kleinman (1980) notes, for example, that when "curing the disease" cannot be achieved, "healing the illness" may still be attainable. For example, in cases of cancer or AIDS, when all possible treatment options have been exhausted, and have produced no results, a practitioner may still provide comfort and reassurance to the patient, on his path towards death. The issue of help for dying people has been elaborated on by a Swiss-born psychiatrist, Elizabeth Kübler-Ross, in her book, *On Death and Dying* (1997). This important aspect may be neglected in biomedicine, where succumbing to death is likely to be perceived as the doctor's failure.

Because humanistic medicine creates space for individual experiences, religion and spiritual practices may emerge as important aspects of the healing process. Later in the book, I will explain how spiritual beliefs may be a significant source of coping mechanisms. When the spiritual needs of the patient are given enough value, the practitioner is more open to cooperation with representatives of this domain, such as ministers, priests, and lamas. Clinical practice based on these humanistic principles is being given more and more credit worldwide. Apart from research findings that stress the importance of engaging psychological factors within the treatment modality, this change may be attributed to the growing market of paid health services, in which patients enjoy a greater variety of options, and make decisions to their own satisfaction. For example, where two highly qualified specialists in a given field are available, the patient may choose the one whom he or she perceived as kinder, more open and attentive. Healthcare services are often assessed in the setting of a medical institution, where the patient may scrutinize various aspects of hospitalization, including administrative quality, rapport with personnel, and the quality of communication, diagnosis, and treatment. Under these circumstances, technocratic institutions and practitioners may experience a decrease in the number of referrals, unless they are sensitive to all their patients' needs and treat them as valued customers or, being highly specialized and having no competition in their area of expertise, they can enjoy a secure position on the healthcare market.

In the context of the present study, there were numerous examples of the two medical models described above. Patient narratives often included references to "the Western model of medicine," yet it was not always clear to what extent institutions and practitioners represented the biomedical or humanistic model. Although the technocratic attitude towards medicine is largely incompatible with traditional Asian values, for the sake of consistency, I will use the term "Western model of medicine" when referring to the diagnostic and treatment methods developed in Europe and America, and incorporated in medical clinics functioning in Asia. Western medicine was represented by health professionals working at hospitals, and in private clinics run by biomedical doctors.

2.1.3 Holistic Model

The term "holistic" is commonly used to describe a systemic approach to treatment, one that is rooted in Hippocrates's philosophy and various forms of ethnomedicine. According to this view, Man is seen as a single psycho-physical unit, incorporating all his experiences, emotions, and thoughts. Man is also viewed as part of the ecosystem. Wrona-Polanska (2000) explains that individual responsibility for maintaining one's health and recovery is crucial, and in the process of treatment, all factors that come from the biosphere, socio-sphere, and culture should be considered. A healthy lifestyle, including an appropriate diet and physical activity, is also stressed.

The holistic model of Man goes far beyond the technocratic vision of body as machine, or even the biomedical one, which sees the body as an organism. In the holistic approach, the body can be seen as being composed of elements—earth, air, fire, and water—or as a unique energy field. Holism assumes the oneness of body-mind-spirit, however abstract the notion of "spirit" may be. For example, Davis-Floyd and St. John (1998) note that there is a consensus between most healers that there exists something like a spirit or soul, which is part of a human being and continues to exist even when the physical body vanishes. According to this view of human beings, the only moment when dualism or separation between the physical and spiritual creeps in is the moment of death.

Taking into account the concept of a spirit or energy, the holistic model uses terms such as energy, *ch'i,*[2] *prana,*[3] energy channels, *chakras,*[4] or meridians.[5] Modalities of treatment that deal with this energetic aspect have been developed within the holistic paradigm. They include acupuncture, homeopathy, intuitive diagnosis, Reiki, hands-on healing, magnetic field therapy, therapeutic touch, flower remedies, massage, reflexology, and chiropractic therapy. The traditional systems of Chinese or Tibetan medicine (elaborated on in this book) and the Indian Ayurveda[6] can also be classified as part of this category. Holistic healers often incorporate the spiritual aspect into the process of healing. They hold a notion that individual health can be influenced by subtle energies. Not only the body has its energy field (sometimes called an *aura*), but emotions or thoughts are viewed in terms of vibrations (Brennan 1988; Myss 1996). For example, negative energy is attributed to anger, jealousy, sadness, or anxiety, and positive vibrations are associated with love, compassion, and joy. Whereas health is understood in terms of inner balance, a sense of fulfilment, and self-realization, disease is associated with energetic imbalance or blockage.

The renowned British scientist and physician Edward Bach (1886-1936) began his research in the field of bacteriology, and through his findings became a holistic healer. He saw the causes for disease in terms of negative states of mind, such as Restraint, Doubt, Fear, Over-enthusiasm, Restlessness, Ignorance, Indecision, Impatience, Indifference, Terror, Weakness, or Grief. In his essay "Free Thyself," he explained: "We have so long blamed the germ, the weather, the food we eat as the causes of disease; but many of us are immune in an influenza epidemic; many love the exhilaration of a cold wind, and many can eat cheese and drink black coffee late at night with no ill effects. Nothing in nature can hurt us when we are happy and in harmony, on the contrary all nature is there for our use and our enjoyment. It is only when we allow doubt and depression, indecision or fear to creep in that we are sensitive to outside influences" (quoted in Howard and Ramsell 1990, p. 51).

Like many modern holistic practitioners, Bach saw the healer's duty in terms of helping patients gain a proper understanding of their health and innate qualities, and motivating them to express their creative potential. Proper understanding relates to the idea that patients are responsible for their own health and should actively participate in the healing process, in making medical decisions, and in applying treatment. To awaken the body's natural healing potential, practitioners often advise on changing dietary habits, using nutritional supplements or nontoxic pharmacological products, or meditation, relaxation techniques, psychotherapy, and exercise. The role of the practitioner is more that of an educator or advisor, who teaches clients to be more independent, to access their inner resources and wisdom, and to learn to perceive and respond to their own needs. It is the client, however, who must make his or her own choices, such as the decision to give up smoking, follow a healthy diet, find a less demanding job, and stand up for his or her basic personal rights.

Using these means to restore equilibrium is often perceived as truly challenging and may thus be rejected by the client. Most patients, brought up in a context where biomedicine is commonly used, would prefer to take a pill, as an easy option with instant results, no matter how quickly the problem returns. In the holistic model, however, far-reaching objectives are preferred to the mere elimination of symptoms. For example, in biomedicine, a person with a skin disorder might immediately be offered some ointment or steroids to eliminate the problem. On the other hand, a holistic healer would start by asking the patient about dietary habits, work overload, or any other stressors, to determine which factors might aggravate the symptoms.

In addition to this, a holistic practitioner might also analyze what advantages a person may have as a result of the symptoms. For example, by being ashamed of displaying an ugly rash on the face in public, a person may avoid social contact. Subsequently, this isolation may protect him or her from other life challenges, which might normally evoke tension due to lack of confidence, or uncertainty and fear. Such challenges may involve looking for a job, finding a partner, or leaving home and starting a new life as an independent adult. This explains the notion that somatic and psychological symptoms, apart from producing stress, can also be ascribed specific informative, adaptive, and transgressive functions—they reflect inner conflicts, help one adjust to various changes, and sometimes trigger self-development, transformation, and going beyond one's boundaries (Pietkiewicz 2002).

Holistic therapists advocate healing individuals in their whole-life context. This is often referred to as "treating the person, not the disease." It implies looking at various aspects of the client's functioning, and examining his or her professional, social, or intimate life, aspirations, and needs, as well as reasons for any frustration. In the healing process, according to Edward Bach, the client is about to awaken qualities that are inherent in his or her mind, such as Love, Understanding, Sympathy, Tolerance, Peace, Wisdom, Steadfastness, Forgiveness, Gentleness, Courage, Strength, and Joy. To remedy negative experiences of the mind, Bach used flower remedies prepared according to methods used in the homeopathic pharmacopoeia. Particular essences addressed specific emotions or personality features. The founder of this method explained the mechanism in which the remedies worked in terms of flooding one's nature with a particular virtue one needed, raising one's vibrations, and opening up channels for the reception of one's Spiritual Self.

With the holistic model, inner wisdom (or "body wisdom") and intuition are highlighted as important sources of information, inspiration, and as solutions for various problems. The use of intuition also applies to the practitioners. Whereas in biomedicine physicians are often trained to rely on textbooks, diagnostic tests, technology, and the experience-based advice of experts, in the holistic model, value is given to direct insight and following one's own quiet inner voice. The postulate of oneness does not only refer to the body-mind-spirit energy field. It also involves a concept of synergy with a therapist. Even though it is appropriate to have well-established boundaries, it may be necessary to loosen them for a time, so that the practitioner can get a feeling for the client and synchronize with his or her rhythm. Establishing that specific connection could be compared to what Milton Erickson referred to as *pacing*, when inducing a hypnotic trance in his client. This requires a certain level of openness, flexibility, and empathy from the therapist.

Most holistic practitioners specialize in one or two modalities. When necessary, they might refer the person to other specialists. This reflects an idea that healers should know their own limitations, do their best in offering services, and give the client enough freedom to chose alternatives. While the boundaries between various modalities of treatment may blur at times, biomedicine (or the technocratic model) and the holistic model can be viewed as extremes along one dimensional continuum. Many biomedical health practitioners regard themselves as holistic, and acknowledge the importance of a multidimensional approach when treating disease, yet they would never use alternative therapies on their own patients. These are the more humanistic biomedical practitioners. There are examples of humanistic physicians who work in a highly technocratic context, yet do their best to express kindness and patience towards those in their care. They take the time to explain medical procedures to the patient, and respect his or her decisions—even a decision not to comply with the doctor's treatment. Under growing pressure from healthcare recipients to make medicine more humanistic, such expectations have grown and become more explicit, especially due to the emergence of competition within the healthcare sector. More and more private clinics and health insurance companies now encompass complementary alternative modalities into their treatment packages. A rising interest in complementary methods is also expressed by the growing number of health spas and wellness centers where practitioners of various modalities offer their services.

In this study, the holistic model of medicine is represented by the traditional Tibetan system of medicine.

2.2 INTERDEPENDENCE BETWEEN CULTURE AND HEALTH

Culture strongly affects physical and mental well-being, and can influence health in either positive or negative ways. Culture may thus be analyzed as a salutary, pathogenic, or pathoplastic agent. The salutary function of culture is defined by how it promotes healthier behaviors, contributes to the formation of personal identity, and provides social support. In the interpretation of illness and health behavior, culture also becomes a meaning-making device.

The pathogenic aspect of culture, which refers to how it contributes to health deterioration, and its pathoplastic aspect, which refers to the ways in which a disorder may be manifested in different cultures, are defined by Katsavdakis (2001). To describe the pathogenic effect of culture, I will examine how cultural values, norms, or traditional behaviors can negatively affect mental or physical health, along with the risk factors associated with migration and social and psychological adjustment (e.g., acculturative stress). The pathoplastic factor may be explained by means of the phenomena popularly classified as culture-bound syndromes.

2.2.1 Culture as a Salutary Agent

Various aspects of culture may have a positive effect on health. The following illustrations refer to the role of culture in promoting healthy behaviors, in strengthening personal identity, and in providing social support. From the perspective of biomedicine, a balanced diet, abstinence from alcohol and tobacco, and getting regular exercises are all important variables in promoting health. According to holistic (or systemic) models, however, psychological well-being is given equal weight in its important to overall health.

2.2.1.1 Healthy Behaviors

Some cultures are associated with promoting healthy behaviors. Gomes et al. (2004) compared Asians and Whites and examined the purported health-risk and health-protective factors attributed to each group. These included anthropometry,[7] soy consumption, smoking, alcohol consumption, physical activity, general health status, and disease conditions. The major Asian subgroups examined were the Chinese, Japanese, Filipinos, Koreans, Pacific Islanders (Native Hawaiians and Samoans), Southeast Asians (Vietnamese and Hmong), and people from the Indian subcontinent. The authors report that Asians, when compared to Whites, consumed considerably more tofu or soy milk. They drank less alcohol, and fewer Asians had ever smoked or were currently smokers. While the authors found certain variations within particular groups, they also reported better health among recent immigrants from Asia compared with those born in the U.S. They propose two explanatory hypotheses: "(1) persons who immigrate tend to be healthier and more robust than those who do not (i.e., the "healthy migrant" effect), and (2) other cultures tend to subscribe to and practice healthier lifestyles than those of the mainstream American culture" (p. 1981).

In the traditional Tibetan system of medicine, much attention is given to dietary, sleep, and work behaviors. While Tibetan doctors urge their patients to follow a healthy and balanced lifestyle, and to refrain from smoking, Tibetans are known for practicing a number of unhealthy behaviors (see Section 2.3.1, "Unhealthy Lifestyles.")

Several studies have linked certain cultural characteristics with attitudes towards violent behavior. According to Yick (2000), "traditional cultural values serve as a protective buffer against stressors engendered by immigration" (p. 263). Yick studied the predictors of physical violence between spouses or other intimate partners in Chinese American families. He found that the more acculturated subjects were slightly more than twice as likely to have been a victim of severe physical violence by a spouse or intimate partner. Similarly, Mexican Americans and Puerto Ricans born in the United States were more likely to assault their wives. On the other hand, members of the Tibetan community in India and elsewhere are discouraged from exhibiting violent or disruptive behaviors. Traditional Buddhist principles, which have become equivalent to the law in Tibetan communities, strongly promote harmony, kindness, and respect.

2.2.1.2 Culture and Identity

Another common example of the beneficial role of culture refers to the concept of identity. Mol (1979) says that the term "identity" connotes sameness, wholeness, boundary, and structure. He refers to it as "wholeness-maintenance," juxtaposing two human tendencies: the tendency towards sameness and the tendency towards change. According to Mol, these two should balance each other, because: "too much change means disintegration and too much sameness means loss of adaptability" (p. 14).

Kim and Kim (1998) describe personal identity as "the total sum of my being and the entirety of what I am . . . the totality of my physical, mental, emotional, social, legal, cultural, and conscious and unconscious thought processes and feelings" (p. 116). While some aspects of personal identity are given and beyond one's control, others can be acquired and cultivated. Kim and Kim (1998) describe the various dimensions and components of identity as: Physical Identity, Legal Identity, Professional/Occupational and Achievement-Related Identity, Psychological Identity, Cultural Identity, and Ideological/Political/Religious Identity.

Physical Identity is determined by factors such as date of birth, birth order, gender, physical appearance (including facial features, skin color, hair and eye color), and genetic factors (such as hereditary dispositions and diseases). These outer features are visible and can be easily distinguished or categorized. Even though some features may be modified (facial features, through plastic surgery; weight, hair color) many remain unchangeable (choice of biological parents, ethnicity, and family lineage).

Legal Identity is defined by the laws of the nation in which one resides, and includes one's legal status in that country. Date and place of birth, legal name, married name, and status as a citizen, permanent resident, illegal alien, or foreign exchange student, are all possible components of Legal Identity. Professional/Occupational and Achievement-Related Identity describe self-identity in terms of academic or professional achievement, degrees, or titles, all of which can enhance self-esteem and determine perception of oneself and others.

Psychological Identity is affected by the nature and quality of relationships with parents, siblings, and extended family, all of which play a crucial role in developing one's ethnic identity as well. Positive psychological experiences may strengthen one's self-esteem, self-concept, or self-affirmation, whereas negative experiences (for example, experiences with prejudice, discrimination, or victimization, along with feelings of alienation, marginality, and insecurity) may result in self-denial, self-hatred, or ambivalence. Ideological/Political/Religious Identity relates to social, political and spiritual/religious beliefs, actions, and behaviors.

Cultural Identity involves the transmission of cultural tradition, values, customs, rituals, and family stories from generation to generation. Berry (2001) explains that the concept of cultural identity "refers to a complex set of beliefs and attitudes that people have about themselves in relation to their culture group membership; usually these come to the fore when people are in contact with another culture, rather than when they live entirely within a single culture" (p. 620). Berry also distinguishes between two dimensions that relate to how one thinks of oneself: identification with one's heritage or ethnocultural groups (ethnic identity) versus identification with the larger or dominant society (civic identity). These two can be independent of each other, however, so that more of one does not imply less of the other. Berry (2001) also stresses that they are "nested," meaning that "one's heritage identity may be contained within a larger national identity; for example, one can be an Italian Australian" (p. 621).

Ethnicity, as distinct from ethnic identity, is another important concept for the purposes of this study. Pires and Stanton (2000) define ethnicity as "an automatic characteristic of racial group membership and a process of group identification in which people use ethnic labels to define themselves and others" (p. 44). As explained by Anderson and Kagawa-Singer (1996): "ethnicity refer to the traditions, values, perceptions, and practices we share through identification with a group of individuals who have in common a geographic and/or racial origin, a language and dialect, a religious faith, or some combination of these" (pp. 219–220). Pires and Stanton (2000) present ethnicity as a three-dimensional construct that results from the interaction of: 1. ethnic origin (natural identification with the original group into which one is born); 2. ethnic identity (individual or group affiliation with a specific ethnic group; it requires recognition by this group); and 3. ethnic intensity (degree of association with an ethnic group).

According to Chan and Rossiter (cited in Pires and Stanton 2000) ethnicity is the result of: 1. biological and physical characteristics; 2. actual and perceived personality traits; and 3. cultural values and norms. The term "ethnic identity," on the other hand, refers to the individual's natural identification with a specific ethnic group[8] (Pires and Stanton 2000). Ethnic identity involves aspects such as self-identification, feelings of belonging and commitment to a group, and a sense of shared attitudes towards one's own ethnic group.

Ethnic identity may be distinguished from ascribed ethnicity (i.e., ethnicity perceived by others). Phinney et al. (2001) note: "Ethnic identity is likely to be strong when immigrants have a strong desire to retain their identities and when pluralism is encouraged or accepted. When there is pressure toward assimilation and groups feel accepted, the national identity is likely to be strong. In the face of real or perceived hostility toward immigrants or toward particular groups, some immigrants may downplay or reject their own ethnic identity; others may assert their pride in their cultural group and emphasize solidarity as a way of dealing with negative attitudes" (p. 494). The authors also note that children who are exposed to negative stereotypes about their own ethnic group may develop conflicting or negative feelings about their own ethnicity.

Ethnic identity is not static, as it can change over time in response to social, psychological, and contextual factors. Behaviors, beliefs, values, and norms are usually constructed around one's ethnic identity (Phinney et al. 2001). Kim and Kim (1998) maintain that individuals who identify themselves with their ethnic background have a more solid sense of who they are, and that their psychological well-being is much enhanced. Cetrez (2005) notes that culture gives the context for identity embedding and negotiation. According to Anderson and Kagawa-Singer (1996): "culture provides a blueprint that guides our behaviour, helps us to determine our values and beliefs, and enables us to evaluate and make sense of our world. . . . Culture passes from the generation of our ancestors to future generations, linking past, present, and future through this heritage" (p. 219), and thus becomes a valuable source of one's identity.

Miranda and Fraser (2002) use the term "social interest," which refers to belonging, identification, or contribution, and "involves a feeling that the person has a place within a group and an orientation toward care for the welfare of the group to which he or she belongs" (p. 425). The authors maintain that this social interest provides a frame of reference for mental health. Miranda and Fraser also refer to the concept of "lifestyle," which "provides the structure and the character and the design for the way in which the person lives. The patterns, actions, decisions, and ability to adapt are manifested in the lifestyle" (2002, p. 426). This particular lifestyle is recognized as a factor providing stability, unity, individuality, and coherence to a persons's psychological functioning (Miranda and Fraser 2002).

The issue of Tibetan national identity has been touched upon in the literature, as well as in the popular press. Von Somm (1999) reports that Tibetan lay youth who attend secular schools often feel alienated from certain aspects of their religious tradition. Their relationship to tradition is less experiential, less embodied, and often ambivalent. However, they are familiar with the concept of Tibet and the imagined community, since they start every school day by singing the Tibetan national anthem. The same author notes: "Tibet is a mental concept, standing for an imagined community and history, which constitutes a national identity" (1998, p. 343). This image has two conflicting sides: on the one hand it is the paradisical, sacred land of the elders' memories, almost unchanged for more than a thousand years. On the other hand, it becomes more and more confounded by the reality of the occupied land, partly due to loosened restrictions on crossing the Indo-Tibetan border. This has enabled some Tibetans to visit the motherland, where they may be bitterly disappointed. As Von Somm (1998) explains: "Testimonies of Chinese oppression strengthen identification with the idealized image of Tibet. Interaction with "native" Tibetans, on the other hand, challenges this idealized notion of a pure, unchanged and traditional sacred country" (p. 344).

Thargyal (cited in Von Somm 1998) refers to the Buddhist teachings[9] as a specific part of culture with which Tibetans identify themselves. He says: "Chos is considered as the only source of Tibetan identity, culture and otherness" (p. 342). However, apart from Dharma, there are other specific ethnic markers (e.g., typical livelihoods, architecture, arts and crafts, traditional garments, decorations) that strengthen ethnic identity among Tibetans and support their psychological well-being (Kolas 2004). Topden Tsering (2004) observes that certain ways of dressing up may be an important way for exiled Tibetans to mark their affiliation with a specific group and a separate identity, so that they blend in and yet stand out. Penny-Dimri (1994) observes, for example: "In the Tibetan Plateau villagers prefer long sleeves on the shirts or blouses worn inside their *chuba* (particularly when they dress up for celebrations). . . . The braided hairstyles and coral, turquoise and amber ornaments attached to the hair of Amdo herding women from northern Tibet have become signs of 'Tibetanness'" (p. 244). She also notes that similar garments are worn by tour guides, and by the staff of guest houses and other tourist enterprises in Tibet.

Religion can also serve as a marker of ethnic differences. Kolas (2004) explains that in Tibet, placing a picture of a reincarnate lama or a white *khatak* scarf in the front window is a way for Tibetans to strengthen their sense of identity. In this way, they can:

> "openly display their beliefs and values as well as their ethnic identities, although they would probably tell you that whatever is hanging from their rear-view mirror

> is 'for luck.' The knots on the khatag scarf are not there to shorten it, but have a very special meaning. The knots have been tied by a guru at Songtseling during a special occasion. During particular religious holidays people congregate outside the chamber where the lama sits, at the top floor of the main temple. They buy a khatag scarf just outside the room, and bring it into the room with them, presenting the scarf to the lama together with a donation of money, as they kneel in front of him. The lama will then either hang the scarf over the worshipper's shoulders, or, if asked, tie knots on it before returning it. On their way out worshippers also receive a red (occasionally yellow) knotted string" (pp. 190–191).

Tibetans' characteristic physical features also constitute a part of their physical identity. Chinese researchers from the Central Institute for National Minorities[10] describe this population: "Tibetans have straight and black hair, brown eyes, with eye fold, their exterior angle of the eye being higher than the interior angle, straight nose, nostril elliptical, medium-thick lips, with protruding lips and cheekbones, wide and flat face, and sparse body hair" (online). In the host country Tibetans can be definitely identified.

Tsering Gellek (2001) reports on the psychological advantages of identifying oneself as a refugee: "Many Tibetans, regardless of the time spent in host countries thus willfully call themselves refugees. The lack of distinction between refugees and those born in exile is institutionalized by the fact that most Tibetan refugee agencies do not make any distinction between Tibetans who have been born in exile and those who are refugees. The politicized ambiguity of a refugee identity has been useful to the diasporic community in at least two ways: first it retains the political definition of Tibetans as a people without a homeland; secondly, by way of the first reason, it consciously directs development of nationhood by evoking (and re-invoking) the shared image and experience of refugeehood" (p. 12). This can be beneficial on a psychological level, by creating an identity for Tibetan refugees, and on a more practical level it can help them to obtain special welfare payments or sponsorships.

2.2.1.3 Culture as a Means of Social Support

Culture is also a means of social support. Tseng (2001) notes: "Family members, friends, colleagues, neighbors, or various social organizations can be the resources of support. The support can be given at the psychological level, such as empathy, emotional encouragement, or advice, or at a mechanical and practical level, such as providing a loan, introducing the migrant to a social network, offering assistance in the search for a job, and so on" (p. 702). The way resources are utilized depends on culture: In some societies people feel more comfortable relying on family members or personal friends, whereas in others, it is the public and social institutions (e.g., banks, employment and welfare offices, the legal system) that are more likely to be approached for help.

Anderson and Kagawa-Singer (1996) observe that in some cultures, "family" has a much broader meaning in comparison to the popular definition of a nuclear or extended family. It can be structurally open and may encompass other family groups in several different households. The authors note: "If a parent was unable to serve as a caretaker, grandparents, aunts and uncles, and cousins were readily available to carry out the parenting role. . . . Adolescents who had difficulties with their biological parents could seek shelter and advice from other trusted adults" (p. 221). They also point out that among some populations (in the Philippines, for example) this social network is reinforced by shared rituals, gatherings, and celebrations that bring people together. The number of potential caregivers is also broadened in this way.

These expanded kinship ties, along with greater involvement with the community and tradition, also help foster adolescent self-esteem. According to Anderson and Kagawa-Singer (1996): "A sense of community, important work to do, and reciprocal networks of obligation and support all aid healthy transitions from childhood to adulthood. Initiation rituals associated with puberty also help tie the adolescent to the community. Even when these ceremonies involve pain and humiliation, adolescents anticipate them positively because of the associated community solidarity and assigned status as an adult" (p. 222).

Tsering Gellek (2001) notes that Tibetans have managed to develop a good community network in which friends and families help one another. Individuals living in exile can still count on support from the Tibetan government or from monastic institutions, as well as from fellow members of the community. As is characteristic of many Asian societies, traditional Tibetan families are extended families. Yet this family model is becoming more and more challenged by the acculturation process.

Availability of social support is an important factor influencing migrants' adaptation, as it can reduce acculturative stress, and thus has a considerable affect on migrants' health. The Internet is also used as a strategy for coping with culture shock: Ye (2005) notes that the Internet can relieve users of anxiety and depression by providing an escape or social support. On the other hand, it can also inhibit the acculturation process. Ye (2005) analyzed three types of motives for using the medium: information seeking, relaxation/entertainment, and social utility. Those with higher levels of perceived discrimination were likely to use it for relaxation/entertainment purposes, whereas fear predicted using it as a social utility. The existence of culture shock correlated with using native-language Internet and using English-language Internet was positively correlated with English proficiency.

Ye (2005) also notes: "Media preference is another important indicator of acculturation for sojourners. Media consumption includes both ethnic media and host media. While ethnic media promote ethnic identity and preserve a group's original culture, in the long run, heavy consumption of ethnic media may be a barrier to cross-cultural adaptation" (p. 155). While I have found no specific studies on use of the Internet by Tibetans, it is widely available for Tibetans in exile. Numerous cyber-cafés can be found in the larger towns or settlements. In Dharamsala, many Tibetans were observed using these services to make friends and chat with them, flirt, write e-mails, and search for information. This medium is popular among both lay and ordained Tibetans; both adolescents and young adults use it frequently.

Jacobson (2002) describes how the presence of close friends outside the immediate domestic unit is an important variable affecting the adjustment process for Tibetans in exile. This social support helps them cope with distress. In the host country, Tibetans form extensive communities that enable them to make friends and cultivate allies. Furthermore, cultural heritage equips Tibetans with various coping strategies, which may manifest as techniques to help them calm down and create meaning in stressful situations. Mercer and Ager (2005) highlight the importance of using traditional rituals and divination in dealing with mental health problems. Tibetans, especially the elderly ones, often visit lamas and ask for advice when important decisions are to be made. However, the authors note that the newcomers can be at a disadvantage when traditional approaches are used in coping with mental health problems. This is due to the fact that they have little understanding of the traditional rituals they follow or have them performed by unqualified monks. Those who do practices "blindly" (that is, those who do not understand the rituals' meaning and significance) may fail to see any results, and after some months they may give them up, saying that Buddhism is useless (Mercer and Ager 2005).

Having analyzed the various salutary aspects of culture, researchers have found an association between culture and healthy behaviors. In the literature, culture is also described as a positive factor affecting one's identity and providing social support. I will now discuss the pathogenic potential of culture: its negative effects on health.

2.3 CULTURE AS A PATHOGENIC AGENT

Some aspects of culture can have a potentially negative effect on health measures. For example, certain lifestyles connected with stress, work overload, and improper diet, may lead to deteriorating health. Among the Tibetans, the trauma they experienced as refugees can have a devastating effect on their health and well-being. Furthermore, the migrants' adjustment to the host culture is usually associated with strong acculturative stress and identity confusion, which can also affect their mental and physical functioning.

2.3.1 Unhealthy Lifestyles

The negative impact of culture on health may manifest itself in the adoption of unhealthy behaviors—which may then become the norm in society. These behaviors may include the consumption of junk food or fast food, indulgence in smoking, drinking alcohol, taking drugs, overwork and other stressful activities. Some studies have focused on culture as a factor that mediates body image and eating behaviors.

For example, White and Grilo (2005) report that dieting behaviors and a preoccupation with thinness as risk factors for eating disorders may differ across cultures. They found a significant difference between Caucasian, Latin American, and African American female adolescent psychiatric inpatients in terms of factors that contribute to eating and body image disturbances. Although reports of binge eating were similar in these ethnic groups, Caucasian girls were more dissatisfied with their body shape and weight than African American girls, and revealed more severe levels of body image disturbance (BID) in comparison to the other groups. The authors explain: "The current findings suggest that a variety of psychological and demographic factors exert influence on body image, and that the relative influence of these factors differs as a function of ethnicity. For Caucasian and Latina American girls in this study, BID was predicted by negative self-esteem only, whereas for African American girls, negative self-esteem, peer insecurity, and anxiety contributed to BID. This finding suggests that for African American girls, the emergence of BID is contingent on a complex interaction of psychological and social difficulties" (White and Grilo 2005, p. 83).

The relationship between culture and eating disorders is also mentioned by Littlewood (2004), who says:

> "Most arguments about eating disorders now recognize something 'cultural' as essential in their etiology; whether body imagery or women's social and family experience. . . . 'Fear of fatness' has accompanied economic and public health changes associated with industrialization: improved nutrition and a general access to food beyond physiological requirements; the development of eating as a leisure activity, with a dislocation of palativeness from nutritiousness through the development of 'cuisine' and the commodification of cooked foods; lower mortality rates but reduced fertility; and an increase of women in the labor market competing against men. . . . In contrast, relative plumpness in

> women in nonindustrial societies, while rarer, has been said to demonstrate health and prosperity" (pp. 597–598).
>
> Lester (2004) notes that eating disorders have long been considered "the consummate culture-bound syndrome of Western (post)industrial modernity" (p. 607). Emergence of eating disorders in unexpected places is often conceptualized in terms of "Westernization" or "modernization," meaning that it is interpreted as evidence that Western culture has been exported (Lester 2007). Furthermore, Littlewood states that: "specific disorders associated with eating disorders (e.g., self-starvation, bingeing and purging, body image disturbances, intense fear of gaining weight) become meaningful expressions of particular cultural features: heightened consumerism, media saturation, an ethos of independence, and an idealization of self discipline, coupled with the constant seduction to 'supersize' everything" (p. 607).

While I found no information in the literature describing the attitude of Tibetans towards weight, they suffer less from obesity than do Indians. Yet the subjects of this study expressed the pathogenic influence of culture in terms of wrong dietary behaviors. High intake of butter and other animal fats by Tibetans resulted in cardiac disease and hypertension, while their large consumption of dried meat was also seen as having negative health effects.

Substance abuse and deviant behavior, as cultural factors, may also lead to health deterioration. McQueen, Greg, and Bray (2003) refer to a number of studies that show an association between high levels of acculturation and alcohol or drug use among adults (as among Mexicans or other Hispanics in the United States): "Adult Mexican men who migrate to the United States appear to adopt the more frequent drinking patterns preferred by Americans but maintain their high quantities per occasion, which is more common in Mexico" (p. 1738).

Hyman and Dussault (2000) investigated the relationship between low birth-weight and the acculturation process, including risk factors such as smoking, alcohol, and excessive dieting, on a sample of 17 Southeast Asian women resettled in Canada. Dieting during pregnancy, inadequate social support, and stressful life experiences positively correlated with higher levels of acculturation. Although none of the subjects reported smoking or drinking alcohol during pregnancy, and most claimed that their diet in Canada resembled the one followed in Southeast Asia, several were more preoccupied with thinness, even during pregnancy. Responses cited by the authors included the following: "In my country, women ate well to have a healthy baby, but here, many women I know are on diets, even when they are pregnant, they don't eat a lot" (27-year-old Vietnamese woman). "Women who have been here a long time, from wealthy classes, are very obsessed with their weight. Perhaps they ate less during their pregnancy because they wanted to maintain their figures" (35-year-old Vietnamese woman). The subjects also reported a lack of appropriate support during pregnancy, either due to an individual's nature ("not interested in making friends," "doesn't like to discuss worries with people") or lack of time to see or talk with friends and family (p. 358).

On the other hand, surprising differences were found among women low in acculturation, as they reported fewer psychosocial concerns about social support and stress; availability of family member support and perceived levels of social support were much higher in this group. Moreover, many respondents reported high levels of stress connected with their financial situation. Greater needs were associated with adopting a new lifestyle (for example, a higher demand for products such as cosmetics required more money). Many also shared a belief that they were obliged to work hard, despite their pregnancy. The authors cite a 34-year-old Laotian subject: "She works very hard for a manufacturer. She is always standing. I encouraged her to apply for maternity leave but she worked until the end of her pregnancy. She was afraid to ask, but also didn't want to go to the CLSC,[11] even if she was sick" (Hyman and Dussault 2000, p. 358). Inability to speak the language of the host society was the most frequently reported source of stress in the group low in acculturation.

No formal research is available on substance abuse in the Tibetan community in exile. However, the Central Tibetan Administration (online)[12] reports that in 2003 a survey was done to analyze the extent of substance abuse in India. In the wake of this study, the Department of Health initiated a three-year plan whose goal was to eradicate substance abuse among Tibetans in India. The project encompasses community meetings, awareness programs, and health talks given by specialists. A Center for Substance Dependence, HIV/AIDS, and HRD[13] has been established in McLeod Ganj (Dharamsala) (Kunphen).[14] This may suggest that problems associated with alcohol or drug use and sexually transmitted diseases have been reported among Tibetan exiles in India. It may be hypothesized that although acculturation in India results in stress and may be conducive to higher intake of harmful substances (drinking alcohol, chewing tobacco, smoking cigarettes), it is also associated with better education opportunities and availability of health education programs. In the course of my field work, I collected various kinds of leaflets, posters, and booklets, which suggested that numerous health campaigns have been undertaken, in order to raise sexual and hygienic awareness, provide information on risk factors, and inform Tibetans about the major symptoms of psychiatric disorders.

2.3.2 Acculturative Stress

One of the most distinct examples of the negative impact of culture on health refers to the concept of acculturative stress. Smart and Smart (1995) list alternative terms to describe the psychological impact presented by the cultural adjustment, namely: "culture stress," "culture shock," "culture fatigue," "role shock," and "language shock." As Gil, Vega, and Dimas (1994) explain: "acculturative stress can occur as a result of the acculturative process, and includes issues such as language problems, perceived discrimination, perceived cultural incompatibilities, commitment or lack of commitment to culturally prescribed protective values/behaviors, such as familialism and cultural pride. . . . Social-stress models of acculturative stress include mediating factors that may affect an individual's ability to adapt successfully to their environment . . . negative outcomes occur when stressors exceed the individual's coping resources, or mediators" (p. 44).

Culture shock is indicated by psychological and social problems, or even breakdown. Although frequent among migrants, acculturative stress is not inevitable. Its severity depends on a number of factors: it is higher among refugees in comparison to immigrants, and in large, monocultural societies versus multicultural ones. Greater acculturative stress is also associated with separation and marginalization attitude, whereas integration is least stressful. Psychological variables, such as an individual's appraisal of the acculturative arena, his or her coping abilities, identity confusion, and the relationship between expectations and aspirations and realistic possibilities are also crucial (Kagitcibasi and Berry 1989). Phinney et al. (2001) report that bicultural orientation is conducive to better school performance, whereas those who expressed marginalized identities showed the lowest levels of psychological adaptation.

Emigration apparently involves a number of significant changes in all areas of life: in one's work, social relations, community networks, and lifestyle. Adjustment in the host country requires special efforts to find a place to live, obtain a job, arrange for education, establish a social network, and be accepted by the members of the host community. Specific features of socioeconomic status (e.g., education and income) are also important as resources for coping in the host society. When these factors are missing, migrants often develop feelings of loss and their effective coping resources are reduced.

Migration is also frequently connected with experiencing loss—of one's family, friends, possessions. Smart and Smart (1995) note, for example, that the most significant aspect of acculturative stress for Hispanics resettled in the United States is the loss of social support, such as family ties and close interpersonal relationships. "Anticipated losses" that involve the mere threat of separation rather than actual separation should also be taken into consideration as a source of great stress. Decreased social support (of family or friends) among immigrant students in a study by Oppedal, Røysamb, and Lackland (2004) was also associated with reductions in host and ethnic competence. This on, the other hand, had a negative effect on mental health.

Abbott et al. (1999) found that stress associated with low levels of English language proficiency, perceived rejection by locals, and living without one or both parents can be associated with experiencing major problems and mental disorders. Hovey (2000) observes that family closeness, hopefulness for the future, and financial resources are crucial factors that shield individuals against acculturative stressors. These stressors included discrimination, language inadequacy, lack of social and financial resources, stress and frustration associated with unemployment and low income, feelings of not belonging in the host society, and a sense of anxious disorientation in response to the unfamiliar environment. Hovey (2000) reports a relationship between family intactness and acculturative stress among Mexican immigrants in Los Angeles. He explains: "The strength of family closeness as a predictor is not surprising. The family is a core feature of Latino culture and has traditionally been important in providing emotional support for its members" (p. 498). Similar attitudes to family support may be associated with Asians.

Vinokurov, Trickett, and Birman (2002) note that besides the problems typically associated with acculturation, such as perceived discrimination, language difficulties, family conflicts, homesickness, and perceived pressures from others to assimilate, additional stresses have been associated with adolescents. These include the inability of parents to help their children with school problems, intercultural dating, perceived discrimination from school personnel, or the culture-broker role of children. Discrimination at school may involve jokes about the ethnic minority or a teacher's forbidding them to use the mother tongue. The authors also mention the "culture-broker role" of adolescents in their families, which refers to having to translate for family members or having to accompany family members to appointments. This was also mentioned by Vang and Flores (1999), who explain that: "young people are faced with having to make decisions for adults on many occasions. They are expected to act as interpreters or instructors and are placed in positions of prominence in their families before tradition deems it appropriate. In this manner, the traditional family structure is often challenged and sometimes destroyed" (p. 11).

Torres and Rollock (2004) report an association between acculturative stress and depression in adolescents and adults. They note however, that it is influenced by variables such as familial and social support, employment, discrimination, role ambiguity or strain, and attitudes toward acculturation. Tseng (2001) notes that: "migration, which is psychologically stressful, might be one of the precipitating factors in the development of certain minor psychiatric disorders, such as anxiety or psychosomatic disorders, but it is not the main reason for the development of major psychiatric disorders (i.e., psychoses), such as schizophrenia" (p. 697). Yet migration-related stress may contribute to the development of alcohol and substance abuse, behavior disorders, depression, or suicidal behavior. Takeuchi and Adair (1992) explain: "The discrepancies between minorities and dominant group members create a social environment characterized by alienation, frustration, and powerlessness. Distress, demoralization, and more serious forms of psychopathology are likely to result from this environment" (p. 112).

On the other hand, in their study of Ghanaian migrants in the Netherlands, Knipscheer, Jong, and Lamptey (2000) report that the subjects' distress connected with adaptation was more associated with acquiring new skills. As the authors explain: "the consequences of migration are not so much related to loss, tension, or any intrapsychic disturbance, but more to the lack of the essential skills to cope with a new cultural situation" (p. 472). Lack of instrumental skills such as language may, on the other hand, result in feelings of inadequacy, worthlessness, and rootlessness (Ramos 2005). In spite of this, Knipscheer, Jong, and Lamptey (2000) assume that "acculturative stress does not necessarily lead to negative health consequences" (p. 472). Similarly, Dona and Berry (1994) maintain that acculturative stress may become "a positive force that enhances an individual's psychological functioning"(p. 60). The outcome, however, is determined by a number of variables, such as acculturation attitudes, cultural maintenance, acculturative experience, and values. Emigrants who choose a separation, an assimilation, or a marginalization mode are likely to suffer from a higher levels of stress than those with a tendency towards integration. The authors' study of Central American refugees who resettled in Canada shows that Latinos report a lower level of acculturative stress in comparison to Asians. These results are explained in terms of cultural norms that encourage individuals to "controlarse" (i.e., control oneself). The authors explain: "Through control of the self, Latinos keep in check negative feelings associated with unpleasant events or troubles" (Dona and Berry 1994, p. 68).

Acculturative stress is also common among members of the Tibetan community. Buchung (2005) writes: "The interaction with the outside culture has posed a dilemma for the Tibetans, particularly when there was contradiction between traditional Tibetan beliefs and the modern world view" (p. 1). Not only do the challenges experienced by migrants produce acculturative stress, but the stress can also result in identity confusion.

Prejudice and discrimination may result from cultural clashes, and are often a source of considerable strain. Williams and Williams-Morris (2000) characterize racism as "an organized system that leads to the subjugation of some human population groups relative to others. Fundamental to the development of such a system is an ideology of inferiority in which human population groups are categorized and ranked with some being inferior to others. This often leads to the development of negative attitudes and beliefs toward racial outgroups (prejudice), and differential treatment of members of these groups by both individuals and societal institution (discrimination). This definition of racism locates it primarily within organized institutional structures and not in individual attitudes or behavior" (p. 244). The authors distinguish a number of key characteristics of racial prejudice, for example, an explicit desire to maintain social distance from stigmatized groups, discomfort with sending children to schools with varying proportions of minorities, disdain for interracial marriage, discrimination in employing minorities, and the persistence of racial stereotypes. Such expressions of racial prejudice have also been reported by Penny-Dimri (1994) among the Tibetan diaspora, where both Indians and Tibetans revealed a degree of bias against the other group.

Normally, one of the direct expressions of discrimination can be segregated schools, which are often associated with lower test scores, fewer students in advanced placement courses, more limited curricula, fewer qualified teachers, little serious academic counseling, fewer connections with colleges and employers, more deteriorated buildings, higher levels of teen pregnancy, and higher dropout rates. These in turn, may predict poor academic and professional achievement, a higher risk of crime and substance abuse, and poorer psychological functioning. However, as far as schooling is concerned, in some settlements Indians rather than Tibetans were characterized as underprivileged[15] (Penny-Dimri 1994).

Williams and Williams-Morris (2000) continue: "Categorical beliefs about the biological and/or cultural inferiority of some racial groups can attack the self-worth of at least some members of stigmatized racial groups and undermine the importance of their very existence. . . . Several lines of evidence suggest that the internalization of cultural stereotypes by stigmatized groups can create expectations, anxieties and reactions that can adversely affect social and psychological functioning" (p. 255). The authors refer to other studies that show an association between internalized racism and lower self-esteem, less ego identity, poorer socio-emotional development, and symptoms of depression (Williams and Williams-Morris 2000).

Berry (2001) observes that individuals who experience prejudice and discrimination (for example, when their physical features set them apart from the host society) may refrain from assimilation as a way of avoiding rejection. He also notes that less discrimination is usually experienced by individuals who seek to assimilate and who undergo greater behavioral shifts. Smart and Smart (1995) explain that in some cultures people are susceptible to discrimination on the basis of their external features, such as the color of their skin or the texture of their hair. For example, individuals may be superficially classified into a category: "white" or "colored." The latter may apparently have a pejorative connotation. For example, light-skinned, young, and educated migrants (in comparison to dark-skinned, older migrants with little education) are likely to experience a more favorable situation in the United States.

Verkuyten (1998) reports that perceived discrimination elevates depressive symptoms and is related to increased aggression, sadness, anxiety, and egotism. He shows a distinction between personal and group discrimination in relation to self-esteem: "perceiving discrimination as an individual member of a group is not the same as perceiving discrimination directed at the group as a whole. I found a positive, but moderate, correlation; the participants reported a higher level of group discrimination than personal discrimination. . . . The social-psychological distinction between the personal and group levels is important because perceived personal discrimination was related to personal self-esteem, but not to ethnic self-esteem, whereas perceived group discrimination was related to ethnic self-esteem, but not to personal self-esteem" (Verkuyten 1998, pp. 490–491).

Noh and Kaspar (2003) note that the health consequences of discrimination vary according to the individual's personal coping mechanisms. The authors refer to the study by Krieger, who found that Black women residing in the United States who responded passively to racism had higher blood pressure, whereas those with a more active approach (such as talking to others or taking action) had lower blood pressure. Noh and Kaspar (2003) also observe that: "members of collectivistic cultures, including Asians and Latin Americans, exhibit a preference for resolving interpersonal conflicts in a way that reflects concern over consequences for others. The avoidant pattern of conflict resolution found among Asian Canadians was consistent with their traditional cultural norm of evading conflicts and preserving interpersonal relationships" (p. 232).

Although stereotypes in relation to both groups exist in Tibetan communities, many Tibetans seem to have developed a strong ethnic pride and openly resist assimilation (Penny-Dimri 1994) This can be understood as a way of coping with uncertainty, feelings of loss, and identity conflicts. No studies have been found on racial discrimination and its effect on health in a Tibetan population.

2.3.3 Identity Confusion

Culture has been identified as an important variable affecting personal identity, as well as one with various effects on health. It can also play a disintegrative role: Various studies that concentrate on emigrants' psychological well-being report that the subjects felt confused in terms of their ethnic identity. This can be particularly noticeable among young migrants, who may be more vulnerable to cultural confusion if they have not had a chance to establish firm personal and cultural identity. This also pertains to the children of migrants born in the host country; it may also be common among refugees as a group.

Anderson and Kagawa-Singer (1996) note the danger of losing parts of one's cultural heritage in the acculturation process, and explain numerous stresses experienced by the emigrant youth: "Many aspects of culture can be lost in the process of acculturation into mainstream society. These losses leave holes in the fabric of everyday family and group life that are poorly filled by the dominant culture. Adolescents become confused if they feel they must choose one or the other . . . complete assimilation is often prevented by discrimination. . . . The acculturation process in many ethnic families is initiated first among the children and teenagers who must adapt to the expectations and norms of the dominant culture expressed in school rules and in their interactions with teachers and peers. These children often have to lead double lives: one in school and one at home. They frequently speak different languages, eat different foods, and interact with others in radically different ways at home and at school" (p. 223). The authors also give an example of American Indian children who could neither speak their native language at school, nor practice their indigenous religion. Upon arriving home, they would perform a ritual cleansing to "rid them of their white man's ways" (1996, p. 223).

Similar experiences were described by Ausubel (1960), who studied the Maori community in New Zealand. This population consists of Polynesian people who migrated there circa 1350 A.D. He writes: "Maori pupils tend to lead two distinct lives—one at school and one at home in the *pa* [a nucleated Maori settlement or village]. There is little carry-over from school to home, but probably much more in the reverse direction. Conflict between home and school standards exists until middle adolescence and is resolved by the dichotomization of behavior: each standard prevails in its own setting. Thereafter, parental values, reinforced by increased contact with the Maori adult community, tend to predominate over the influence exerted by the school and the wider *pakeha* [European] culture" (p. 625).

In the same work, Ausubel describes a number of cultural differences between Western and other societies in terms of values, parent-child relationships, and expectations: "With the onset of adolescence in Western culture, children are expected to strive more for primary status based on their own efforts, competence, and performance ability and to strive less for derived status predicated on their personal qualities and on their dependent relationship to and intrinsic acceptance by parents, relatives, and peers . . . adolescents are expected to be less dependent than children on the approval of their elders, to play a more active role in formulating their own goals, and to relate more intimately to peers than to parents. They are also under greater pressure to persevere in goal striving despite serious setbacks, to postpone immediate hedonistic gratification in favor of achieving long range objectives, and to exercise more initiative, foresight, executive independence, responsibility, and self-discipline" (p. 617).

In contrast to this Western picture, Ausubel (1960) talks about the values present in a traditional Maori society, in which culture is less concerned with personal ambition and self-enhancing achievement, and instead places greater stress on tasks-oriented motivation, kinship obligations, enhancement of group welfare and prestige, and the social values of attaining common objectives by working in co-operation. He writes: "Valuing personal relationships, derived status, and kinship ties above material possessions and occupational prestige, helpfulness, generosity, hospitality, and sociability count for more in his eyes than punctuality, thrift, and methodicalness . . . he is less accustomed than the *pakeha* [European] to a regular and steady employment . . . he finds dull, monotonous labor less congenial than the *pekeha* does . . . the concept of thrift for vocational or economic purposes is more foreign to him . . . he does not value work as an end in itself, as a badge of respectability, or as a means of getting on in the world" (p. 624).

Another example of conflicting cultural differences is shown by Speller (2005), who compares Asian and American values: "Asian values are centered on the concept of interdependence in a collectivistic society. As a result Asian cultures emphasize concepts such as emotional self-control, humility, filial piety, family recognition through achievement, and the integration of the mind and body. Contrastingly, American society glorifies the individual, encouraging self-sufficiency and independence. American culture tends to value emotional self-expression, expression of pride, a duty to satisfy personal needs, self-recognition through achievement, and the separation of mind and body" (p. 71).

Exposure to conflicting values (those of the culture of origin and of the host culture) may result in confusion and attempts to constitute one's own "independent" identity, dissociating oneself from either culture as described by Bourhis et al. (1997). I presume that perhaps this is conducive to marginalization or (already described as one of the attitudes towards acculturation). Marginalization may then be understood as a way of coping with conflicting values. Still, in many cases this confusion may lead to psychological or psychiatric disturbances. Oh, Koeske, and Sales (2002) note, for example, that higher levels of depression among Korean American students are associated with perceived parental traditionalism. Faced with conflicting values (those of the culture of origin and of the host culture), Korean adolescents experienced discomfort and stress. Similar issues relating to identity conflicts in a Tibetan context are discussed by Tobten Tsering (2005). Family conflicts, or separation from family members that spring from the discrepancy between the acculturation level of the children and that of their parents, may also result in a higher risk for alcohol use or deviant behavior (McQueen, Greg and Bray 2003).

Adjustment to social rules of the dominant society can sometimes be perceived as disloyalty to one's own heritage. Subsequently, individuals cannot feel comfortable in either culture. This may lead to emotional despair, alcohol and drug use, and even suicide. Yeh et al. (2003) also note that whereas some migrants identify with their ethnic background, others may feel that they do not belong to either culture. The authors stress that maintaining strong identification with at least one culture was associated with better psychological well-being.

Oh, Koeske, and Sales (2002) reported that higher acculturation of Korean immigrants in the United States was associated with lower levels of depression due to decreased acculturative stress. On the other hand, higher levels of depression was also associated with greater assimilation into American culture. The authors referred to this phenomenon as the "depression-inflating effect of identity shedding" (p. 521). Operating in parallel cultures is said to carry the risk of increased stress and depression. The study shows that "unfettered assimilation to the host culture is not fully adaptive;" although it reduces acculturative stress, it "increases depression by eroding a sense of Korean identity and participation in traditional practices. . . . Abandonment of one's Korean identity and traditions may place the immigrant at risk of depressive symptoms" (p. 522).

The study of ethnic minority youth in the Netherlands by Vollebergh and Huiberts (1997) shows that allochthonous pupils in autochthonous ("White") schools report more emotional problems. Students were classified as "allochthonous" if: a) both parents were born outside the Netherlands in a non-Western country (Turkey, Morocco, Surinam, Asian and African countries), and b) both parents were born in the same country. Autochthonous pupils in autochthonous schools (with no pupils from different ethnic backgrounds) had lower stress and greater levels of well-being. The authors also found out that allochthonous subjects who identify with their own ethnic group (and not with the host culture) are more vulnerable to negative ethnic attitudes and attitudes towards living in the Netherlands: "the more negative they consider being a member of their own ethnic group, the higher the level of stress" (p. 255). Unfortunately, no research has been found on Tibetan children and schooling. Yet material collected during the course of my field work implies that there is a significant tendency to send Tibetan children to Tibetan schools (e.g., Tibetan Children's Village). No examples of Tibetan children going to Indian schools have been found. On the other hand, single cases of Indian children attending Tibetan schools have been reported.

Gil, Vega, and Dimas (1994) investigated the differences between individuals of Hispanic origin born in and outside the United States. They refer to a review of 30 other studies on acculturation among Hispanics living in the United States, which were carried out by Rogler et al. (cited in Gil, Vega, and Dimas 1994). The authors identify some key theoretical relationships. First of all, they assume that individuals low in acculturation, who experience high levels of stress, are likely to have negative self-esteem, to experience conflicts, to feel cut off from their culture of origin, as well as from their supportive networks, and to lack the knowledge and skills they need to cope with their new environment. Secondly, it is assumed that those low in acculturation, with lower levels of stress, are likely to have better mental health and adjustment. They might also benefit from the mediating effects of traditional cultural values (e.g., family support) and be less susceptible to negative stereotypes and prejudices present in the host culture and directed towards Hispanics, due to knowledge and pride in their native culture.

The authors observed that Hispanics born in the United States were likely to have low self-esteem stemming from acculturative strains and low family pride, regardless of acculturation level. But high acculturation had a strong degenerative effect on family pride among those who were born outside the United States. The authors explain this by stating that: "bicultural respondents are better equipped to negotiate the home and external environments than others, thereby minimizing the conflicts in either domain" (p. 52). Additionally, language conflicts are reported as being more important for foreign-born adolescents with high levels of acculturation. Those born in the United States, who had a low level of acculturation, reported higher levels of perceived discrimination in comparison to the foreign-born individuals. The authors explain that both groups may have had differing expectations of American society.

My field observations have led me to believe that Tibetans are more likely to use the integration pattern of acculturation. I also noticed the separation pattern on the part of some elderly Tibetans, as well as those living in remote settlements, where the influence of the host culture and exposure to Western culture was diminished. These people are less exposed to cultural stereotypes and use a whole repertoire of coping strategies, characteristic of their ethnic group. The positive impact of these strategies relates to the cited "benefit from the mediating effects of traditional cultural values."

The problem of identity confusion among the Tibetan diaspora is illustrated by Von Somm (1998), who notes: "Tibetan life in India is dominated by the counterpoised concepts of 'modern' and 'traditional.' Social customs, religious rituals, arts, and crafts belong to the latter, as well as to Tibet itself. Tibet is a mental concept, standing for an imagined community and history, which constitutes a national identity" (p. 343). But Von Somm also points out that there are significant differences between idealized Tibetan self-representation and the Western myth of Shangri-La. Dechen Khando and Sither (2004) note that young Tibetans in exile often struggle with a commercialized picture of "Tibetanness" created by Western society and imposed on them. The authors observe that Tibetans who socialized in Western societies were often dismissed as "not being Tibetan." The authors quote a respondent, who said: "We're expected not to eat meat, drive a car, throw a hip Tibetan New Years Party or even to initiate activism on political campaigns. Instead, we're expected to wear our Tibetan *chuba* to every event—to look Tibetan and exotic. We are frustrated by these kinds of stereotypes that are projected onto us" (online).

Von Somm (1998) also touched upon this issue of the construction of a Tibetan identity and the concept of "Tibetaness." He comments: "What counts as distorted or as real tradition, as authentic "Tibetaness," is a matter of negotiation and a product of mutual influence" (p. 341). Yet this Western *imaginaire* of Tibet—an exotic image, based on early travel literature and ethnic stereotypes—is very much influenced by the Tibetans themselves. Von Somm (1998) explains: "In order to gain access to financial and political help, Tibetans have felt the need to satisfy Western ideas of Tibetan culture. The modern concept of Tibetaness is mediated between Tibetan refugees and Western supporters" (p. 344). The situation described above can produce tension and inner conflict, and thus may become a pathogenic factor.

In conclusion: Culture may have many different pathogenic aspects, and may contribute to unhealthy lifestyles. In addition, the acculturation process may have many negative effects, including stress derived from prejudice and discrimination, and from identity confusion. The pathoplastic role of culture refers to how it mediates the expression of pathological symptoms.

2.4 CULTURE AS A PATHOPLASTIC AGENT

The pathoplastic influence of culture on health is expressed through the concept of culture-bound syndromes. *The Diagnostic and Statistic Manual of Mental Disorders* (DSM-IV-TR) defines the term: "culture-bound syndrome denotes recurrent, locality-specific patterns of aberrant behavior and troubling experience that may or may not be linked to a particular DSM-IV diagnostic category. Many of these patterns are indigenously considered to be 'illnesses," or at least afflictions, and most have local names" (p. 898). These symptoms are usually limited to specific societies or culture areas and relate to localized, folk-diagnostic categories.

DSM-IV (2000) identifies and explains a number of culture-bound syndromes, for example: *amok, ataque de nervios*, bilis and colera, *boufée delirante,* brain fag, *dhat,* falling-out or blacking-out, ghost sickness, *hwa-byung* (or *wool-hwa-byung*), *koro, latah, locura, mal de ojo, nervios, pibloktoq, qigong* psychotic reaction, rootwork, *sangue dormido* (sleeping blood), *shenjing shuairuo* (neurasthenia), *shen-k'uei* (in Taiwan) or *shenkui* (in China), *shin-byung,* spell, *susto* (fright or soul loss), *raijin kyofusho,* and *zar*. The International Classification of Diseases (ICD-10) provides additional references to these well-known culture-bound categories, listing names of similar syndromes observed in various parts of the world (Finerman 1998).

Guarnaccia and Rogler (1999) note that a given culture-bound syndrome could be associated with different psychiatric diagnostic criteria by various researchers. For example, some categorized *koro* as somatoform disorder, whereas others perceived it as an anxiety disorder. The authors maintain that in order to understand the syndrome's phenomenology, one needs to examine feelings associated with the syndrome, the physical sensations, emotions and thoughts of the person experiencing the syndrome, how the syndrome affects the person's orientation towards time and place, how it is acted out or performed, and how the person's significant others recognize the suffering associated with the syndrome.

Once the full symptom profile has been defined—not just the predominant symptoms—another issue that needs to be considered is the location and social context of the sufferer. It is crucial to identify which factors provoke the syndrome, along with the social and psychiatric history of the sufferer, including their life history and any traumatic events. The following is a discussion of both recognized and potential (as yet unreported) culture-bound syndromes embedded in Asian and other cultures.

Dhat

One of the culture-bound syndromes that has received much attention in numerous studies is concerned with male sexuality in Asian populations. Dewaraja and Sasaki (1991) explain that according to the Chinese and Ayurvedic medical systems, excessive loss of semen is regarded as unhealthy, because it weakens the body and is considered detrimental to mental and physical health. Asian people are thus biased against losing semen, which is believed to be a precious substance. According to these Eastern medical systems, large amounts of nutrition are required to produce a small quantity of semen. Manjula et al. (2003) comment: "It is commonly believed that 40 drops of butter produce one drop of blood and 40 drops of blood produce one drop of semen" (p. 702).

In India, the discharge of semen is associated with severe anxiety and hypochondria, a whitish discoloration of the urine, and feelings of weakness and exhaustion. This syndrome is known by the folk-diagnostic term *dhat* (DSM-IV-TR 2000). Manjula et al. (2003) explain that the syndrome mostly affects young and sexually ignorant men, whose families often exhibited extremely conservative attitudes toward sex. Syndromes that include similar symptoms are known as *jiryan* (in India), *sukra prameha* (in Sri Lanka), or *shen-k'uei* (in China).

Koro

One interesting culture-specific sexual disorder reported originally in China, Malaysia, and Indonesia is *koro*. The onset of its symptoms is associated with periods of imagined "sexual excesses," including frequent masturbation or nocturnal emissions. The psychological symptoms involve: 1. a belief or delusion of retraction of the penis into the abdomen, 2. intense panic with physical signs of anxiety, and 3. the use of mechanical means to prevent penile retraction (Fishbain, Barsky, and Goldberg 1989). The perception of involution of the penis is accompanied by a fear that this phenomenon will eventually result in death. Those who were convinced that their penises were shrinking (or gradually disappearing) would frequently use rubber bands, string, or clothespins to prevent them from retracting. This often resulted in severe organ damage. Other sufferers might let their parents or friends clutch the organ and pour cold water over it as a form of treatment.

Chowdhury and Bera (1994) offer this description of one of their patients: "he discovered that his penis had seemingly gone inside the abdomen beyond grasping or holding. At this feeling of 'penis loss' he shouted for help and experienced a premonition of impending bodily catastrophe, even death. His friends came hurriedly and 'dragged out' the receded penis manually. He was in a state of acute psychogenic shock with excessive sweating, palpitation, extreme dryness of mouth and speechlessness. He was taken to a nearby pond with his penis held by one of his friends and he was put into the water up to the level of his umbilicus for more than 2 hours" (p. 1018).

There were also cases of mothers who used similar remedial measures to protect their babies from penis loss. Bartholomew (1999) writes: "Some parents tied string to their sons' penises to reduce or stop retraction, a practice that occasionally produced penile ulcers. Authorities even went to the extent of measuring penises at intervals to allay fears. A popular local remedy was to have the 'victim' tightly grasp the affected body part, drink lime juice and be dowsed with buckets of cold water" (p. 47). Bartholomew also describes symptoms of *koro* among women, who feared that their breasts or vaginas were being sucked into their bodies. The syndrome evokes much clinical interest, as it resulted in large epidemic episodes with thousands of patients affected by *koro*. The poor and uneducated were most susceptible to it. They attributed the onset of *koro* syndrome in men to the influence of certain spirits of the dead, especially fox maidens who were searching for penises—which were believed to give them power. In Thailand, on the other hand, the symptoms emerged in the context of anti-Vietnamese sentiment and rumors about the alleged deliberate contamination of food and cigarettes with a *koro*-inducing powder. Bartholomew (1999) reports: "the poisoning rumors became self-fulfilling as numerous Thai citizens recalled that previously consumed food and cigarettes recently purchased from Vietnamese establishments had an unusual smell and taste" (p. 47).

A similar syndrome to *koro* was also reported in Nigeria, where people believed in magical genitalia loss. Bartholomew (1999) writes: "A major Nigerian episode of 'vanishing' genitalia in 1990 mainly affected men, but sometimes women, while walking in public places. Accusations were typically triggered by incidental body contact with a stranger that was interpreted as intentionally contrived, followed by unusual sensations within the scrotum. The affected person would then physically grab their genitals to confirm that all or parts were missing, after which he would shout a phrase such as 'Thief! My genitals are gone!'" The "victim" would then completely disrobe to convince the quickly gathering crowds of bystanders that his penis was actually missing. The accused was threatened and usually beaten (sometimes fatally) until the genitals were "returned." While some "victims" soon realized that their genitalia were intact, "many then claimed that they were 'returned' at the time they raised the alarm or that, although the penis had been 'returned,' it was shrunken and so probably a 'wrong' one or 'just the ghost of a penis'. . . . In such instances, the assault or lynching would usually continue until the 'original, real' penis reappeared" (p. 47).

Women "victims," on the other hand, were seen holding on to their breasts, either openly or discreetly (crossing the hands across their chests).

There is a typical symptomatic aura associated with *koro* syndrome. These symptoms may include anxiety, sweating, nausea, headache, transient pain, pale skin, palpitations, blurred vision, faintness, insomnia, or delusional thinking. Patients who suffered from *koro* were often preoccupied with masturbation and nocturnal emissions, or perceived sexual inadequacies or excesses. Many felt unconfident in sexual relationships. In certain regions where epidemics of the syndrome were reported, a number of cultural beliefs were also associated with *koro* (Bartholomew 1999).

The symptoms of *koro* or *suk-yang* (shrinking penis) have been reported in different parts of the world, including Malaysia, the Indonesian archipelago, Singapore, Thailand (where it is known by the Thai term *rok joo*), in India (where it is known as *jinjinia bemar*) (Hawley and Owen 1998) and in Egypt (where it is known as *rabt*) (Finerman 1998). Some authors maintain that they have also observed it in Western countries. Fishbain, Barsky, and Goldberg (1989) present two cases of Black patients in Miami, Florida, who believed in and feared the retraction of their penises, along with other symptoms. Kennedy (1991) shows another example of a White man who "became increasingly anxious and preoccupied with the fear that his penis was retracting. He had also had fears of genital retractions 6 years earlier when he used a vibrator two or three times for masturbation. He recalled panic-like symptoms when masturbating 3 or 4 years earlier and alluded to God's punishing him for his behaviour" (pp. 1278–1279).

Susto

Another type of culture-bound syndrome refers to the belief in "soul loss," which is common among some Latinos living in the United States, as well as in their native regions in Mexico and in Central and South America. It is known by various terms, including *susto, pasmo, tripa ida, perdida del alma,* or *chibih,* and describes an illness attributed to a frightening event that is believed to cause the loss of one's soul. Masyk (1998) explains that the concept of the soul in these instances is different from the Christian one. It refers to the ancient Mesoamerican concept of *tonalli,* which denotes the vital force as it informs the relationship between man and the universe.

The *tonalli* is located on top of one's head, and is believed to be connected to the world of the gods by an invisible thread. Any damage to this thread, by either natural or supernatural means, could produce fatal consequences. Children are believed to be especially susceptible to soul loss, because the ossification of their skulls is incomplete, and also because they are more easily frightened. Other situations associated with the risk of losing one's soul involved the wrath of the gods due to sexual excesses, sleep, sickness and death, or cutting the hair on the back or crown of the head, from which the tonalli could escape (Masyk 1998). The symptoms of *susto* include strain in key social roles, and in extreme cases appetite disturbances, inadequate or excessive sleep, troubled sleep or dreams, feelings of sadness, lack of motivation, and feelings of low self-worth or dirtiness. Patients also complained of symptoms including muscle aches and pains, headaches, stomach-aches, and diarrhea (DSM-IV-TR 2000).

Masyk (1998) maintains that susto could be "the result of an individual's inability to adequately fulfill the role expectations of the society into which he/she was socialized. . . . [It] provides the victim with a socially-sanctioned avenue of escape from intraculturally-induced stress" (p. 190). O'Nell (cited in Masyk 1998) observed another interesting relationship between the onset of the syndrome and fear of losing control over one's hostile feelings towards others, particularly in a culture where marked sanctions against violent behavior are present. Castro and Eroza (1998) note that syndromes like *susto* can generally be acknowledged in Latin American communities, and form a means of coping with traumatic, threatening, and dangerous situations.

Syndromes similar to *susto* were also reported in Bali (*kesambet*), China (*ching* or *haakts'an*), and New Guinea (*mogo laya*), as well as among refugee Hmong children who came to the United States from Laos. These children suffered from *ceeb* (pronounced "cheng"), an illness from fright (Capps 1999). Baer et al. (2003) also describe the syndrome called *nervios,* and explain that among Puerto Ricans, Mexicans, Mexican Americans, and Guatemalans, there is an overlap in aspects of *nervios* and *susto,* for example, crying, shaking, and sleep difficulties. Baer et al. (2003) note: "Causality of *nervios* is attributed to anger, grief, birth control pills, other illnesses, the birth of a child, anxiety, problems, susto, and other stressful occurrences. . . . Reported symptoms include headaches, despair, facial pain, trembling, and anger. . . . Treatment most commonly comes in the form of 'nerve pills' bought in local stores or alternative home remedies" (p. 317).

The departure of *tonalli* is also believed to create an empty space in the skull, which is observed as a cranial depression (*fallen fontanelle*, or *caida de la mollera* in Spanish). This is a folk illness attributed to children who accidentally strike their heads. Castro and Eroza (1998) describe the symptoms: "This condition has three basic signs. By simple visual inspection, individuals may notice that a baby's head is depressed, and thus claim that its fontanelle has fallen. More often, a baby's sudden inability to suck or having difficulty in swallowing are considered signs that the fontanelle has fallen, independently of any other physical evidence to support this diagnosis. Accompanying these signs is the third criterion, the presence of diarrhoea, which serves to confirm the presence of this illness" (p. 221). Castro and Eroza (1998) also note that there may be individuals in a community who have an alternative meaning-making system or paradigm, transmitted by means of education. The non-believers were observed to "display permanent ambiguity in their scepticism, which allows them to be ever ready to believe in these illnesses, should it be necessary" (p. 225).

Other Culture-Specific Syndromes

Some authors present cases that could be regarded as possible culture-bound syndromes, even though they are not yet classified as such in either the DSM-IV-TR or the ICD-10. There are also cases in which patients presented symptoms similar to those of a culture-bound syndrome, but in a different cultural context than the syndrome itself (e.g., the example of *koro* in a Caucasian man). To solve the argument as to whether or not a particular syndrome is culture bound, it is necessary to analyze the pathological picture in its wider, cultural context rather than simply looking at the symptoms.

Grigsby et al. (1999) describe patients in the Piedmont region of the U.S. state of Georgia who consumed significant amounts of chalk—the syndrome known as pica. DSM-IV-TR (2000) describes pica as: "eating of one or more nonnutritive substances on a persistent basis for a period of at least 1 month" (p. 103). The substances may include paint, plaster, string, hair, or cloth, animal droppings, sand, insects, leaves, or pebbles, and clay or soil. Grigsby et al. (1999) report that kaolin (white dirt, chalk, or white clay) ingestion is a common type of pica in the Georgia Piedmont area. These patients may continue to indulge in eating kaolin even when it causes medical complications, such as constipation, anemia, or colon rupture.

Shome, Bhutia, and Gautam (1993) describe another local phenomenon that may be classified as "culture-bound trichotillomania." According to DSM-IV-TR (2000), trichotillomania is the recurrent pulling out of one's own hair, often resulting in noticeable hair loss. Patients suffering from this syndrome may pull out their axillary, pubic, or perirectal hair. Shome, Bhutia, and Gautam (1993) describe the behavior of a monastic sect of the Jain community in India, who "remove all their hair on the head by manually plucking it out, called 'Locha.' This method of getting rid of the hair is peculiar to the Jains and is regarded by them as an essential rite. This is done to denote detachment from physical pain. This practice enjoys social sanction and is performed in a ceremonial manner by the monk or his disciples" (p. 674).

Beng-Yeong Ng (1998) presents a case of a patient with *wei han zheng*, a culture-bound syndrome of frigophobia in Singapore. Frigophobia refers to fears of cold-temperatured foods, which, according to the indigenous systems of medicine, are believed to be cold or yin in nature. The author describes the key symptoms: "core features include a morbid fear of cold (*pa-leng*), fear of loss of vitality, excessive fear of the wind (*pa-feng*) and the need to wear excessive clothing" (p. 582). The patient's fears were rooted in cultural conceptualizations of illness, and she sought help from traditional healers, who provided her with Chinese herbal medicines and dietary advice.

Hikikomori is a form of acute social withdrawal reported extensively in Japan. The syndrome usually affects adolescents and results in school non-attendance, along with isolation that may last for a number of years. In addition to avoiding strangers, individuals with *hikikomori* maintain minimal contact with their families. Ng (1998) described such a person: "He slept during the daytime and stayed awake at night watching satellite television or playing video games. Food was left at his door and he returned the trays when finished. When family members were away during working hours or at sleep at night, he was noted to tiptoe into the kitchen to replenish his supplies for his room" (p. 193). The family believed that the young man's behavior was instigated by spirit possession, so they consulted an indigenous healer for help.

Taijin kyofusho is another syndrome from Japan that resembles a social phobia. According to DSM-IV-TR (2000): "This syndrome refers to an individual's intense fear that his or her body, its parts or functions, displease, embarrass, or are offensive to other people in appearance, odor, facial expressions, or movements" (p. 903). Suzuki et al. (2003) describe the four sub-types of the syndrome: the phobia of blushing (*sekimen-yofu*), the phobia of a deformed body (*shubo-kyofu*), the phobia of eye-to-eye contact (*jikoshisen-kyofu*), and the phobia of one's own foul body odor (*jikoshu-kyofu*). The authors note that whereas *sekimen-kyofu* meets the criteria of a social phobia, *shubo-kyofu* relates more to the dismorphic disorder in DSM-IV classification. The remaining two subtypes could not be referred to any of the DSM-IV syndromes. Suzuki et al. (2003) further maintain that because *taijin kyofusho* incorporates diverse clinical entities, "it is difficult to make a firm conclusion as to whether all four subtypes of *taijin kyofusho* are culturally bound or whether some of the subtypes are virtually specific in Japan" (p. 1358).

Greenberg, Stravynski, and Bilu (2004) describe a syndrome that relates to social phobia, but is rooted in the context of the Jewish culture. They describe the concept of fear of the congregation (*aymat zibur* in Hebrew) as a culture bound syndrome of ultra-orthodox Jewish communities: "*aymat zibur* is used in the Talmud to refer to the feelings of those fulfilling a public function in prayer (the *hazzan* or the priest blessing the people) who act as intermediaries between God and man. The term is synonymous with respect for the congregation, in that fear is the emotion expected of one who has this onerous task" (p. 296).

Aymat zibur relates to two aspects of religious performance: 1. teaching Torah or speaking publicly on a religious topic, and 2. leading prayers or performing a religious ritual in public. Whereas the former is an expression of prestige, the latter is expected of every adult male. Greenberg, Stravynski, and Bilu (2004) show an example of a man who was "called to the Torah" in the synagogue. While standing on the podium and reading the text he heard a disparaging comment made by the man who was responsible for leading the prayers. The speaker felt hurt by the remark. Subsequently, he became anxious about going to public prayers and if he was called, he would start choking while saying the blessings and not be able continue. The problem worsened over time—the man would avoid all synagogues and would not visit his parents and parents-in-law on the Sabbath. Greenberg, Stravynski, and Bilu (2004) explain that the man understood his problem as a spiritual one: "The problem has afflicted him because of his sins, and for this reason he has visited the tombs of the righteous, hoping their prayers will help him" (p. 298).

Another examples of *aymat zibur* refers to a man suffering from strong anxiety when his daughter became pregnant, because if she gave birth to a son, he would have to attend a public circumcision in the synagogue. The same man also feared his parents' death, as he would be expected, by tradition, to lead public prayers for a whole year. When leading prayers, he would blush, choke, and feel his legs trembling. Other symptoms of performance-type social phobia have included difficulties eating in public, or using a public lavatory.

Some syndromes, even though they may be viewed in terms of psychopathology, are valued and desirable in the culture of origin. For example, Greenberg, Stravynski, and Bilu (2004) quote El-Islam: "Being bound to the home, which is a sign of severe agoraphobia in the West, is a sign of virtue in a Muslim housewife; the Koraan addresses women in the verse 'stay in your homes and do not misbehave like the early pagans'" (p. 294). Another example could be a Muslim man who avoids social contact while studying the scriptures intensively. He would be called *"zaddik"* (a righteous person) by the community and he would receive more help from its members. Greenberg, Stravynski, and Bilu (2004) write: "Interactional social phobia in the ultra-orthodox community emerges as a condition that may be very isolating yet may be accorded religious status and accolade. This is not to suggest that every *zaddik* has social phobia; rather that among those whose immersion in study is for spiritual betterment may be those whose primary motivation is avoidance of anxiety-provoking social contact" (pp. 295–296).

Culture can thus provide individuals with socially accepted ways of expressing certain conflicts or disorders. Somatization is one good example of this. Miranda and Fraser (2002) note: "somatization not only may be present as part of a certain syndrome but also may constitute a culturally adequate form of expression for the disorder . . . somatization may be part of the syndrome and what most cultures sanction as the appropriate manner of its expression" (p. 423). Bhui (1999) says: "The findings that 'Asian' peoples rarely present in primary care with depression, and that they are thought to present somatic manifestations of distress more often has led some to conclude that the somatic symptoms are manifestations of depression that goes undetected. . . . Such hypotheses have been confirmed by studies in India, China and Africa . . . where the expression of emotional distress is stigmatized in society, somatic expressions become manifest; that is they are culturally sanctioned and legitimate the patient seeking the sick role" (p. 141).

Lin, Carter and Kleinman (1985) maintain that Asian refugees and immigrants may be particularly predisposed to somatization. They observe that this mechanism is most often associated with the less educated, those of lower socioeconomic status, or those with rural backgrounds, as well as among ethnic groups that discourage the direct expression of emotional distress. In China, for instance, patients were often reported to express symptoms of depression and other psychological problems through a somatic idiom. One of the reasons for such behavior was an attempt avoid the severe stigma attached to mental illness in Chinese and many other Asian cultures (Lin, Carter, and Kleinman 1985).

Dewaraja and Sasaki (1991) report a similar situation in Japan: "it is common for patients to explain their subjective feelings of distress and anxiety in the vocabulary of stress or overwork . . . patients express their distress to the therapist on the basis of their own belief systems regarding the causes of illnesses" (p. 19). Escobar (2004) reports that in Nigeria and India the most common somatic symptoms include "feeling of heat," "peppery and crawling sensations," "numbness," "burning hands and feet," or "hot, peppery sensation in head." In Western countries these symptoms are very rare, however. Escobar (2004) explains: "patients tend to develop symptoms that are "medically correct," that is, symptoms that physicians expect and understand . . . somatic symptoms are easier to recognize and their scrutiny proves less intrusive that that of psychological constructs. Thus, they can be reliably elicited with little resistance offered by the subject because they tend to be less stigmatizing than psychological symptoms" (p. 10).

This concludes the section on culture-bound syndromes as a specific expression of culture's pathoplastic influence on health. It has been shown that similar expressions of certain culture-specific disorders can be found in different societies, where they are designated with folk names. It follows that some culture-specific disorders might be recognized in the Tibetan population. For example, it might be possible that some cases of ghost possession would resemble *susto* in some respects. Because certain of my Tibetan interview subjects reported a particular concern with losing sperm (or specifically, "energy drops," referred to as *tigle*), and because they consider frequent sexual intercourse (more than once a week) to be unhealthy, I thought there might also be cases in which individuals would develop symptoms similar to those of *dhat.* But neither my own research nor the literature supported this.

2.4.1 Culture as a Meaning-Making Device

In this section, I will describe culture as a meaning-making device for illness interpretation and health behavior. A firm grasp of the issues discussed here is essential to understanding the qualitative material presented later. First, I will explain the concept of disease versus illness, followed by a short presentation on the comparative frameworks for theories about illness. Then, I will concentrate on how various cultures determine the perception of illness, including folk categories and explanatory models. I will also cover the related issues of help-seeking behaviors and help-seeking pathways.

2.4.4.1. Idiom of Health and Ill-Health

Whether an individual is classified as healthy or unhealthy is as much determined by cultural norms as it is by contemporary definitions of health. Kleinman (1980) stresses that culture has a significant influence on how symptoms are understood, what value they are given, and how they are assessed (whether they are perceived as normal, abnormal, or even extraordinary—that is, when symptoms are perceived as an expression of spiritual attainment). Kleinman makes a useful distinction between disease and illness, a definition whose use has become popular in the social sciences. Both are said to express different interpretations of a single clinical reality, or different aspects of a plural clinical reality, and should be regarded as explanatory concepts, not entities. Whereas disease refers to a malfunctioning of biological or psychological processes in an individual, illness refers to psychosocial experience and meaning attributed to the symptoms of disease. Illness describes personal, interpersonal, and cultural reactions to disease or discomfort, and is shaped culturally.

Kleinman, Eisenberg, and Good (1978) explain: "Modern physicians diagnose and treat diseases (abnormalities in the structure and function of body organs and systems), whereas patients suffer illnesses (experiences of disvalued changes in states of being and in social function; the human experience of sickness)" (p. 251). It is also significant that illness may occur in the absence of disease or when the disease is in remission. Conversely, the experience of disease may be accompanied by minimal or no illness. Grzymala-Moszczynska (2004) explains that in many cultures it is insufficient to simply cure the disease (that is, to eliminate the symptoms by means of Western models of medical intervention) in order to perceive the treatment as complete. Certain religious means are also necessary to heal the illness, and so a special ritual may also be performed for the patient.

The understanding of health problems in terms of their etiological origin is also culturally determined. Garro (2000) describes three comparative frameworks for theories about illness. First, she refers to Murdock's typology: natural causation and supernatural causation. The former refers to "any theory, scientific or popular, which accounts for the impairment of health as a physiological consequence of some experience of the victim in a manner that would appear reasonable to modern medical science" (Murdock, cited in Garro 2000, p. 306). This category comprises four distinct types of theories: 1. infection, 2. stress, 3. organic deterioration, and 4. accident. It also refers to the biomedical model described earlier.

The supernatural causation theories are not recognized by modern medical science as valid and include three types: 1. mystical causation (encompassing fate, ominous sensation, contagion, and mystical retribution), 2. magical causation (sorcery, witchcraft), and 3. animistic causation (soul loss, spirit aggression). Such theories can be expressed within the holistic model in which the psychological and spiritual domains are given credit, alongside physiological explanations. Another framework presented by Garro (2000) refers to Foster's classification of naturalistic versus personalistic systems. The naturalistic one explains illness from a systemic point of view. Disease is understood in terms of imbalance between natural forces or conditions (e.g., cold, heat, dampness) and body elements. On the other hand, in personalistic systems, causes of illness are attributed to "active, purposeful intervention of an agent, who may be human (witch or sorcerer), nonhuman (ghost, ancestor, evil spirit), or supernatural (a deity or other very powerful being)" (Garro 2000, p. 307). Examples of these can be found in the qualitative material gathered in the present study. The third framework created by Young distinguishes between "externalizing" and "internalizing" systems. An expression of internalizing systems can be found in biomedicine, which relies upon physiological explanations and conceptions of internal mechanisms.

2.4.4.2 Folk Categories and Explanatory Models

To understand how the perception of illness is constructed by individuals, it is useful to refer to two more theoretical concepts of illness, namely folk categories (or local categories) and explanatory models. Both concepts are used in the area of cross-cultural psychiatry, where emphasis is placed on mental health. Personally, I find the concept of explanatory models especially useful in explaining patients' behaviors, irrespective of health problem type—be it mental or purely physical.

Folk categories refer to ways in which people in different societies recognize and label mental illness (Tseng 2001). An example of folk categories is presented by Jegede (2005), who elaborates on the idiom of health and illness among the Yorubas community in Nigeria: "In the Yoruba belief system, 'aisan' depicts 'not well.' To be well does not only mean biological well-being but the holistic condition of the individual and the society. . . . Diseases are considered as abnormalities in the structure and functioning of the body organs. For the Yorubas, ill-health is an external factor to the body, thus accepting of biomedical illness, but a wide range of people's constraints concern the parts of human life that cannot be reached by these tools. . . . The Yorubas believe that mental illness can result from four perspectives—natural source, such as those resulting from accidents or drug use, supernatural or mystical source, such as those resulting from the anger of the gods, preternatural source, which is usually caused by witchcraft, and lastly the inheritable ones. The Yorubas believe in the germ theory in the etiology of disease. Every departure from approved way of behaviour, especially those on the extreme, is considered as mental illness thus depicting social instability and in this situation pathological condition" (p. 120).

Jegede further explains *ware*—a local category for an illness that describes symptoms such as non-conformity to an approved way of life—especially when the afflicted person's behavior is extreme. Considering the above, local categories refer to a general notion people in a given society have about healthy and unhealthy behaviors. The way in which people make meaning of their symptoms is largely determined by culture. The concept of folk or local categories is apparently interconnected with the culture-bound syndromes discussed earlier.

Explanatory models, on the other hand, refer to particular episodes. Kleinman (1980) defines explanatory models (EMs) as "the notions about an episode of sickness and its treatment that are employed by all those engaged in the clinical process" (p. 105). EMs refer to five areas that they attempt to explain: 1. etiology, 2. time and mode of onset of symptoms, 3. pathophysiology, 4. course of sickness (including both degree of severity and type of sick role—acute, chronic, impaired, etc.), and 5. treatment. Kleinman designed eight generic questions (cited in Aull 2005, p. 284) to elicit the patient's story about his or her health problems:

1. What do you think has caused your problem?
2. Why do you think it started when it did?
3. What do you think your sickness does to you? How does it work?

4. How severe is your sickness? Will it have a short or long course?
5. What kind of treatment do you think you should receive?
6. What are the most important results you hope to receive from this treatment?
7. What are the chief problems your sickness has caused for you?
8. What do you fear most about your sickness?

EMs held by the practitioner determine how he or she understands and treats sickness. On the other hand, EMs held by the patient and family influence their understanding of the particular episode of illness, help-seeking behavior, and evaluation of treatment. Kleinman (1980) also stresses that:

> "Explanatory models need to be distinguished from general beliefs about sickness and health care. As we have seen, such general beliefs belong to the health ideology of the different health care sectors and exist independent of any prior to given episodes of sickness. EMs, even though they draw upon these belief systems, are marshaled in response to particular illness episodes. They are formed and employed to cope with a specific health problem, and consequently they need to be analyzed in that concrete setting. In practice, laymen either do not volunteer their EMs to health professionals or, when they do, report them as short, single-phrase explanations because they are embarrassed about revealing their beliefs while in formal health care settings. They fear being ridiculed, criticized, or intimidated because their beliefs appear mistaken or nonsensical from the professional medical viewpoint" (p. 106).

Bemak, Chung, and Bornemann (1996) explain how practitioners' explanatory models determine treatment. They compare the perception of the mental health problem and effective intervention strategies held by traditional Western healthcare providers and representatives of a Hmong community:

> "a Hmong refugee may believe in animism or spirits as the cause of emotional imbalance and may be visualizing and hearing a deceased relative. Traditional Western psychotherapists correlate these symptoms with psychosis and employ counseling techniques and medication that focus on the symptomatology (the 'hallucination') to treat the underlying psychosis. Indigenous healing methods would approach the same symptoms from a different cultural belief system, incorporating the concept of the deceased relative and spirit as an important and relevant personal and spiritual communication potentially contributing to the stabilization of the individual and even the entire family" (pp. 245–246).

In their study of explanatory models of psychosis among community health workers in the state of Tamil Nadu (South India), Joel et al. (2003) note that indigenous beliefs about mental illness often contradict the concepts present in the biomedical model; for example, where chronic psychosis is not recognized as a disease condition but as a result of black magic, possession by evil spirits, or poverty. McGuire (1987) notes: "Social scientists have tended to view 'non-scientific' medical systems in modern society as remnants of primitive or peasant, old-country traditions, or as characteristic of uneducated, lower-class persons who cannot afford modern 'scientific' medical treatment" (p. 365). This attitude has been characterized as an expression of ethnocentrism on the part of Western health professionals and researchers.

Joel et al. (2003) also maintain that individuals can hold diverse and contradictory beliefs simultaneously: some may hold beliefs about black magic and evil spirits as the cause of their illness and still seek professional help from a therapist, or be hospitalized and treated for schizophrenia. The authors also observe that: "non-biomedical beliefs about chronic psychosis can delay early recognition of disease, prevent early institution of medication, interfere with medication compliance and follow-up resulting in poor outcome" (p. 68). At least one non-biomedical belief about psychosis was recognized among the majority of health workers in their study.

Yeo et al. (2005) present an interesting account of community beliefs that Chinese-Australians held regarding cancer. In examining how their respondents understood their health conditions, the authors reported that whereas many included narrative terms that seemed to match Western biomedical explanations, most of them also maintained traditional folk beliefs—despite high levels of acculturation and belief in biomedical explanations for illness. The authors report: "Explanations included the following: (i) psychological factors (personality, being unhappy, inability to express emotions or holding them in); (ii) stress (e.g. migration, unpleasant experiences, many deaths in the family); (iii) foods, diet (low fiber, high salt, pork, high fat, too much meat, salted fish); (iv) drugs, alcohol, smoking; (v) chemicals or radiation (e.g., dry-cleaning chemicals, pesticides, petrol fumes, greenhouse gasses, genetically modified foods); (vi) hormonal factors (pregnancy); (vii) breast feeding (mild getting stuck) or not breast feeding; and (viii) physical strains (wearing tight-fitting brassieres, lifting)" (p. 179). The non-Western explanations included a belief that ill-health was due to imbalance of the positive and negative life force (yin-yang) in the body. Meanwhile, many respondents held traditional beliefs about the causes of cancer, and referred to such concepts as:

1. karma (*yeh*): cancer resulting from bad karma of oneself or one's ancestral line (for example, if a family member was a butcher who made a living by killing other beings "there was blood on the hands of a generation");

2. retribution (*bao ying*): cancer as a form of retribution for the misdeeds of the previous generations;
3. fate (*ming yun*) or Heaven's or God's will: cancer believed to be a lesson from God (for example, to increase one's faith, understand in-depth the suffering of others);
4. geomancy (*feng-shui*): fate influenced by the natural surroundings (seen as a contributing factor), for example, the family house faced a wrong direction or statues of the gods were not placed in the right locations;
5. touched evil (*zhong chia*): illness caused by offended spirits (e.g., if an individual walked over someone's grave, urinated on the graves, or said inappropriate things about the dead);
6. misfortune and bad luck (*shui wan, dong hark*): cancer as a result of bad lack due to a family curse or other people's jealousy of the family's wealth and good fortune;
7. offending the gods or deities requiring prayers or offerings for appeasement (e.g., the earth god, kitchen god, Monkey God);
8. black magic (*kong-tau*): spells invoked through human intervention;
9. incompatible astrological sighns (*pazi buhe*) between partners (Yeo et al. 2005).

Songwathana and Manderson (1998) studied the perceptions of HIV/AIDS among village women in southern Thailand. They reported that perception of the disease was mediated to a large extent by television and radio. It was associated with dirt, danger, and death. At the same time, it was believed to be "a disease of karma" (*rok khong khon mee kam*) and a "woman's disease" (*rok phuying*) associated with prostitution. Perceptions and meanings of AIDS derived from three broad modalities: biomedicine, traditional Thai medicine, and religious beliefs (Buddhist and Muslim). Many respondents held folk beliefs related to blood, which was thought to be one of the main components of the body. Infected with germs, blood was believed to change its color from red to black and become poisonous. Death resulting from AIDS is perceived as bad death (*tai mai dee*) and its circumstances are regarded as dangerous and polluting. While AIDS infection was often associated with sexual activities or needle sharing, some respondents attributed it to bad karma (e.g., due to telling lies, being promiscuous, gambling). Animistic explanations of the causes of the disease were also reported, which referred to beliefs of *tuuk kong* (a kind of black magic and sorcery), angry spirits, neglected ancestors, or malicious human beings.

Aull (2005) notes that in some societies one is discouraged from speaking freely before authority figures, and is expected to adopt a stoic response to illness. Cross-cultural collision may arise when the practitioner and the patient represent different cultures. Aull says: "When the culture of the physician and other health-care workers who are treating a "case" is markedly different from the culture of individuals in the society of which the sick person is part, how can the physician/listener understand the life world of the teller, especially when the interpretation of a set of symptoms is totally different in the two cultures (and especially when there is little time to review and ponder over interviews)?" (p. 283). Aull (2005) presents an example of a patient from a Hmong community who was treated for epilepsy. But both the patient and her family understood the cause of the disease in terms of "life-soul loss"—"the spirit catches you and you fall down" (p. 283). Such individuals would normally be expected to become shamans as they were believed to have a gift of seeing supernatural things. Subsequently, the patient became ambivalent about administering her medicine to suppress seizures, was confused by the changing medicine regimen and side-effects, and would not adhere to it.

> Haar (1987) presents an interesting example of an interaction between explanatory models of a patient, a clergyman, and health workers. He quotes a pamphlet written by Archbishop Milingo about an African woman who displayed serious psychiatric symptoms (according to DSM-IV), and after being unsuccessfully treated at mental hospital, sought help from the priest:"There was a woman who had suffered for five months. She sometimes could spend months on end without eating anything. She could only drink water or soft drinks. She feared her child because she did not consider him a human being. She constantly heard voices speaking to her. She was treated at a mental hospital, but to no avail. On the 2nd April 1973 she came to my office. She explained her problem. I told her we should pray together. She came back on 8th April 1973 and once more explained everything systematically to me. I brought her to my residence where I heard her Confession, then we celebrated Mass. But in spite of all this the voices continued to be heard and she still feared her own child. At that time I did not know how Satan behaves once he is in possession of someone. I contemplated various ways of helping the woman when suddenly an idea glowed in my mind, 'look three times intently into her eyes and ask her to look three times intently into yours. Tell her to close her eyes the third time and order her to sleep. Then speak to her soul after signing her with the sight of the cross.' I carried out this instruction systematically. The woman was overshadowed by the power of the Lord. She relaxed calmly and so I was able to reach her soul. I prayed as much as I could, then I woke her up. We both did not know what had happened to us."
>
> On reflection Milingo realized "that the Lord was leading me to the healing of the disease that is common among people, MASHAWE. This disease cannot be treated in a hospital" (pp. 478–479). Ritchie (2004) explains that in African culture there is a widespread belief in illness caused by witchcraft and sorcery. The symptoms of *mashawe* described by Ritchie (2004) include anxiety attacks, grave fear, the symptoms of nervous breakdown. and even death. They are

compared with phobic or dissociative states. However, Ritchie's explanation of *mashawe* symptoms does not include hearing voices (as in the case presented by Archbishop Milingo), which would indicate another, more severe disorder according to DSM-IV.

Aull (2005) points out that explanatory models can be affected by acculturation. For instance, the hot-cold theory as describing the causes of symptoms among Puerto Rican families in New York prevailed among the elderly (non-U.S. born) and uneducated. In my study of the Tibetan diaspora, I have made similar observations, and have analyzed acculturation as an important variable affecting illness behavior and help-seeking pathways.

How patients communicate their EMs is also affected by their culture. For example, Snodgrass et al. (1993) note that in Asian cultures, where individuals are expected to be obedient to their elders and to conform to the expectations of those in authority, patients may shape their responses in such a way as to please the practitioner. Kleinman, Eisenberg, and Good (1978) note: "How we communicate about our health problems, the manner in which we present our symptoms, when and to whom we go for care, how long we remain in care, and how we evaluate that care are all affected by cultural beliefs. Illness behavior is a normative experience governed by cultural rules: we learn 'approved' ways of being ill" (p. 252). Furthermore, what meaning patients and family make of their symptoms may directly affect illness behavior—the key issue explored in the present study.

As demonstrated in the examples cited above, culture affects the patient's perception of health problems, while the idiom of health and ill-health is constituted by cultural norms and beliefs. A distinction has also been made between two concepts that describe different aspects of suffering, namely disease (which refers to the biomedical diagnostic criteria) and illness (which is a psychological response to the disease and the mental suffering associated with it). Specific labels known as folk categories are assigned to mental disorders in various cultures. Explanatory models, on the other hand, refer to individual perception and understanding of a particular episode of illness. The concepts of folk categories or explanatory models have been drawn from studies of cross-cultural psychiatry, and are usually used in reference to mental illness. I found them useful, however, in understanding how any kind of suffering, including somatic diseases, can be experienced across different cultures.

2.5 ILLNESS BEHAVIOR

Illness behavior is yet another theoretical concept important to this study. It is defined as the behavioral reactions of individuals who become ill. As Tseng

(2001) explains: "it covers a set of sequential behaviours, including how the person recognizes, perceives, and interprets the discomfort or suffering and reacts against it; how he seeks help, attention, or treatment from others; how he communicates and presents his problems or illness to his family, healers, and others; how his role changes when he is sick, including how he is cared for by family members, friends, or others; how he reacts to therapy prescribed or treatment offered by healers, including compliance and adherence to it; and how he accepts or reacts to the results of treatment and the prognosis of his disorders" (p. 165). In other words, it is a very general concept that refers to folk categories and explanatory models, help-seeking behavior, and help-seeking pathways.

2.5.1 Help-Seeking Behavior

Help-seeking behavior is a component of illness behavior, and describes how the patient and his or her family seek help to cope with the illness. Help-seeking behavior is determined by a number of factors, including the nature and severity of the illness, the degree of motivation to seek help, the explanatory models of the illness, awareness of the possible treatment methods, their availability, the patient's financial status, and other economic factors.

Pillay (1996) presents six major categories of variables defined by Cummings, Becker and Maile that affect help-seeking behavior. These are:

1. accessibility of healthcare (includes patient's ability to pay for health services, awareness of the available services, and availability of healthcare per se);
2. attitudes towards health (including beliefs in the benefits of treatment, and beliefs about the quality of medical care provided);
3. threat of illness (involves the patient's perception of his or her symptoms and beliefs about susceptibility and the consequences of disease);
4. knowledge about the disease;
5. social interactions, social norms, and social structure;
6. demographic characteristics (including social status, income and education).

Pillay notes that the crucial factor in determining whether the patient will seek treatment is personal and cultural beliefs. Cultural beliefs will also determine preferred methods of treatment. Cambodians, for example, often adhere to their "philosophy of syncretism or complementarity of Buddhism and folk religion" (Uehara 2001, p. 524), which determines their help-seeking behavior. Uehara (2001) comments:

> "To be health restoring, treatment must be directed at the true causes of suffering and affliction . . . appropriate treatment is differentiated by type of affliction

> and degree and severity of suffering. For example, while self-remedies such as pinching, cupping and coining are seen as appropriate for milder conditions (caused, for example, by a temporary disturbance in family life), more serious afflictions (caused, for example, by the invasion of a malevolent spirit) require more potent treatment from a specialist or *kru khmer* who possesses the ability to cure illness. From the Khmer perspective, a wide range of treatments are culturally permissible, including those based on alternative medical belief system (such as the Western biomedical model)" (p. 524).

Addington et al. (2002) studied help-seeking behavior among psychotic patients, and enumerated the factors that may delay them in using medical services. These include: the severity of the illness, level of substance abuse, homelessness, individual propensity to seek help, accessibility of services, and the stigma associated with the disease. The authors observed that some patients may deny that they have a problem, and hope that they can get better on their own. They further explain that: "in the early stages individuals are concerned about a range of symptoms. But it is not until symptoms become severe (e.g., psychotic or suicidal) and individuals are presenting to psychiatry or emergency services that they actually make a successful contact and receive the appropriate care" (p. 363).

Considering the above, there are many different variables associated with illness-behavior, such as the availability of healthcare, the patient's attitudes towards and knowledge about the illness, its severity, cultural norms, and the patient's personal characteristics.

2.5.2 Help-Seeking Pathways

The term "help-seeking pathways" refers to "the sequence of contacts made with individuals and organizations by the distressed person and the efforts of his or her significant others in seeking help, as well as the help that is supplied in response to those efforts" (Tseng 2001, p. 170). For example, Knipscheer, Jong, and Lamptey (2000) studied how various ethnic minorities utilize mental health facilities. Whereas Hispanics and Asian Americans in the United States showed a tendency towards underutilization, African Americans were likely to overuse mental health services. This may be explained in terms of their attitudes towards the mental health system: African Americans often sought help in mental health institutions for practical problems. These may have included administrative matters (such as difficulties with the law, or requests related to social services and housing), or non-psychiatric medical problems. The authors concluded that African Americans view the mental health system as a referral service rather than as a resource for providing individualized psychological help.

Knipscheer, Jong, and Lamptey (2000) show another example of cultural differences in terms of expectations addressed to health services agencies. After a plane crash in Amsterdam in 1992, crash victims who were of non-native ethnicity sought immediate financial assistance at health institutions. Meanwhile, their service providers were more focused on the patients' psychological trauma and related mental problems. Those who sought help were not aware of the separation between material and psychological assistance in the Dutch system. Because their expectations were not met, they felt abandoned when social welfare workers could not address their material problems.

Chung and Lin (1994) compared the help-seeking behaviors and pathways adopted by Vietnamese, Cambodian, Laotian, Hmong, and Chinese-Vietnamese refugees in their home countries and in the United States. In all the groups studied, the authors reported a dramatic shift from using traditional medicine in the home country, to a higher use of mainstream services in the United States. Respondents in all five groups reported using dual healthcare systems in both Asia and the United States. The authors explain the observed changes in terms of the degree of exposure to Westernization and the availability of Western medicine. English proficiency and youth were also recognized as predictors for using Western medicine in the United States (Chung and Lin 1994). I have made similar observations about this shift in the course of researching Tibetans in exile.

In their study of Asian youth, Yeh et al. (2003) reported: "in Asian culture, people tend to seek help from intimates, including friends and family, rather than a stranger, such as a counselor. . .it is assumed that Japanese immigrant youth would feel uncomfortable sharing their difficulties and feelings with a counselor" (p. 493). Some studies also highlight a common tendency among Asians to express emotional distress through somatic symptoms. This is often the case among Tibetans. Crescenzi et al. (2002) observe: "The high levels of anxiety and depression in the Tibetan community is consistent with our clinical experience. Patients typically seek help by presenting headaches, stomach pain, body-aches, fits, medically unexplained paralysis, feelings of unhappiness, palpitations, insomnia, discomfort with anger, and difficulties concentrating and learning" (p. 374).

Beiser, Simich, and Pandalangat (2003) note that it is essential for immigrants and refugees to recognize health problems, and to be aware of the available services and perceive them as useful and appropriate, in order to actively seek help. According to their report, among Tamil immigrants in Canada the help-seeking behavior varied considerably according to the nature of the health problem; that is, the propensity to seek help was influenced by the distinction between "physical" and "psychological" complaints. Respondents were asked about their potential responses to hypothetical situations, such as: "feeling sad most of the time," "experiencing fear without any reason," or "having suicidal thoughts." The results show that 62.7 percent, 66.6 percent, and 51.2 percent, respectively, answered that they would rather not seek help. Asked about somatic symptoms (chest pain, problems with vision, and toothache) only 1.4 percent, 1.5 percent, and 2.1 percent, respectively, reported that it was unlikely that they would seek help. In Chapter Seven, "Presenting and Analyzing the Quantitative Data," I will demonstrate a parallel situation, in which a particular model of treatment is likely to be chosen by Tibetans, according to the nature of the disease and the severity of its symptoms.

As mentioned previously, illness behavior can be affected by a number of variables; for example, the availability of health services or the degree of acculturation. Chung (2001) notes a dramatic shift in the pattern of help-seeking behavior among Cambodian refugees in America. Whereas traditional medicine was frequently sought in Cambodia, refugees report a more frequent use of mainstream services in the United States. This may be due to the fact that few traditional care providers had emigrated to America, many of them (including monks) having been killed by the Pol Pot regime. Nevertheless, many Cambodians (especially women) in exile still reported seeking traditional methods as a preferred way of treatment, or used a dual healthcare system of both traditional and Western practices in the United States. These preferences were associated with lower education and literacy levels (Chung 2001).

Speller (2005) describes a number of barriers to seeking help among Asian immigrants to the United States. She points to the need for bilingual Asian-American healthcare providers, due to the language barrier among the immigrant population. Other barriers include the high cost of treatment, as many Asian-Americans live below the poverty level and have no health insurance, as well as lack of awareness of the available services. Speller also notes: "Asian American view emotional distress as a sign of weakness, resulting from a lack of discipline or will power" (p. 72).

In Tibet, the pathogenesis of disease was often understood in terms of the influence of malignant forces (such as evil spirits and ghosts, or the serpent deities known as *nagas*.) For that reason, Tibetans would traditionally seek help from a lama or a healer and would use spiritual methods to cope with health problems. Pathak (2003) notes: "It was believed that the causation of ailment was due to the effect of supernatural intrusion or possession by ghosts on the morbid person, which was responsible for the imbalance of body constituents. The tradition of various types of offerings to appease the angry deities or the nature worship such as sun, moon, stars and so on was the only resort for the caring of ill-health in Tibet" (p. 46). In another study, Pathak (2004) investigates illness behavior among Tibetans living in exile, where two main systems of medicine are available: the Western allopathic or biomedical model, and the traditional Tibetan system of medicine. According to Pathak's findings, Tibetans older than age 50 report Tibetan medicine to be effective for all kinds of ailments, and Tibetan medicine is preferred by 80.2 percent of the older generation for chronic ailments. According to the respondents in Pathak's study, even though treatment with herbal medicines takes longer, it provides a permanent cure. They also stressed that Tibetan medicines are comparatively cheaper than Western medicines and methods, and are also safer in that they produce no side effects. However, according to some respondents Tibetan herbal pills needed further improvement. Furthermore, fifteen per cent of elderly Tibetans consulted indigenous healers to treat conditions such as severe headaches, psychological disturbances, or epilepsy.

Like their elders, the younger generation affirmed that traditional Tibetan medicine is good for chronic ailments, even though the duration of treatment is longer. On the other hand, Delek Hospital and other Western allopathic clinics or private practitioners were consulted by 80 percent of respondents younger than 50 years of age, for all kinds of ailments. While they sought the fast recovery attributed to Western medicine, so as not to miss time from work or school, a significant number of Tibetan youths also visited the Tibetan Medicine and Astro Institutes, which offer traditional Tibetan medical services. Some of the young respondents also consulted faith healers in Dharamsala (Pathak 2004). The qualitative material I gathered during the course of my own research confirmed these findings.

Various authors have discussed the potential threat of stigmatization as an additional factor affecting help-seeking behavior. For example, Knipscheer, Jong, and Lamptey (2000) report the situation among Ghanaians: "the search for a cure of a serious illness is usually a collective family affair. Mental disorders are often socially stigmatized . . . traditional healers and the spiritualist church are the most frequently utilized modalities for mental healing" (pp. 472–473). Ghanaians did seek out professional, Western healthcare when their symptoms were severe. The same authors note that although some studies in Ghana show that traditional healers are more effective than biomedical health professionals in treating mental disorders, some individuals might avoid talking about these traditional healers for fear of embarrassment (2000). Bhugra (2004) refers to a study of South Asian women in London who chose to consult religious preachers and go to religious places for comfort and reassurance instead of seeking help from their general practitioner, which carried a stigma in their communities.

In many other studies, religion has been reported as an important factor affecting help-seeking behavior and pathways: sometimes to the detriment of health. Koenig (2004) observes that religion can interfere with disease detection and treatment compliance. Ferraro and Albrecht-Jensen (1991) show examples of the adverse effects of religion on health, for example, individuals who are Jehovah's Witnesses or Christian Scientists may refrain from blood transfusions or other types of medical treatment. Koenig (2002) also refers to a study by Ehman et al. (1999), who surveyed 177 consecutive adult outpatients visiting a pulmonary clinic. About 45 percent of the subjects reported that their religious beliefs would influence their health behavior (for example, medical decisions) if they became gravely ill.

In another study, Koenig (2004) points to the fact that religious beliefs play an important role in patients' decision-making, regarding the use of chemotherapy and other life-saving treatments. While in some cases, these beliefs are reported to be in conflict with medical care, religion is often a popular and significant strategy in coping with illness. Koenig (2002) shows that attending church was associated with greater social support. In a later study, he reported that religious people, who often have greater social support, may be encouraged by other members of their spiritual community to seek help and treatment (Koenig 2004).

As an example of how these concepts are expressed in a clinical setting, I will refer to a case study by Jacobson (2002) that shows how different explanatory models interact with one another and how they affect illness behavior. Jacobson describes a similar context to the one presented in this work—namely, the Tibetan community in India. A Tibetan refugee woman in her seventies reported suffering from severe "life-wind" (Tib. *srog rLung*) illness for a period of 2 or 3 years. The patient had a long history of traumatic experiences (being robbed by Chinese troops, escape and subsequent financial losses, displacements, death of three of her children and her husband). Her symptoms included "anxiety," "heartbeat" (Tib. *snying phar*), the sensation of a rope around her neck, severe headaches, as well as occasional difficulty in walking. The patient recognized her "anxiety" in the chest as a respiratory impairment. Jacobson (2002) reports: "She complained of a combination of depressive and anxious symptoms in which various somatic dysphorias and disabilities played a large part. Against the background of this waxing and waning syndrome she also suffered acute episodes of panic and less frequently of anger" (p. 259). The symptoms presented by the patient were classified according to DSM as 296.32 Major Depression, moderate and recurrent, without psychotic features, with atypical features (duration of episodes would not meet two-week criterion) and 300.02 Generalized Anxiety Disorder, with Panic Attacks (with duration of onset apparently slower that 10-minute criterion).

Jacobson (2002) further relates how patients' explanatory models were affected by their caregivers' explanatory models (EMs): "a diffusion of illness names and simplifications of classical theory into the discourse of lay Tibetans (who are with rare exceptions illiterate in classical Tibetan) occurs through the brief explanations which *emchi* provide in response to their patients' infrequent and tentative questions. Lay and professional understandings of medicine are therefore distinct but closely related" (p. 267). The Tibetan doctor (*emchi*)[16] diagnosed the woman's illness as life-wind concurrent with blood-wind disorder. The "wind" or *"rLung"* disturbances are associated by an average Tibetan with feelings of sadness and anxiety, which may be combined with disruptions of heartbeat, breathing, and other somatic dysphorias. The patient herself referred to her illness using three terms: "The first was *'ngangtra' (dngang skrag),*[17] of which 'anxiety' is the most accurate English gloss. In this, she was using a word that denoted a common affect and also a specific symptom to name an entire illness. The second was 'wind,' which is the name of a basic pathodynamic and can also indicate non-medicalized, temporary disturbances of 'wind.' At yet other points she referred to her affliction as 'blood-wind' and reported that her neighbors had also applied this term to it. Like 'wind,' the latter refers to a pathodynamic which is presumed to underlie the illness, i.e., an excess of 'blood' and 'wind' at the same time. The metonymic principle underlying each of these three terms is common in lay talk about illnesses" (269).

To treat her "wind" imbalance the patient sought help from many allopathic doctors, including Tibetan and Indian biomedical physicians. She was treated with injections and medicines alternately with no success, until she felt "rough" in her body, became discouraged, and abandoned the allopathic treatment. She was then advised by a Tibetan doctor, who decided that the disease was karmic and advised her to use religious practices and go on a pilgrimage. In addition to this, the patient began to consult practitioners in the traditional Tibetan system of medicine. She was treated with "golden needle"[18] therapy, and immediately reported some benefit. But because her doctor died unexpectedly before the entire treatment was finished, the patient visited another doctor, from whom she received thirty-four additional golden needle treatments as well as moxibustion[19] therapy (for an explanation of these treatment methods, see Chapter Five, "The Traditional Tibetan System of Medicine in Tibet and in Exile"). After some time, however, the woman became reluctant to use these methods due to the pain she experienced during therapy. Subsequently, the efficacy of these treatments in relieving her symptoms waned. Despite that, the patient continued taking Tibetan herbal medicines and engaged herself in religious coping strategies (which included *mani* mantra recitation, circumambulating of holy places, taking "blessed pills," annual pilgrimages to Bodhgaya, and sponsoring monks to perform rituals prescribed by her lama).

Further examples of how Tibetans make meaning of their health problems, what help-seeking behaviors they adopt (when and under what circumstances), and their help-seeking pathways will be described in Chapter Seven: "Presenting and Analyzing the Qualitative Data."

NOTES

1. Whereas *transference* refers to people unconsciously transferring feelings and attitudes from a person or situation in the past to a person or situation in the present, *countertransference* is an unconscious response to the former. For example, a hospital patient who perceives his or her parents as uncaring, indifferent or even hostile , may develop similar attitudes towards hospital personnel, who represent caregiving figures. In a clinical setting, many patients are likely to regress to their childhood feelings, attitudes, and expectations. Subsequently, some may perceive physicians as powerful, all-knowing, omnipotent—just as many small children perceive their parents. However, patients are not likely to verbalize these attitudes *expressis verbis.* Some of them may also expect to receive special attention and care. Secretly or sometimes more explicitly, they desire to be "special patients" or "the only patients" to their doctor. They may attempt to please the therapist by offering gifts or by acting in a way that they think the practitioner expects them to act. When these expectations become frustrated and remain unconscious, the patient may feel rejected, uncared-for, unloved, or even worthless. Obviously, it is impossible for healthcare providers to fulfill immature, childlike desires and become the best parents for their patients. Why should they? It is not their role. The real problem begins, however, when he or she starts to think so. When a doctor responds to transference by trying to satisfy these desires (this is where *countertransference* starts), it inevitably leads to confusion of roles, frustration, and emotional tension. Many doctors will obviously fear that.

2. Ch'i (or Qi) energy in traditional Chinese culture and medicine refers to a 'life force' that is believed to be present in all living beings and circulates through the body through a network of channels (meridians). Health practitioners using this ethnomedical modality would concentrate on diagnosing the energy flow, blockages, or disturbances. Treatment often involves introducing changes into one's lifestyle, dietary habits, taking herbal medicines, or accessory therapy (e.g., acupuncture) to harmonize the energy flow.

3. *Prana* is a Sanskrit word that refers to life force of living organisms and vital energy involved in all natural processes. It is believed to flow through a network of

subtle energy channels (nadis) and concentrate in places, called chakras. The concept is used in Indian ethnomedicine (Ayurveda) and Yoga.

4. *Chakra* is a Sanskrit word that denotes 'circle' or 'wheel,' and refers to concentration of the spiritual energy. Theories of chakras have become widely incorporated in many healing modalities used in the West. They are used to describe the holistic concept of the 'bodymind'—the unity of the physical, mental, and spiritual in a humans.

5. *Meridian* is a term used in traditional Chinese medicine that refers to channels through which the Ch'i (or Qi) energy circulates through the body.

6. *Ayurveda* refers to an ancient system of medicine practiced in India.

7. "Anthropometry" literally means "measurement of humans." In physical anthropology, it refers to the measuring of representatives of the human species in order to develop understanding of the physical variations among races. The characteristics of body dimensions an important consideration in clothing design, ergonomics, or architecture. Body dimensions can be affected by a number of factors, such as lifestyle, nutrition and dieting habits, and are subjected to change (e.g., growing obesity in the American population).

8. Aboud and Skerry (cited in Pires and Stanton 2000) characterize an ethnic group as "a socially or psychologically defined set of people who share a common culture or cultural background, often because of similarity of race, nationality, or religion" (p. 46).

9. Tib. *chos*

10. China Tibet Information Center. (online document). A Brief Description of the Historical Relations Between Ancient Tibetan Culture and the Chinese Culture. Available at: http://www.tibet.cn/english/zt/TibetologyMagazine/..%5CTibetologyMagazine/2003120044211152145.htm

11. CLSC (*centre local de services communautaires*) refers to local community health centers—free clinics which are run and maintained by the provincial government in Canada.

12. Source: http://www.tibet.net/en/health/heasp.html

13. Human Resources Development (HRD) includes: 1. Social reintegration program, 2. Vocational training & Developing career skills, and 3. Aiding & seeking employment.

14. Source: http://www.kunphen.org

15. Tibetan and Indian children are usually sent to separate schools. However, I have found single examples of an Indian child being admitted to a Tibetan school.

16. In some texts it is also spelled as '*amchi*' or '*amchee*'. I shall use the latter form.

17. It is spelled like this according to the Wylie transliteration scheme.

18. Tib. *khab gser*

19. Moxibustion refers to applying moxa, which usually contains mugwort, to warm, and thus stimulate, certain acupuncture points.

Chapter Three

Religion and Health

3.1 Interdependence between Religion and Health
3.2 Religion and Mental Health
3.3 Overview of the Research Findings
3.4 Religion as a Salutary Agent
3.5 Mechanisms for Religion's Effects on Health
3.6 Religion as a Source of Coping Strategies
3.7 Religious Coping in Empirical Studies
    3.7.1 Predictors of Religious Coping
3.8 Pathogenic and Pathoplastic Functions of Religion

3.1 INTERDEPENDENCE BETWEEN RELIGION AND HEALTH

Although religion can be regarded as a specific aspect of culture, I have given it special attention in this study and thus will analyze it separately. In this section, I will discuss some of the general points of interdependence between religion and health, followed by an overview of research findings on the effect of religion on mental and physical health. In particular, I will concentrate on examples of the salutary function of religion, with a specific emphasis on religion as a coping strategy.

In a short historical analysis, Vanderpool (1980) points out that health used to be defined as the absence of disease, and that disease was caused by distinct, identifiable entities. Religion, on the other hand, was regarded a relic of a superstitious, antiquarian past, and rejected. It was maintained that disease can be conquered apart from religious, ethnic, and social influences. However, the services and insights of hospital chaplains and social workers have been increasingly utilized since the second and third decades of the twentieth century. This may result from the trends to "humanize" medicine. The more inclination there is towards the humanistic and holistic models of healthcare, the more credit will be given to experiences and needs associated with the psychological or spiritual domain.

Vanderpool (1980) also identifies six major areas of interaction between religion and health:

1. Religion has an influence on human health due to the fact that it shapes human mental and emotional states. The author relates findings in the areas of psychiatry, psychosomatic medicine, and biofeedback, which indicate that physical well-being is greatly influenced by emotions and mental attitudes. Religion is also seen as a source of coping strategies. It helps individuals overcome situations of crisis, cope with stress, and deal with loneliness. Religion can also positively influence one's ability to enjoy life. The suitability of pastoral counseling is also mentioned.
2. Religion also informs and shapes the general values of medicine and can be referred to when important medical decisions are to be made; for example, regarding euthanasia or abortion. Furthermore, Vanderpool says: "numerous ethicists—not to speak of the medical institutions of a number of religious groups—maintain that decisions about the rightness and wrongness of medical procedures and policies must necessarily include religious components" (1980, p. 11).
3. Religion can also provide unique explanations of health and disease. As Vanderpool explains: "concepts of health and disease have shifted over time from rather exclusive theological explanations for illness and health to empirical, scientific ones. Nevertheless, theological explanations for disease and health continue to be espoused literally and almost exclusively by a number of usually smaller religious groups, and theological explanations are still regarded as valuable and meaningful supplements to scientific explanations by probably the majority of patients and physicians" (1980, p. 12). In some cultures, the causes for sickness can be explained in terms influence of malignant forces, demon or spirit possession, or punishment by God. Even though such explanations may be rejected by scientifically trained healthcare professionals, they still exist in many ethnic-religious communities. The Tibetans studied here are one such example. It is also significant that religion can support individuals in their search for meaning when faced with sickness or some other crisis. It helps them find answers to questions, such as: "Why did this happen to me?" Vanderpool points out that the religious explanations "are not regarded as conflicting with scientific, empirical knowledge but rather are held as valid and true

explanations that transcend the limits of empirical medicine" (1980, p. 12). This area of interaction between religion and health will be closely examined in the present study.

4. Religion can offer ways of reducing stress, and of developing a sense of peace, security, and well-being. This function of religion can be utilized in therapy. Meditation and prayer are often seen as salutary in their functions. Furthermore, when disease is believed to be spiritual or due to possession by evil spirits, religion provides certain methods of coping. Special religious beliefs and rituals are then utilized by the priests, shamans, or spirit healers. Moreover, popular rites of healing that involve catharsis, forgiveness, and supplication to a higher power are believed to be theologically and psychologically effective.
5. Another area of interaction between religion and medicine refers to "health behavior," a sub-discipline within the field of preventive medicine. Health behavior addresses issues including hygiene, dieting, proper patterns of work and recreation, sexuality, and substance use. According to Vanderpool (1980), religion is a critical, largely unappreciated or unknown factor even though it encompasses important points of reference to health. He writes: "This is a vast range of issues that are closely linked to religious taboos and prescriptions. A mere listing of topics indicates the degree to which religious traditions are closely linked to health behaviour: vegetarianism of Seventh-Day Adventists, prohibitions of abortion and birth control by Roman Catholics, strictures against homosexuality by traditional Jews and Christians, emphases on work and success among assorted Calvinists, and taboos regarding blood among Jehovah's Witnesses" (1980, p. 14).
6. Finally, Vanderpool (1980) touches upon the issue of death and dying. He highlights the changes that have occurred in medicine in relation to this topic: the development of the funeral industry and the increased numbers of deaths in modern hospitals that take place under the supervision of physicians and nurses (euthanasia, or "medicalized dying"). Still, religion remains relevant when it comes to shaping our understanding of death. It provides comfort, reassurance, and consolation, and restores hope. Religion also affects ideals concerning treatment of terminally ill patients, and influences policies about informing patients of their medical condition.

Bogdan de Barbaro (2002) notes that religious (or metaphysical) themes are very popular in the area of psychiatry and psychopathology. Patients with severe episodes of depression can experience delusions of guilt, punishment, and damnation; obsessive-compulsive disorders may involve obsessive religious thoughts and also the narratives of schizophrenic people are often saturated with religious symbols. Barbaro (2002) stresses that healthcare professionals are required to be specially sensitive and respectful of such topics. In some cases they may find it reasonable to refer the patient to a theologian or priest for a consultation.

Another interesting point of interdependence is mentioned by McGuire (1987), who elaborates on the issue of ritual and symbolism in healing practices. She points out the importance of "religious language"—defined as "speech events and words that are themselves believed to have special efficacy—that is, inherent power, a power separate from and in addition to their cognitive aspect, their meaning" (p. 66). With respect to the Christian religion, this may involve the command of a healer or exorcist (e.g., "Heal!" or "Be gone evil spirit!"). Special mantras may be used in other cultural contexts. Moreover, the recitation of prayers and special visualizations can be invoked by practitioners as a "protective cloak." Symbols that mediate healing power can also be used. These may be concrete objects, such as crystals, metals, cloths, shapes, numbers, colors, or nature symbols (fire, water, air, earth, sun, moon, stars, etc.). McGuire (1987) says: "Some adherents held that healing power could be sent, through such objects, over distance or time. A prayer group would, for example 'fill' or 'soak' a piece of cotton with healing power; the cotton could then be taken by anyone elsewhere to where healing was needed. Similarly, they saved the healing power 'stored' in blessed oil or salt for future healing uses" (p. 369). Many such examples can be found among Tibetan Buddhists, in which objects are assigned tantric power.

The relationship between religion and health is widely discussed in the literature. Some studies concentrate on the question: How does religion (and issues of the mind in general) affect the physical body? This problem is often challenged by research in the area of psychoneuroimmunology (PNI) and psychosomatics. PNI investigates the interconnection (or communication) between the four information-processing systems in humans: 1. the mind, 2. the endocrine system, 3. the nervous system, and 4. the immune system. Ray (2004) explains that from the biopsychosocial perspective, the mind is understood as an activity of the brain:

> "Our thoughts, our feelings, our beliefs, and our hopes are nothing more than chemical and electrical activity in the nerve cells of our brains. It is literally true that as experience changes our brains and thoughts, that is, changes our minds, we are changing the biology. . . .We know that our beliefs influence the biology of our bodies. When an experience is psychological, not physical, it is all in the mind. However, because the mind is a part of the functioning brain, the body responds to the brain regardless of whether the beliefs and ideas are imaginary or based in reality, or whether they are positive or negative. What a

> person thinks does make a difference—sometimes it is good for him or her, sometimes it is bad" (2004, pp. 31–32).

Jones (2003) gives an example of the religious practices, such as meditation or prayer, which can elicit a "relaxation response." This relates to reduced muscle tension, lowered activity of the sympathetic nervous system, lower blood pressure and heart rate, and changes in brain-wave patterns.

3.2 RELIGION AND MENTAL HEALTH

There is also substantial evidence as to the association between religion and mental health—one of the interests of psychiatry and the psychology of religion. Batson et al. (1993) point to some methodological problems in this regard. According to the authors, the relationship between religion and mental health is complex and can be confusing, as it depends on how researchers define both phenomena. Grzymala-Moszczynska (2004) notes that most studies measured religiousness quantitatively, often in terms of having or not having some religious affiliation. Mental health, on the other hand, was often defined by specific, desirable characteristics (for example, proper social behavior). Because there was little reflection upon a wider context for these properties in an overall healthy functioning, the results were quite narrow. For example, they might only indicate a relationship between religiousness and positive personality features, such as the ability to overcome a sense of powerlessness, or between optimism and better family relations. The findings might also indicate a relationship between religiousness and neurotic features of character, such as anxiety, or else they might show no relationship between religiousness and personality traits (Grzymala-Moszczynska 2004).

In their meta-analysis of literature findings, Batson et al. (1993) stress the necessity of characterizing precisely what is meant by religion and what is understood as mental health. They analyze a number of studies according to the applied definition of mental health and type of religiousness, and use a three-dimensional analysis of individual religion: as means, end, and quest. The extrinsic, means dimension is defined as "the degree to which an individual's external social environment has influenced his or her personal religion. [Extrinsically motivated individuals] would presumably be motivated by a desire to gain the self-serving, extrinsic end of social approval" (1993, p. 169). This refers to Allport's definition of extrinsic motivation: "Persons with this orientation may find religion useful in a variety of ways—to provide security and solace, sociability and distraction, status and self-justification. The embraced creed is lightly held or else selectively shaped to fit more primary needs. In theological terms the extrinsic type turns to God, but without turning away from self" (Allport and Ross 1967; cited in Batson 1993, p. 161).

The intrinsic, end dimension is characterized as "the degree to which an individual's religion is a result of internal needs for certainty, strength, and direction" (Batson et al 1993, p. 169). It refers to people who use religion to find clear answers to their existential questions. Allport and Ross explain that it refers to living one's own religion and finding one's master motive in it. They add: "Other needs, strong as they may be, are regarded as of less ultimate significance, and they are, so far as possible, brought into harmony with the religious beliefs and prescriptions. Having embraced a creed the individual endeavors to internalize it and follow it fully" (Allport and Ross 1961; cited in Batson et al. 1993, p. 161). On the other hand, the authors point out that this can also relate to characteristics of a fanatical, rigid true believer. Finally, Batson et al. 1993) present the quest dimension, which is defined as "the degree to which an individual's religion involves an open-ended, responsive dialogue with existential questions raised by the contradictions and tragedies of life" (p. 169). It describes a spiritual quest in which the individual needs to "absorb new points of view into his truth system" in the "continual search for more light on religious questions." (Clark 1985, cited in Batson et al. 1993, p. 166).

Mental health is described by means of seven different conceptions:

1. as absence of mental illness (that is, where none of the psychopathological symptoms defined by the *Diagnostic and Statistical Manual of the American Psychiatric Association* are present);
2. as appropriate social behavior (an individual does not require psychotherapy as long as he or she behaves appropriately, which, on the other hand, is culturally biased);
3. as freedom from worry and guilt (refers to freedom from the psychological conflict between the ideal and real self, as well as freedom from anxiety and guilt);
4. as personal competence and control (refers to a postulated need for competence, as well as psychological theories of motivation which assume that individuals will feel motivated only when they feel uncomfortable in some way);
5. as self-acceptance and self-actualization (describes health in terms of one's ability to accept oneself as one is and beyond—the apex of psychological health or self-actualization as defined by Maslow);
6. as personality unification and organization (describes health as having a unified and hierarchically organized structure of personality; there can be

a core system or master-sentiment, for example, religious sentiment, and other ones arranged in subordination to it);
7. as open-mindedness and flexibility (associates mental health with the ability to adapt to new information and experiences) (Batson et al. 1993).

Having analyzed the studies according to the concept of religion and mental health applied by various researchers, Batson et al. (1993) note a negative correlation between the amount of spiritual involvement and mental health when the extrinsic, means dimension is analyzed, and a generally positive relationship between religion and mental health, in light of the intrinsic, end dimension and the quest dimension. The intrinsic, end dimension is positively correlated with: greater absence of illness, more appropriate social behavior, greater freedom from worry (but not guilt), greater personal competence and control, greater unification and organization, and negatively with greater self-acceptance, self-actualization or greater open-mindedness and flexibility. A positive relationship is observed between the quest dimension and mental health understood as greater open-mindedness and flexibility, greater self-acceptance, and possibly between the quest dimension and greater personal competence and control. Batson et al. (1993) finish their analysis with a conclusion that it is equivocal to say whether religion is a force for mental health or sickness because it depends on the particular dimension of religion being analyzed and how mental health is defined.

3.3 OVERVIEW OF THE RESEARCH FINDINGS

Religion, just like culture, may be analyzed in terms of its salutary, pathogenic, and pathoplastic functions. In this short overview of the research findings, I will present examples of the correlation between religion and specific health variables, concentrating on the salutary aspect of religion, in which it promotes a healthier lifestyle, provides context for social support, and becomes a source of coping strategies.

3.4 RELIGION AS A SALUTARY AGENT

According to Sosis and Alcorta (2003), the potential benefits of religion include improved health, survivorship, economic opportunities, sense of community, psychological well-being, assistance during crises, mating opportunities, and fertility. Oman and Thoresen (2002, p. 366) review a number of studies and report that there is a positive correlation between religious involvement and lower all-cause mortality, longevity, lower blood pressure, and incidence of physical disability. Ferraro and Albrecht-Jensen (1991) show that people who are spiritually involved (that is, who pray and participate actively in their religion) have better health, regardless of age.

In his study of religious beliefs and practices among hospitalized patients with congestive heart failure (CHF) and chronic pulmonary disease (CPD), Koenig (2002) observed a positive relationship between religious activities and attitudes and lower severity of illness, physical disability, or shortness of breath, fewer prior psychiatric problems, and lesser psychotropic medicine use. The author explains that: "Private religious activities such as prayer, meditation, and scripture study, may provide a sense of comfort and peace that enabled patients with CHF or CPD to relax and function better" (p. 273). Moreover, religiousness and spirituality consistently predicted greater social support, fewer depressive symptoms, better cognitive function, and greater cooperativeness (Koenig et al. 2004). A relationship between religion and improved physical health can also be observed.

Much research has been done on the effects of religion on mental health. Kendler et al. (2003) report a relationship between the lifetime risk for nine disorders and various aspects of religiosity. They distinguish between five "internalizing" disorders (major depression, phobias, generalized anxiety disorder, panic disorder, and bulimia nervosa) and four "externalizing" ones (nicotine dependence, alcohol dependence, drug abuse or dependence, and adult antisocial behavior). They also identify seven factors of religiosity: 1. general religiosity, 2. social religiosity (relates to what others term "religious social support"), 3. involved God, 4. forgiveness, 5. God as judge, 6. unvengefulness (relates to forgiveness versus revenge), and 7. thankfulness.

The authors observe a correlation between two factors (social religiosity and thankfulness) and reduced risk for both internalizing and externalizing disorders. The following four factors—general religiosity, involved God, forgiveness, and God as judge—are associated with reduced risk of externalizing disorders, and one factor (unvengefulness) correlates positively with reduced risk for internalizing disorders (Kendler et al. 2003). Oman and Thoresen (2002) refer to studies that indicate a positive relationship between religious involvement and lower depressive symptomatology, greater well-being, and less spousal abuse, or reduced alcohol and substance abuse. Koenig (2001, 2004) also reports that religious beliefs and practices are associated with lower suicide rates, less anxiety, less substance abuse, less depression and faster recovery from depression, greater well-being, hope, and optimism, higher morale, more purpose and meaning in life, higher social support, as well as greater marital happiness and stability.

3.5 MECHANISMS FOR RELIGION'S EFFECTS ON HEALTH

Despite extensive research supporting the notion of a positive correlation between religion and mental health, it is not entirely clear how (in what mechanism) it affects physical health. To answer the question: "Does religion (or spirituality) cause physical health benefits?" Oman and Thoresen (2002) analyze four potential interpretations or mechanisms according to which "religion causally influences health by:

1. any mechanism, including well-established factors such as social support and improved health behaviors;
2. additional mechanisms, such as enhanced positive psychological states (e.g., faith, hope, inner peace) acting through psychoneuroimmunologic or psychoneuroendocrinologic pathways;
3. offering psychological strength for acquiring or maintaining positive health behaviors; or
4. causally influencing health by distant healing or intercessory prayer" (p. 365).

Health behaviors—the first mechanism—refers to the fact that members of some religious communities are encouraged to abide by strict behavioral norms, such as abstaining from smoking tobacco and drinking alcohol, and maintaining healthy dietary habits and proper exercise. Two examples of religious sects that take this view are the Church of Latter-Day Saints (the Mormons) and the Seventh-Day Adventists. Flannelly, Weaver, Larson, and Koenig (2002) report lower all-cause death rates for American and European clergy compared to people of similar age in the general population. This may be connected with healthier behaviors, such as abstinence from smoking. A number of researchers, including Oman and Thoreson (2002), also connected the adoption and maintenance of these positive health behaviors with religious beliefs and practices.

Hummer et al. (2004) found that: "Individuals who attend religious services more often and/or who belong to specific denominations are less likely to initiate, or to continue, smoking or be heavy users of alcohol and drugs compared with people who attend less regularly or who belong to less conservative denominations or none at all . . . religiously involved individuals are less likely to carry or use weapons, fight, exhibit violent behavior, and partake in risky sexual behavior compared with their less religious counterparts. Furthermore, persons who are religiously involved may encounter fewer day-to-day stressors, such as marital and family problems, legal hassles, and on-the-job troubles, which may result in health benefits and lower mortality risks over the life course" (p. 1227).

Grzymala-Moszczynska (2004) explains that religion can control or inhibit pathological thinking and behavior via a moral code that the individual respects. Religion can also be a source of escape mechanisms for those who find it hard to cope with everyday life challenges; for example, it may enable a structured, monastic life with opportunities to undertake retreats at certain intervals. Finally, religion can play a therapeutic role in and of itself. Tibetans who follow the traditional Buddhist principles will be discouraged from involvement in disruptive behavior, and from eating, drinking, and smoking to excess. Instead, they will give special credit to being in control of their minds and bodies, and to maintaining a healthy distance from life's problems.

Social support relates to the greater contact with co-religionists experienced by people who are spiritually involved. They have larger and stronger social networks available to them, as a source of greater emotional support. Sosis and Alcorta (2003) stress the fact that religion promotes group solidarity and enhances adaptation. They refer to Durkheim, Douglas, Radcliffe-Brown, and Turner, who claimed that "collective rituals enable the expression and reaffirmation of shared beliefs, norms, and values, and are thus essential for maintaining communal stability and group harmony" (2003, p. 265). In a Tibetan Buddhist community this principle is exemplified by special emphasis on the role of the Sangha (the community of practitioners, and the "Noble Sangha"—the teachers and spiritual masters). Finally, Tsering Gellek (2001) found that religious institutions played a significant role in establishing social networks and providing emotional comfort, reassurance, and guidance.

Psychological strength—the third mechanism—focuses on religion as the source of strategies for coping with adverse life situations. Oman and Thoresen (2002) report that religiously involved people experience better mental health and more positive psychological states, such as joy, hope, or compassion. At the same time, these individuals have a reduced level of negative emotional states (fear, sadness, anger).

The final mechanism—the "Superempirical" or "psi" influences—refers to laws that are "beyond current modern scientific understanding." Religious coping is known to be an important and valuable strategy in dealing with life's adversities, including health problems. Considering the above, religion can affect health indirectly—through pathways such as health behaviors, social support, and psychological states (Oman and Thoresen 2002). An association between religion and health behavior was also observed by Van Ness, Kasl, and Jones (2002), who investigated the relationship between women's religious involvement (measured by frequency of church attendance) and their decision to have breast cancer screening—mammography and clinical breast examination. They found out that higher levels of organized religious behavior correlated with higher rates of cancer screening among White women, which gave an opportunity of earlier detection and treatment. While

African-American church-going women, on the other hand, had lower rates of breast cancer screening, the authors explain this in terms of lower levels of physician recommendation for this procedure.

Koenig and Larson (1999) note an association between participation in and affiliation with a religious community and lower use of hospital services by medically ill older adults. They presume that religiously active people may be more successful in coping with their physical illness because of the religious community's support. According to the authors, people who attend church frequently and are involved in a caring community are more likely to have their health problems diagnosed and treated earlier. To support this view, they refer to a study by Levin & Markides, which shows that religiously involved older people see their physicians more frequently. Still another explanation is that religious adults are simply healthier than their non-religious peers (Koenig and Larson 1999).

Soothill et al. (2002) report that religious patients identify fewer psychosocial needs in comparison to those without faith. On the other hand, they express a greater need for opportunities for personal prayer, support from representatives of their religious group, and from a spiritual guide. The authors also observe: "The patients with faith indicate that they place less reliance on and have fewer expectations of health professionals, express much less need for information, have less concern about maintaining independence in the face of illness, and point to less need for help with any feelings of guilt or help in considering sexual needs, compared with the patients without faith" (pp. 260–261). In the present study, I observed similar attitudes to those described by Soothill et al. (2002) among religiously involved Tibetans.

3.6 RELIGION AS A SOURCE OF COPING STRATEGIES

One of the most significant examples of the salutary function of religion refers to the concept of religious coping. In general, "coping" is a term that refers to a "search for significance in times of stress" (Pargament 1997, p. 90). Significance, on the other hand, is understood as a phenomenological construct that involves feelings and beliefs associated with worth, importance, and value, and that is associated with caring, attraction, or attachment. It is object-oriented, that is, people look for "significants" (objects of significance). Significants do not necessarily involve only the sacred. Other forms are also popular, for example, material significants (money, food, cars, houses, drugs, weapons), physical significants (health, fitness, appearance), psychological significants (comfort, meaning, growth), or social significants (intimacy, social justice). The spiritual significants, on the other hand, may involve the desire for closeness with God, or other types of religious experiences (Pargament 1997).

Coping is a multilayered, contextual phenomenon, a process that involves all dimensions of human functioning: cognitive, affective, behavioral, and physiological. It occurs on familial, organizational, institutional, community, societal, and cultural levels. One of the essential qualities of coping is possibility: "the possibility that the person can rebound from difficult circumstances, that a problem can be anticipated, prevented, or solved, that something good can be found in hardship, or that a devastating loss can be met with some integrity" (Pargament 1997, p. 86). The choice of a coping strategy may not be fully conscious, in other words, when behaviors are very well learned, they do not require much conscious processing. Pargament and Emery (2004) differentiate between coping and automatized adaptive behavior: whereas the former is limited to stressful situations that require effort to manage, the latter is initiated "mindlessly" and with little effort. Hood et al. (1996) point out that coping styles or traits are relatively long-lasting (if not permanent) individual characteristics. Good coping is defined by Pargament (1997): "by what works well for particular people in particular situations and by the degree to which the coping process is well integrated" (p. 91).

Religious behaviors may be involved in coping, but there are also people who handle difficult situations and times of crises without turning to religion. Nevertheless, the coping function of religion is extremely popular, as it serves a number of purposes. Hood et al. (1996) refer to Pollner's suggested reasons for the effectiveness of religion as a coping strategy: "1. lending a quality of order and coherence to stressful situations, 2. countering feelings of shame or anger that are aroused by stress, 3. supporting positive feelings about oneself simply because of having a perceived relationship with the deity, and lastly 4. fostering a tendency to see the self and the world in positive terms" (p. 385).

Pargament, Koenig, and Perez (2000) list five key functions of religion: 1. Meaning, 2. Control, 3. Comfort/Spirituality, 4. Intimacy/Spirituality, and 5. Life Transformation. Meaning refers to one of the major human needs, namely: understanding what is experienced so as to avoid ambiguity, doubt, and uncertainty. According to Argyle (cited in Hood et al. 1996) "a major mechanism behind religious beliefs is a purely cognitive desire to understand" (p. 380). Religion is a system that provides understanding and interpretation. Pargament and Emery (2004) note that people use such religious reframing "to construct the meaning of the event from the perspective of a benevolent religious perspective . . . negative events can be framed as a lesson from God, or part of God's mysterious but ultimately benevolent plan" (pp. 8–9).

Gaining control refers to the desire for mastery and power. Hood et al. (1996) say: "Faith often conveys the meaning that life's difficulties can be overcome. Whether or not a person can control objective conditions may be of less importance than the belief that even insurmountable obstacles can be mastered. In much of life, the sense of control is really an illusion; yet it is one that can be a powerful force supporting constructive coping behavior" (p. 381). The authors also distinguish between interpretive control, predictive control, and vicarious control. Interpretive control usually involves reinterpretation of a situation so that it is less troubling or even seen in positive terms, for example, cancer may be seen as a detour in the road, but not a roadblock. In this way, instead of feeling hopeless one can gain some measure of control. Predictive control refers to the human desire to be able to foretell the future. Individuals will thus seek cues (signs or omens) that will signify a favorable outcome, subsequently fostering hope. Vicarious control is described by means of a situation in which one has lost hope of coping with a problem (for example, in in the event of a serious, life-threatening disease) and turns to a deity, identifies with it, and derives strength through a perceived divine connection (Hood et al. 1996).

Comfort/Spirituality relates to this function of religion, which reduces an individual's apprehension associated with the awareness of the impermanence of all things (for example, that disaster can occur at any moment). Pargament, Koenig, and Perez (2000) note, however, that it is difficult to draw a line between comfort-oriented religious coping and its genuine spiritual function (the desire to be one with a force that goes beyond the individual). Intimacy/Spirituality characterizes the religious function of fostering social solidarity and social identity. Intimacy with others can be maintained by getting involved in religious community events, providing spiritual help to others, and receiving spiritual support from clergy or other members of the in-group.

Life Transformation refers to the aspect of religion that encourages people to progress to a higher spiritual level. Pargament and Emery (2004) note that religious people may be encouraged to let go of old goals and values and seek new ones when necessary. Religion provides other transformational forms of coping; for example, rites of passage, which facilitate transition through critical periods of life. What Pargament (1997) describes as giving up old objects of value and finding new significants relates to the concept of psycho-transgression, that is going beyond one's material, social, and symbolic boundaries (Kozielecki 1997).

Pargament (1997) distinguishes between three religious approaches to responsibility and control in coping: self-directing, deferring, and collaborative. The self-directing style refers to those who rely on themselves rather than

God in coping with a situation. The deferring style describes a situation in which an individual remains passive and defers responsibility to God. Finally, the collaborative approach is characterized by an active involvement of both the individual and God, as partners. For example, one actively seeks a solution to the problem and prays to God for strength and help. Definitions of religious coping methods and a list of subscales were presented by Pargament, Koenig, and Perez (2000) in the "RCOPE Subscales and Definitions of Religious Coping Methods" (see: Appendix). Some of these approaches and subscales will be referred to in Chapter Seven: "Presenting and Analyzing the Qualitative Data."

3.7 RELIGIOUS COPING IN EMPIRICAL STUDIES

Religion has been reported to be of significant benefit to those who suffer from chronic illness or who experience bereavement. Koenig (2001) gives an account of a study of 372 consecutive medical patients who were asked about the most important factor that enabled them to cope with stress. Forty-two percent of these patients reported that religious faith helped them the most. In another study, Koenig (2004) indicates that patients with arthritis, diabetes, kidney disease, cancer, heart disease, lung disease, HIV/AIDS, cystic fibrosis, sickle cell anaemia, amyotrophic lateral sclerosis, chronic pain, and severe or terminal illness as adolescents often turned to religion in order to find comfort, hope, and meaning. Lorenz et al. (2005) reported that in a study of 2266 patients with human immunodeficiency virus (HIV), most of the patients used religious or spiritual means in making decisions and confronting problems. For the disabled, religion allows them to maintain self-esteem and add meaning to situations. It can also be effective in coping with pain, taking into account that physical and psychological pain are often interconnected (Hood et al. 1996).

In one study, Pargament et al. (1998) tested the Brief RCOPE on three study groups: 1. recent survivors of the Oklahoma City bombing, 2. hospitalized, medically ill elderly patients with major illnesses, and 3. college students who faced significant life stressors (for example, death of a family member, health-related problems). In this study, the authors observed a more frequent use of positive religious coping than negative.[1] The positive religious coping was associated with lower levels of psychological distress, greater self-reported growth, and more positive interviewer ratings. On the other hand, higher levels of depression, lower quality of life, more psychological symptoms, and greater callousness toward others correlated with negative religious coping. According to Koenig et al. (2004) "Religious beliefs help patients make sense of their medical conditions and may enable them to better integrate health changes into their lives. Religious practices can help to relax, distract, and counteract the effects of loneliness and isolation that are so prevalent" (p. 559). It has also been observed that the intensity of religious involvement (especially private religious activities) increases when the medical illness grows more severe.

Religious belief has been associated with lower levels of depression. Harrison et al. (2001) found that individuals coping with financial or health stressors (e.g., cancer) who used positive religious coping (in particular, seeking spiritual support, expressing spiritual contentedness, receiving congregational support, benevolent reframing of the stressful event, and collaborative partnership with God) reported the lowest rates of depressive symptoms. In her review of studies on coping styles, Yangarber-Hicks (2004) reports a relationship between the collaborative approach and greater involvement in recovery-enhancing activities, increased empowerment, and a decrease in depression. An association has also been observed between the deferring coping style and improved quality of life. Pleading, on the other hand, has been considered a maladaptive coping style, associated with greater distress.

Religion has also been found to rate as important later in life, which may support the findings that people become more religious as they grow older. Pargament and Emery (2004) report a positive relationship between religion and well-being in elderly people: "many older adults also experience an increasing number of losses of assets that are central to their identity, including roles, relationships, aspects of health, cognition, and functional ability. In some sense, the elderly experience the loss of pieces of themselves, including the loss of whatever they hold sacred. These losses, in combination with concerns about death, becoming a burden to one's family and friends, and adapting to changes in physical, functional, recreational, and social status may lead to grief, loneliness, anger, and depression" (p. 4). Religion then becomes a source of strength and solace. It can explain why religious coping is more frequent among older adults in comparison to younger adults.

The authors also note that religiousness correlates positively with disability, becoming a source of personal stability and identity: "Being part of a sacred tradition may provide elders with a sense of continuity in the midst of rapidly unfolding changes of late life. . . . Religious involvement helps define who the individual is and who the individual is not . . . although physical appearances and material affluence may change, the person continues to be defined by his/her spiritual character" (p. 6). Bosworth et al. (2003) show a relationship between religious involvement among elderly people and depression: "religious practice and positive and negative religious coping are related to depression outcome among on-going treated geriatric depressed patients . . . positive religious coping predicts longitudinal levels of depression in this group" (p. 910). They also draw the conclusion that patients should be inquired about and supported in their religious faith, especially when they are undergoing emotional distress.

Religion can also protect individuals who experience acculturative stress. In a study of African immigrants, Kamya (1997) noted that most individuals who belonged to this ethnic group believed in a Supreme Being who controlled the natural order of things. Some respondents also believed in spirits or spiritual beings who worked in concert with the Supreme Being. They frequently indulged in prayers for obtaining or restoring life energy, shielding them from impending dangers, or for recovery from illness. The authors explain that "spiritual well-being and the role of religion in immigrants' lives may enhance loyalty and attachment to their culture of origin" (p. 159). This stress-buffering role of religion is also exemplified by the qualitative material in the present study.

Many people reported prayer as an important and effective coping strategy. Pargament (1997) says that among other coping strategies (for example, seeking information, resting, following a treatment regimen, taking prescription medication, and visiting doctors), prayer is one of the most frequent strategies used in coping with medical problems. In their study on the use of prayer by coronary artery bypass patients, Ai, Bolling, and Peterson (2000) found that those individuals who used this strategy experienced better postoperative emotional health. These patients reported that pursuing private or public religious activities was a way of coping with physical and emotional problems following surgery. Those who prayed had a significantly lower level of depression. Differences between age groups were also observed: whereas patients older than 65 were more likely to use prayer if religion was important to them, those younger than 65 were more likely to use this coping strategy if they had lower incomes, better preoperative health, and more education. Prayer was also identified as a frequently used coping strategy among Tibetans in the present study. Individuals often repeated short prayers on a daily basis, apart from the regular repetition of mantras.

To sum up, it has been shown that many patients refer to religion in times of crisis. Religious coping is frequently used in case of chronic illnesses, pain, and other situations in which the patient meets stressful circumstances. Religion helps them maintain self-esteem and make meaning of the difficult situation. It also gives strength, hope, and reassurance in critical periods of life, when existential questions regarding the sense of life come up. It helps individuals deal with impermanence, bereavement, or one's own death and dying. Religion can also shield people from acculturative stress, which was thoroughly discussed in Chapter Two. Prayer has been identified as an important and effective strategy, one that helps individuals deal with each of these situations.

3.7.1 Predictors of Religious Coping

A number of variables determine the ways in which people cope with difficult life events. Pargament (1997) maintains that the choice of religious coping is affected by personal factors (for example, demographics, personality, religion), situational factors (types or numbers of stressors, time since a stressful event), social factors (cultural, congregational). Various studies on religiousness, especially the use of private prayer, show that this strategy is more likely to be used by women, ethnic minorities, the retired, the disabled, the mentally and physically ill, those imprisoned, those with less education, and those with lower incomes (Cohen and Koening 2003). According to Batson (1993) women, in comparison to men, are "more religious," pray more often, attend worship more frequently, express more support for traditional religious values, and view religion as more important.

Ethnicity has also been recognized as one factor associated with the use of religious coping. Pargament (1997) notes that coping is embedded in culture: "Coping plays itself out against the backdrop of larger cultural forces. . . . Culture has to do with the underlying blueprints of a society, blueprints that influence and pattern the 'complex whole' of social life. . . . In the language of coping culture shapes events, appraisals, orienting systems, coping activities, outcomes, and objects of significance" (p. 117). Similarly, Koenig (2001) notes that the rate of using religious coping can vary in different parts of the world; for example, in Sweden a much lower level of religious involvement is observed.

Ellison and Levin (1998, cited in Pargament, Tarakeshwar, Ellison, and Wulff 2001) note that the relationship between religion and well-being was especially significant among older, less educated, southern, and African-American groups. Taylor, Chatters, Jayakody, and Levin (1996) show that the African-Americans demonstrated higher levels of both public and private religious behaviors. They were also more likely to endorse positive statements or attitudes that referred to the strength of personal religious commitment (for example, the importance of religion, religious comfort, and of being religious-minded). Ferraro and Koch (1994) report a higher level of religiosity among Black individuals and women. Black people were also more likely to experience health problems and use religious coping. In another study, Taylor et al. (2000) reported: "Black ministers, to a greater extent than white ministers, were involved in crisis intervention and in counseling individuals with diagnosed mental illnesses. Compared with their white peers, black clergy placed greater emphasis on using religious practices (for example, church attendance) as a method for treating emotional problems" (p. 77). Ellison (1993) writes:

> "Throughout much of American history, religious institutions have occupied an important position in black society. Black churches have provided centers for community gatherings and for the development of social and political leaders, various programs of mutual aid and community uplift (e.g., burial societies), and stimulated education . . . participation in church-related activities brings individuals together with others who have similar status characteristics as well as common religious beliefs. For church members, regular interaction with these like-minded others may reinforce basic role identities and role expectations. Through formal and informal involvement in their church communities, these persons may gain affirmation that their personal conduct and emotions with regard to daily events, experiences, and community affairs are reasonable and appropriate" (p. 1029).

Ellison reported that Black people used religion to cope with stressful events and conditions, such as poor health, poverty, and racism (1993). Ellison also notes that several studies looked into "the role of religious institutions and practices in shielding black Americans from the harsh psychosocial ramifications of continued deprivation and structural exclusion" (p. 1032). Ellison (1993) reports a correlation between the self esteem of Black Americans and their involvement in church communities as well as private religious activities. Religious coping "cushions the harmful effects of certain types of adversity on black self-esteem. This stress-buffering pattern is particularly evident with regard to states of the physical body, its attractiveness and its health" (p. 1043). The study of Culver et al. (2002) also shows that African American and Hispanic women with early stage breast cancer exhibit a higher level or religious coping in comparison to Whites. Considering the above, some ethnic minorities are reported to use religious coping more often than Whites.

The fact that use of religious coping can be related to the severity of the symptoms (or suffering) is exemplified by Rogers et al. (2002), who studied coping strategies among 379 individuals with persistent mental illness. They found out that individuals with more severe symptomatology were more likely to use religious coping in comparison to those who had less severe symptoms. The authors offer this explanation: "The experience of more severe symptoms may not only render nonreligious methods of coping as inadequate to afford a sense of control and meaning, but they may also necessitate a perspective beyond oneself that can only be garnered through prayer, meditation, or other religious strategies. . . . Individuals who suffer from relatively minor depressive symptoms and small degradations in cognitive impairment may be less confronted by their limitations, have access to more resources for coping, and thus experience a reduced need for religious coping" (pp. 163–164). Osborne and Vandenberg (2003) also maintain that the extent to which one engages in religious coping depends on situational and denominational variables. They note: "religious coping is particularly helpful in boundary situations, such as serious illness, trauma, and death, which require confronting human limitations, vulnerability, and finitude" (p. 112). This explains why the use of religious coping is more associated with threatening situations (such as being in a storm without a life-jacket) and loss (such as the death of one's father), rather than challenge (say, performance-based job promotion).

The study by Osborne and Vandenberg (2003) also confirms that denominational differences can influence religious coping style. According to this study's findings, Catholics, in comparison to Protestants, displayed greater difficulties in adjustment when faced with an uncontrollable situation. The authors concluded that "their practices and beliefs may predispose them to greater religious discontent when confronting these type of situations" (p. 120). They also note, however, that one of the important limitations of their study was that it was done in a monocultural context (subjects were predominantly White and highly educated).

Koenig, George, and Titus (2004) report that religious activities are prevalent in older, hospitalized patients, with women, nonwhites, and older patients reported as being more religious and spiritual. An individual's concept of God is an essential factor in choosing a particular religious coping style. Individuals who perceive God as benevolent, omni,[2] guiding, and stable are likely to surrender their situation to God. Maynard, Gorsuch, and Bjork (2001) explain: "individuals feel most comfortable giving over the ultimate outcome of their situation to a God who they believe cares for them and has the power to know, act on behalf of, and guide the individual in times of distress" (p. 72). When they perceived God to be a stable, guiding force, they felt comfortable adopting the deferring coping style, whereas the self-directing style was associated with the false, deistic, and worthless image of God. The self-directing style would not correlate with the Benevolent, Omni, Guiding, and Stable categories. As the authors explain: "individuals prefer not to try to solve problems on their own in the presence of a deity who they perceive to possess the qualities necessary to assist in times of distress" (p. 72).

Predictors of religious coping styles may include personal, situational, and social factors. It was shown, for example, that there are links between the use of religion and ethnicity (some groups refer to religion more frequently than others), poor health, poverty, and discrimination. Religious coping is more likely to be used in boundary or crisis situations, and when the symptoms of illness are more severe.

3.8 PATHOGENIC AND PATHOPLASTIC FUNCTIONS OF RELIGION

While there are many examples of the salutary effects of religion, negative influences have also been reported in literature. The pathogenic function of religion, discussed by Grzymala-Moszczynska (2004) is related to the fact that religion can become a source of stress, one that may trigger and develop the pathology of an individual. Two possible examples of this are glossolalia (the utterance of unfamiliar words in a series, also known as "speaking in tongues," or obsessive thoughts about guilt and sin. Koenig refers to a study by Soranson et al. (1995, cited in Koening 2001), which examined the relationship between mental health and the religious affiliation, church attendance, and self-rated religiousness of 261 teenage mothers (228 of whom remained unmarried) living in Ontario. After observing higher depression scores among Catholics, individuals from other conservative religious groups, and mothers who attended religious services more frequently, they concluded that "religion may foster feelings of guilt or shame, erode feelings of competence, self-worth, and hopefulness, and encourage withdrawal of community support from those who do not conform to social norms" (p. 70).

Pargament, Koenig, and Perez (2000) also note cases in which religious coping is ineffective and causes dysfunction. They report an association between Punishing God Reappraisals, Demonic Reappraisals, Spiritual Discontent, Interpersonal Religious Discontent, and Pleading for Direct Intercession, and greater levels of distress. Pargament and Emery (2004) explain: "Negative religious coping activities reflect a general religious orientation that is, itself, in tension and turmoil, marked by a shaky relationship with God, a tenuous and ominous view of the world, and a religious struggle in the search for significance. Negative religious coping methods include: questioning the powers of God, expressions of anger toward God, and expressions of discontent with the congregation and clergy" (p. 11). Pargament et al. (2003) define three types or dimensions of hypothetically ineffective religious coping, which characterize a conflict between an individual and his or her interpersonal and ideological systems: 1. Wrong Direction, 2. Wrong Road, and 3. Against the Wind. The Wrong Direction is described in terms of "involvement in goals or values that reflect an imbalance of self-concerns and concerns that go beyond oneself" (p. 1337). An individual exhibits either "Self Neglect" (overemphasizes religion, congregational or spiritual values, and neglects other needs), "Self Worship" (overemphasizes personal goals and values and neglects religious or spiritual ends), or "Religious Apathy" (devalues both self and others, loses interest).

The Wrong Road dimension is described by Pargament et al. (2003) as "religious coping strategies that are inappropriate to the demands of critical life events or to the specific ends sought through coping" (p. 1338). It refers to a situation in which someone forms faulty appraisals or situations based on his or her religious beliefs and practices and neglects other potentially appropriate explanations—that is, he or she attributes negative life events exclusively to punitive deities. Examples of this might include someone who believes that his relative's cancer is caused by his own sins, or who refuses medical attention and leaves her health exclusively in the hands of God. Pargament et al. (2003) explain four patters within the Wrong Road dimension: "God's Punishment refers to the use of religion to punish oneself for a stressful situation. Religious Passivity describes the use of religious coping efforts that defer or externalize all of the responsibility for coping to God or the congregation. Religious Vengeance involves the use of religion to inflict pain or punishment to others. Finally, Religious Denial refers to the use of religion to deny that the stressful event had any negative consequences for oneself" (p. 1338).

The third dimension, Against the Wind, relates to conflicts with others within a religious system, with God, or within the individuals themselves. This may lead to arguments, rejection, and emotional turbulence. Pargament et al. (2003) characterize four potential patterns: "The first domain, Interpersonal Religious Conflict, describes the experience of religious conflict with family, friends, or fellow congregation members. The second domain, Conflict with Church Dogma, involves the experience of conflict with religious dogma as expressed by the church or the clergy. The third domain, Anger at God, refers to anger at God for the role of the deity in the negative event. The final domain, Religious Doubts, describes the experience of personal religious doubts and confusion in coping with the event" (p. 1339). Furthermore, Pargament et al. (2003) assume: "the efficacy of coping is related to the degree to which a person's beliefs, emotions, relationships and values are integrated in their response to specific stressors" (p. 1345). They report an association between poorer mental health and Religious Apathy, God's Punishment, Anger at God, Religious Doubts, Interpersonal Religious Conflict, and Conflict with Church Dogmas.

Religion can also have a pathoplastic function, in which it becomes an expression of odd, deviant thinking and behavior. Such behaviors are more easily accepted in a religious context. For example, fanatic involvement with actions or manifestations promoting "decency," addressed against ethnic or sexual minorities, or different lifestyles, may be associated with personality disorders, mania, or psychosis. Another example of this is known as *sinbyong* in Korea—a disorder characterized by the appearance of productive symptoms (visual and auditory hallucinations) and strong anxiety, which is interpreted by means of a religious discourse as a calling to become a shaman (Prince, cited in Grzymala-Moszczynska 2004). In some cultures, epilepsy may be interpreted as a shamanistic trance, or a journey into the land of the spirits. (See Chapter Two, Section 2.4.4.2, "Folk Categories and Explanatory Models.")

According to Pruyser (1977, cited in Koenig 2001), people can also use religion to rationalize hatred or prejudice. This is also common among those with excessive dependency, obsessive thinking, perfectionism, exaggerated guilt, or excessive anxiety. Furthermore, religion can be used to satisfy a number of needs. Some of those who become priests or religious community leaders may be motivated by the desire to gain power, social status, or influence.

Examples of the pathoplastic function of religion in a Tibetan Buddhist setting can be exemplified by cases of disruptive behavior that is normally attributed to spirit possession, in which individuals (often young girls) became excessively angry, vulgar, and impulsive.

In this section, religion has been discussed as a pathogenic and pathoplastic factor. It can trigger pathological reactions, create stress, and engender obsessive thoughts and conflicts. Religion can also be associated with guilt and shame. Pathogenic religious behavior also includes situations in which individuals refrained from medical treatment due to their religious beliefs. The pathoplastic function, on the other hand, refers to situations in which odd, deviant thinking or behaviors can be expressed through religion.

This concludes the presentation of the theoretical framework used in this study. In the following chapter, I will describe the religious system prevailing in the studied sample, namely Tibetan Buddhism.

NOTES

1. Whereas "positive religious coping" is associated with aspects, such as benevolent religious reappraisals, "negative religious coping" results in shaky relationship with God, anger at God, discontent with the congregation and clergy.

2. Omni probably refers to features, such as: omnipresent, omnipotent, omniscient, etc.

Chapter Four

Tibetan Buddhism in Tibet and in Exile

4.1 History of Tibetan Buddhism
  4.1.1 Hinayana, Mahayana, Vajrayana: Three Paths of Dharma
  4.1.2 History of Buddhism in Tibet
    4.1.2.1 The Cultural Revolution
4.2 Key Teachings of Dharma
  4.2.1 The Truth of Suffering
  4.2.2 The Truth of the Causes of Suffering
  4.2.3 The Truth of the Cessation of Suffering
  4.2.4 The Truth of the Path
4.3 Coping with Suffering
  4.3.1 Taking Refuge
  4.3.2 Calm-Abiding Meditation
  4.3.3 *Tong len*
  4.3.4 Purification and Two Accumulations
4.4 Dharma in Everyday Life
4.5 Religious Institutions in Exile

The aim of this chapter is to present basic concepts present in Buddhist philosophy. In order to better understand the qualitative material gathered and analyzed in this study, it is essential to become familiar with traditional Tibetan beliefs and the meaning of certain rituals or practices. I will describe them from the *emic* perspective—in other words, from the standpoint of someone who is immersed in this symbolic system. This is an important point, because most of the technical literature in the field of religious studies presents Buddhism from the *etic* perspective. I chose the concepts presented here from a wide range of teachings, selecting the ones that refer to the qualitative material analyzed later. In the interests of congruence, the majority of authors I cite in this section are Tibetan.

The majority of Tibetans are Buddhists. The strong impact of this religion can be observed in their everyday life, as it pervades and affects most of their activities so to create meaning. The Tibetan Centre for Human Rights and Democracy (TCHRD) states: "Tibetan religion is connected to Tibetan identity and, by exerting religious practices, Tibetan people are asserting their cultural and national identity" (TCHRD 2000). Most Tibetans are often familiar with key religious concepts and the major deities. This is the result of religious socialization that usually starts early in a child's life at home, and continues at school and throughout adulthood. It is possible (and socially expected) to attend public teachings where Dharma is expounded upon by numerous lamas. I have selected the following metaphors, teachings, and other examples because they are frequently referred to by Tibetans in daily discourse and in a clinical context.

4.1. HISTORY OF TIBETAN BUDDHISM

The Buddhist tradition is rooted in ancient India. It was founded as a school of religion and philosophy between the sixth and fifth centuries B.C. by Siddhartha Gautama, who was later known as the Shakyamuni Buddha. In the context of the prevailing caste system of Indian society, Buddha propagated the idea of equality of all people in the face of suffering and death, and promised an opportunity to attain liberation from suffering. Buddha's teachings were written down and now constitute the 108 volumes of Kanjur[1] and about 218 volumes of Tenjur (a collection of extensive commentaries by renowned masters).

In the centuries that followed, Buddhism became one of the world's most widespread religions. It developed a pantheon of deities, a system of rituals and ceremonies, and a religious hierarchy (rankings of religious authorities). In his teachings, Buddha explained the reasons for one's suffering in terms of cause and effect—"karma"—which became one of the key concepts in the doctrine. Using the early Indian animistic ideas of the spirit's journey (reincarnation) as a base, Buddhism has created a dogma of transformation of beings, according to which death merely manifests a disintegration of the compound "Dharmas" (i.e., parts or elements that compose the whole) and the beginning of a new combination, determined by the law of karma. On the other hand, Buddhism rejects the existence of a soul as a separate spiritual entity inside humans, as well as essence of things that does not depend on others. It did not, however, reject or condemn any folk beliefs or primitive religions. On the contrary, it aimed at developing and refining them (Rerich, cited in Sieradzan et al.1987). The aim of adopting Buddhist principles is the development of loving kindness, compassion, and wisdom. This process is connected with transcending one's personality, exhibiting more patience and humility, and less egotism in relation to others. Through the practice of sacred Dharma, the practitioner purifies negative karma, produces positive impressions, and accumulates merits, so that the final goal of attaining Enlightenment can be reached.

4.1.1 Hinayana, Mahayana, Vajrayana: Three Paths of Dharma

Three main paths of Buddhism were created, and historically, they have been referred to as The Three Vehicles: Hinayana, Mahayana, and Vajrayana. Although each one is based on different sources of sacred texts, and the corresponding religious, cultural and philosophical systems, in many cases they are drawn from each other. Most teachers stress that it is impossible to practice Mahayana without developing the proper ethics and discipline highlighted in Hinayana teachings. Similarly, it is said to be fruitless or even dangerous to engage oneself in the tantric practices of Vajrayana without the appropriate motivation—which is aspiration to attain Enlightenment for the benefit of all sentient beings, which stems from loving kindness and compassion so much associated with the path of the Bodhisattva Mahayana.

Early in its history, several different schools of Buddhism were created. Although the ancient Indian treatises are the doctrinal core of all forms of Buddhism, what became the key criterion for this division was the attitude of Buddhist leaders towards the religious dogmas, philosophical concepts, and cultural-textual legacy—the interpretation of which is the source of ideological concepts (Androsow, cited in Sieradzan 1987). Because the followers of different schools often argued about certain points of the doctrine, there was a need to call a council, which would aim at straightening out the contradictions, standardizing the theory, and specifying the practice. Despite four such attempts, the councils failed to mitigate the dispute (Rarich, cited in Sieradzan 1987). In the third century B.C., Buddhist teachings crossed the Indian border into Tibet.

4.1.2 History of Buddhism in Tibet

Before the introduction of Buddhism, the first Tibetan kings were said to be the followers of the Bön tradition. This was not an organized religion, but a set of shamanistic and animistic practices. The first contact with the Buddhist tradition dates to the time when Tibetans invaded monasteries and temples in central Asia, and killed a number of monks. Although plunder was the initial purpose of these forays, subsequently the Tibetans were converted, and after some centuries they became zealous practitioners of the Buddhist faith. Officially, Buddhism appeared in Tibet during the reign of the king Lha Thothori Nyantsen,[2] born around A.D. 173. It was not until the reign of Songtsen Gampo[3] (617–698 AD), however, that it was effectively introduced. Songtsen Gampo and his successors—Trisong Deutsen[4] (742–798 AD) and Tri Ralpachen (806–841 AD) are regarded as the three ancestral spiritual kings[5] of Tibet (Dorjee and Giles 2005). During the reign of Trisong Deutsen, one of the most outstanding tantric masters—Guru Rinpoche (Padmasambhawa)—was invited to Tibet. His activities led to significant development of Buddhism during that period. At that time, Tibetans already believed in a host of benevolent and wrathful deities and a number of these existing beliefs were adopted and by the Buddhist faith. Padmasambhawa is credited with subduing all "evil spirits" thwarting the foundation of Buddhism in Tibet (Dorjee and Giles 2005). These spirits and many other deities were believed to become Dharma protectors. Tibetans also "came to embrace the Buddhist view of life, as a continual stream of death and reincarnation. A cycle in which human birth represents the precious opportunity to make the moral choices that will determine one's destiny in the next life: reincarnation in the lower realm of existence, into another human life, or ultimately into nirvana—a state of freedom from the suffering of physical existence" (Spiritual Cinema Circle 2005).

The king—Trisong Deutsen—also sponsored the translation of Buddhist scriptures, inviting translators from India, Kashmir, and China, and sending young Tibetans to study in India. The court's tradition of supporting Dharma activities reached its climax during the reign of Tri Ralpachen, who is praised for his unique contribution to the development of Tibetan Buddhism. He allocated large sums of money for building monasteries and temples—vast structures that became homes for tens of thousands of monks and nuns, publishing centers for all Tibetan society, and libraries for ancient texts. The Buddhist terminology for Tibetan translations was also standardized during that time (Dorjee and Giles 2005).

King Trisong Deutsen was said to be so deeply involved with his religion that he neglected state matters. This resulted in the dissatisfaction of his ministers, who finally murdered him. His successor, Lang-dar-ma[6] (reigned 838–842 AD), was known as a great persecutor of Tibetan Buddhism, who closed the monasteries and defrocked monks and nuns, ordering them to return to lay life. He is presented as a Bön follower, possessed by a demon, and his rule marked the end of the first dissemination of Buddhism in Tibet.

Dharma regained its popularity and strength at the end of the tenth century A.D., when the ruler Tsenpo Khore relinquished his throne and became a monk. Taking the new name Yeshi Ö, he sent twenty-one monks to study in India, two of whom returned to Tibet and became great scholars and translators: Rinchen Sangpo and Lekpe Sherab. In the year 978 they came back to Tibet, accompanied by some Indian scholars. The most significant event at that time was the visit of the famous master Atisia in the year 1042. This is regarded as the second spread of Dharma throughout Tibet.

Several local schools of Tibetan Buddhism were founded in the Land of Snow. In 1071, the Sakya order was established as the first and therefore the oldest of these, combining tantric mysticism with the philosophy of Mahayana Buddhism. In this sect, monks were not required to be celibate, and the religious hierarchy was secured among certain families. The post of abbot, for instance, was hereditary (Yamamoto 2005). The other three major sects were Gelukpa (represented by the Dalai Lamas), Kagyupa (with Karmapas as the lineage lamas), and Nyigmapa.

Historically, the distribution of power and influence of each these schools depended very much on their affiliations with the proper patrons. It is important to note that in the twelfth century, the system of lay patronage over monasteries was developed. When threatened by Mongolian power, Tibet subjected itself to Genghis Khan. Despite this, Tibet was invaded in 1240 by the Mongolian leader Godan, who later met the lama Sakya Pandita and was very much impressed by him. A specific kind of relationship was created: the patron/or sponsor[7] provided military protection, which strengthened the position of the lama. In exchange, the spiritual leader[8] was responsible for the spiritual needs of the patron. This kind of symbiosis between lay people and monastery representatives became characteristic of traditional Tibetan society. It is also reflected in the Tibetan community in exile, where a clear distinction can be observed between the social roles of the two groups, lay people versus monks and nuns.

Over the course of centuries the spiritual and state leadership converged. Tibetans also developed a tradition of identifying individuals who were called *tulku.*[9] One of them in particular was believed to be an incarnation of Chenrezi (the embodiment of loving kindness and compassion) and became known as the Dalai Lama. Among many important figures in Tibetan Buddhism it is important to mention the Fifth Dalai Lama, Ngawang Losar Gyatso (1617–1682), who managed to unite the central, south and west Tibetan provinces and was the first Dalai Lama to rule a united Tibet. Tibetans regard the Dalai Lama as a living Buddha.

The Buddhist philosophy profoundly influenced all areas of life in Tibet. Its principles became part of everyday existence and had a strong impact on the Tibetan sense of morality as well as its the social system, which was newly infused with benevolence, including non-violence and compassion towards all sentient beings. This set a new standard for living, and "the degree to which Tibetans integrated these beliefs into everyday lives grew to be the signature of their culture" (Spiritual Cinema Circle 2005).

4.1.2.1 The Cultural Revolution

Until the twentieth century, Tibet remained isolated and sheltered behind its mountain walls from the influence of the modern world. Problems began when the Chinese invoked past diplomatic ties between Tibet and the Chinese monarchies, and announced that Tibet should be returned to its "Motherland." This was a mere pretext to claim Tibet's strategic location, rich geological resources, and the head waters of key Asian rivers. In 1949, the armed forces of the People's Republic of China began invading Tibet and destroyed much of the country's cultural and historical heritage. Monasteries were plundered and razed, and a great number of monks and nuns were killed. Executions, as well as many other offenses, repression, and persecution were reported. Even though Tibetans made a number of attempts to fight back the Red Guards, they lacked military skills and weaponry. In a series of bloody and hopeless battles, they were outnumbered, and it is reported that more than 1.2 million Tibetans (which exceeded 20 percent of Tibet's entire population) lost their lives. Those who proclaimed allegiance to the Dalai Lama were imprisoned, tortured, or killed (Tsering Gellek 2001).

Before the invasion, an estimated 20 percent of the Tibetan population were monks or nuns, who were housed in 6000 monasteries. Tsering Gellek (2001) writes: "like nuclei of a community, monasteries represented the center of Tibetan life and were the intellectual repository of Tibet's history, scientific and medical knowledge, philosophical debates, law, and any other form of documented cultural knowledge" (p. 4). These institutions were among the primary targets of China's so-called "Cultural Revolution." Most of them were looted and destroyed (Kolas 2004).

Beginning with the initial occupation, Tibet faced increasingly restrictive religious and economic policies. The practice of religion became the main target of criticism by the Chinese authorities (Tsering Gellek 2001; Kolas 2004). Aiming to introduce the Communist social and economic systems, the Chinese subsequently devastated Tibet's culture and people. Tsering Gellek (2001) reports: "The razing of all but a handful of Tibet's 6000 monasteries and the systematic attempt to eradicate Buddhism and its adherents were for Tibetans a violent awakening to the so-called 'modern world'" (p. 5). All types of religious activities were completely "outlawed"

(Kolas 2004). The Tibetan Centre for Human Rights and Democracy (2000a)[10] describes the situation in their brochure: "The 'work teams,' composed mainly of Public Security Bureau (PSB) officials led extended re-education sessions, which disrupts the monastic schedules. Their main purpose is to identify, expel and arrest monks and nuns considered 'unpatriotic,' those who express any opinion contrary to Party's policy or those who don't agree with the five points required by the pledge, which all monks and nuns are forced to sign."

Violence was often used during re-education sessions, when individuals refused to: 1. declare their opposition to separatism, 2. agree to the Chinese version of Tibetan history, 3. recognize the Chinese-appointed Panchen Lama, 4. deny Tibet's independent status, and 5. denounce the Dalai Lama as a traitor of the "Motherland." In some cases the "work team" officers would expel monks and nuns and make them return to their families. Performing any religious rites or joining any other nunnery or monastery was forbidden. Some monks and nuns were also arrested for political activities, including the act of possessing pictures of the Dalai Lama. Basic religious practices were also banned in prison: "Monks and nuns in prison are prohibited to prostrate, make beads out of dough or wear robes. Rather, they are obliged to let their hair grow. The mere act of praying aloud is forbidden, and punishment for breaking this 'rule of silence' includes physical and verbal abuse" (Tibetan Centre for Human Rights and Democracy 2000a).

The picture of the Tibetans' spiritual leader was banned not only from religious institutions, but also forbidden in private homes. TCHRD (2000a) further reports that "approximately 450 Tibetans were fined 500 yuan each for having displayed the Dalai Lama's picture in their homes." Birthday celebrations for His Holiness the Dalai Lama were defined as "propagating acts of splittism and instigating the masses to oppose the Chinese government" (TCHRD 2000a) and subsequently prohibited. Raids, during which Chinese officials confiscated religious belongings (such as altars, thangkas, statues, etc.) were conducted in Tibetan houses in Lhasa. Tibetans were also forbidden to develop "devotional faith, considering the Dalai Lama as an enlightened being, sending their children to schools run by the Dalai Lama, and pursuing the path of the Dalai clique" (TCHRD 2000a). People who violated the statutory law were subjected to severe punishments following rigorous investigation. The Chinese government also abolished the traditional practice of reading scriptures in Tibetan homes. To perform a religious ceremony, special permission had to be obtained. Moreover, age limits for monastery enrollment were introduced: Monks and nuns younger than age 18 and older than age 50 were expelled and denied the right to study or practice religion. According to the Tibetan Centre for Human Rights and Democracy (2000a), this law threatens the survival of Tibetan Buddhism because senior religious people play a pivotal role in the transmission of religious teachings. Although some of the monasteries have been rebuilt since the invasion, these include only the well-known sites and those accessible to tourists. Even though the monks and nuns were "permitted" to practice Buddhism, the right to religious freedom has been severely restricted (TCHRD 2000a).

In 1959, after ten years of unsuccessful negotiations, the Dalai Lama and more than 85,000 Tibetans fled Tibet for India, Nepal, and Bhutan. In these host countries, a number of religious institutions have been established in the newly created Tibetan settlements. Among them are monasteries that have been providing shelter and education for a large number of ordained monks, nuns, and novices. These institutions have become centers for religious life, and a nexus of social networks have been created around them. Plus, the growing interest in Tibetan Buddhism on the part of Western people has also created a new type of consumer market, with increasing demands for religious objects, texts of the practices, and Dharma books.

4.2 KEY TEACHINGS OF DHARMA

The idea behind this chapter is to give the reader a feeling of what is being transmitted to Tibetans in the process of religious socialization. Concepts described here include the main topics being discussed by lamas who give public lectures to the faithful. Many Tibetans who attend these teachings become familiar with them to a greater or lesser degree. Like those who attend these public teachings, readers will become familiar with a number of poplar and renowned scholars and Buddhist masters, both past and present.

Buddhist philosophy is grounded in the teachings that have been expounded upon by Buddha in the place known as Beneres (Varanasi). This set of teachings is referred to as the First Turn of the Wheel of Dharma, and sheds light on the "Four Noble Truths."[11] Just like a doctor, Buddha diagnosed the unenlightened beings, in speaking about the existence of suffering and its genesis. He presented the goal that all sentient beings pursue (the cessation of suffering) and offered a remedy—skilful means (or Dharma) to be chosen according to the needs and predispositions of the practitioner. The aim is to liberate one from suffering and attain Enlightenment: the complete realization of Buddhahood.[12] Becoming a Buddha implies that one's mind becomes thoroughly purified of any emotional obscuration or defilements (Tib. *sangs*) and the enlightened qualities (Tib. *rgyas*) are manifested.

4.2.1 The Truth of Suffering[13]

The First Truth elaborates on the fact that suffering exists in the lives of all beings, who, since beginningless time, continuously are reborn into one of the six realms of the conditioned world—*samsara,* or cyclic existence. Suffering is present in all of these realms, due to attachment, aggression, and ignorance. There are three Lower Realms: 1) the Hell Realm, 2) the Hungry Ghosts Realm, 3) the Animal Realm, and three Upper Realms: 1) the Human Realm, 2) the Demi-Gods Realm and 3) the God's Realm. These six can be subdivided into many different realms. The inhabitants of each realm experience a particular type of suffering, mental state, or condition. From the very first day of life, this cyclic existence is inseparable from suffering.

Tarthang Tulku Rinpoche (1973a) talks about the suffering associated with human existence—suffering of birth, disease, aging, and death: "The bodymind confusion is characterized by pain from its conception. After an agonizing cramp in the womb for several months, the first reaction to birth is a scream. The pains of growth are punctuated by disease of the bodymind and disease follows one until death. Sickness is suffering. Then after the maturation of the bodymind, decay sets in with its accompanying failure of the senses and the brain in senility until the heart can function no longer and the ultimate pain of death must be suffered. This is the pain of the human condition: embodiment. The bodymind is the form of embodiment" (p. 72). The four main types of suffering (birth, sickness, old age, and death) are often accompanied by many others: "suffering of not obtaining what one wants, to be dispossessed of what one possesses, to be separated from loved ones, and to be associated with beings that one does not like" (Kalu Rinpoche 1995, p. 89). Tarthang Tulku Rinpoche (1973a) adds: "even getting what is wanted is suffering when the thrill of possession turns into the grey despondency of regret" (p. 73).

Rinpoche explains that lack of awareness of the causes of suffering and insistent movement in the same direction along the path that caused it compounds suffering. He further explains: "The man who mistakes wealth for the antidote to the suffering of poverty merely replaces one pain by another. The pain of acquisition, of miserliness, of fear of loss may cause a welter of confusion and far greater pain than the original condition. There is no release by replacing one mental state by another, one passion by another, one woman by another, one home by another or one life by another. Change in itself is a cause of suffering. The belief that greater contentment can be found by this kind of alternation is a potent delusion" (Tarthang Tulku Rinpoche 1973a, p. 73).

The phenomenon of suffering is explained in details of the Buddhist teachings. The Sanskrit words *dukha* (or Tibetan '*sdug bsngal*) translated as "suffering" have broad meanings. Three types or levels of suffering can be differentiated.

The first type is "the suffering of suffering," which characterizes the physical and mental pain experienced by all beings. Such sensations accompany experiences like disease, wounds, hunger, cold, or difficult emotions. We can also add to this list the pain of losing loved ones, such as parents or partners.

The second type is "the suffering of change," which relates to the fact that everything is impermanent. According to the Buddhist philosophy, all the conditioned (or compound) phenomena must undergo change or decay at a certain time. Tarthang Tulku Rinpoche (1973a) presents examples of change:

> "The seasons change, day turns into night, the moon has its phases, the seasons are accompanied by life cycles of flora and fauna. So it is with the human body, achievements and values. Nothing lasts. Few human beings have ever lived beyond two or even one hundred years; no hero, prophet, priest or king could escape death. The remains of civilizations remind one of past races and cultures which were inevitably consumed in the passage of time. Culture, customs, and values change from year to year. Wealth changes hands with no apparent cause, and it is impossible to retard the process of change in economic status through miserliness. There is nothing in the realm of human experience, which does not change. Emotional states are totally erratic, depending upon the stimulus and the changing karmic stream. Moods of others can be observed changing without any apparent cause" (pp. 68–70).

The law of change also affects happiness and suffering, as these are merely an illusion—nothing real or substantial, but a result of many interacting conditions. Similarly, things and people who are the source of pleasure finally become the source of suffering, as they are transformed by time and leave us with a feeling of disappointment and loss. Buddhist teachers often remind their disciples that money, academic titles, social status, family, and friends are all things that they will have to lose—if not during their lifetime, then surely at the time of death. Tibetans often use a metaphor of food mixed with poison—it is delicious while being eaten and produces pleasing sensations, but creates pain and suffering after some time.

Impermanence also concerns one's life span. Dilgo Khyentse Rinpoche (2002) taught that: "All birth ends in death. Has there ever been a single being that has escaped death? What is accumulated will inevitably be exhausted. Whatever quantity of goods you have been able to amass will sooner or later be squandered. All assembly ends in separation. . . . Whatever rises must fall: no one has held the same rank forever" (p. 24). Dharma teachings often expound upon the uncertainty of the circumstances of death. Apart from the fact that death is certain, the time of death and the associated circumstances remain unknown. Khenpo Ngawang Pelzang (2004) reminds us: "At death nothing can accompany you. When you die, apart from the sacred Dharma nothing can help you: your food, clothes, home, bed, possessions, parents, relatives, friends, and partner are of no use to you" (p. 60).

Similarly, Tarthang Tulku Rinpoche (1973a) advises contemplation of the impermanence and uncertainty of the time and conditions of one's death: "Knowing that all things will decay and eventually pass away, it is important to realize that the time of that eventual demise is unknown. No one knows the time of his death, whether he will live to a fine old age, whether he will leave a widow and children, whether he will die in his sleep tonight, whether he will be killed on the road this afternoon, or even whether he will live to draw another breath. There can never be certainty" (pp. 68–70).

The third type of suffering refers to the fact that beings are continuously reborn in the conditioned world, a fact that is inseparable from suffering. Patrul Rinpoche (1998) gives an example of a man who feels that everything is apparently fine with him at the moment and does not acknowledge any suffering. In spite of that, he is "immersed in the causes of suffering . . . for our very food and clothing, our homes, the adornments and celebrations that give us pleasure, are all produced with harmful actions" (p. 79). To explain this, Rinpoche gives as an example the production of tea. Large number of small beings such as insects and worms will inevitably lose their lives during this process. It is also connected with the suffering of the animals and people performing their difficult, painstaking work. Thus, "all the factors we now see as constituting happiness . . . are likewise produced through negative actions alone. . . . So everything that seems to represent happiness today is, in fact, the suffering of everything composite" (Patrul Rinpoche 1998, p. 80).

The Dalai Lama (quoted in Powers 1999) describes this type of suffering as an ubiquitous suffering of existence, because it pervades all the transmigrating beings. There is no escape from it, other than attaining Buddhahood—the state that is utterly free of any suffering. Bokar Rinpoche (1996) explains that "suffering of conditioned existence is suffering one undergoes because of the deluded nature of samsara. It ends only when one attains awakening" (p. 55). This is further described by The Second Truth of the Causes of Suffering[14] and the Third Truth of the Cessation of Suffering.[15]

4.2.2 The Truth of the Causes of Suffering

According to Buddhist philosophy the root cause of suffering is basic ignorance and clinging to the "self." Both "I" and everything that is not "I" (in other words, the external world) is similarly experienced as real. The unenlightened beings who perceive phenomena with their senses naturally tend to conceptualize (name and evaluate) what they sense around them. They react accordingly with desire (if they experience a given phenomenon as pleasant or attractive), aversion (if phenomena are perceived as ugly, unpleasant, or painful) or indifference (if things are perceived as neutral). But perceiving phenomena as real and substantial in their nature is merely an illusion, according to Buddhist teachings.

Tibetans often use the metaphor of a dream state. While sleeping, one can experience the dream as real (for example, being chased by a tiger). Then, naturally one might experience emotions (fear or panic), manifest physiological changes (sweating, tachycardia), and wake up with a scream. On waking, one realizes that it has just been a dream. In a similar vein, Buddha presented the concept of the "relative truth" and the "absolute truth." He explained that although phenomena may seem to exist and evoke pain and suffering (relative truth), in fact, from the perspective of the absolute truth, they are like a reflection of the moon in the surface of water—neither real nor substantial. They are merely a combination of different conditions that came together at a certain time in space. Buddhist teachers often use other metaphors to explain this concept, sometimes comparing the phenomena to waves on the surface of an unlimited ocean (of mind), or clouds, rainbows, rain, or thunderstorms that appear in the vast space of consciousness for one moment, and then dissolve back to space. Because phenomena are compound (and so conditioned), they must fall apart sooner or later.

The entire concept is thoroughly explained in *Prajnaparamita sutra* (*The Heart Sutra*) and numerous commentaries to it. This popular Mahayana text expounds on the doctrine of the lack of reality of phenomena—the empty nature of everything:

> "Form—voidness; voidness—form. Form not separate from voidnesss; voidness not separate from form. Similarly, feeling, distinguishing, affecting variables, types of consciousness—voidness . . . all phenomena—voidness: no defining characteristics, no arising, no stopping, no being stained, no being parted from stain, no being deficient, no being additional . . . in voidness, no form, no feeling, no distinction, no affecting variables, no kind of consciousness. No eye, no ear, no nose, no tongue, no body, no mind. No sight, no sound, no smell, no taste, no physical sensation, no phenomena. No cognitive source that's an eye, up to no cognitive source that's mind (no cognitive source that's phenomena), no cognitive source that's mental consciousness. No unawareness, no elimination of unawareness, up to no aging and death, no elimination of aging and death. Likewise, no suffering, no cause, stopping, and pathway mind. No deep awareness, no attainment, no non-attainment . . . through there being no attainment of bodhisattvas,[16] he (or she) lives, relying on far-reaching discriminating awareness, with no mental obstruction. (Because of there being

> no mental obscuration,) there is no fear, gone beyond what's reversed, (thus) nirvana release, complete to the end. In fact, it's by relying on far-reaching discriminating awareness that all Buddhas arrayed throughout the three times are full manifest Buddhas in peerless and perfect full Buddhahood" (Berzin 2004)

Until they have obtained Enlightenment, sentient beings are trapped in the wheel of cyclic existence—they die and are reborn, led by their karma. This in itself constitutes the aforementioned suffering.

Karma

Buddha taught that our existence is a series of continuous births, deaths, and rebirths. Having abandoned the body, the mind moves on, together with "karma"—the impressions gathered in the stream of consciousness: "Fundamental consciousness can be compared to a ground that receives imprints or seeds left by our actions. Once planted, these seeds remain in the ground of fundamental consciousness until the conditions for their germination and ripening have come together. In this way, they actualize their potential by producing the plants and fruits that are the various experiences of samsara" (Kalu Rinpoche 1997, p. 31). It is thus important to engage oneself in actions that aim at developing positive impressions, because karma will determine how the mind will experience reality after death and the circumstances of the next rebirth. Karma determines each life, the condition and form in which one is reborn, as well as the accompanying circumstances. "In general, the collection of imprints left in the fundamental awareness by past actions serves to condition all states and experiences" (Kalu Rinpoche 1997, p. 31).

Kalu Rinpoche (1995) explains the meaning of the word "karma".[17] The Tibetan word *las* refers to actions, including our personality and activities of the body, speech, and mind. In Tibetan, *gyu* means "cause"—according to the Buddhist philosophy, both positive and negative actions leave an imprint that becomes a cause for future actions. The word *'bras* means "result"—the painful or pleasant situations that have been created due to certain actions. This notion of karma "includes the entire gamut of activity, from the cause up to the consequence of an action. Karma is, therefore, activity understood as being the series of causes and results of actions" (Kalu Rinpoche 1997:31). The law of cause and effect implies that actions, according to their nature, are causes engendering defined results. Every thought, word, or the smallest action—even the blinking of an eye—can produce karma. When action is accompanied by specific intention (for example, to harm someone, to cause suffering, or to liberate someone from suffering) the karmic results are especially strong. The results of actions may appear instantly, or else they may be delayed in time. They can also ripen in lives to come.

Bokar Rinpoche (1996) comments: "Once dead, we are like a lamp whose oil is exhausted. Wherever we are reborn, we cannot do it freely, but it is certain that we are led by karma and have no control of our own. It is commonly said that the various manifestations of happenings and suffering are the result of positive or negative acts" (p. 19). That is why the aim of one's spiritual practice will be developing loving kindness and compassion, as well as wisdom. These lead to positive actions and elimination of emotional defilements,[18] which constitute the three mental poisons (desire, aversion, and ignorance). The three mental poisons may result in one of 84,000 negative states that make one engage in actions that produce suffering in oneself and others.

According to the Buddhist philosophy, there are ten kinds of negative (or non-virtuous) actions: three types of non-virtuous actions connected with the body: taking life (killing), taking what is not given (stealing), and sexual misconduct; four types of non-virtuous actions connected with speech: lying, slander (or sowing discord), harsh speech and idle or worthless chatter; and three types of non-virtuous actions connected with the mind: covetousness, wishing harm on others, and wrong view (e.g., that karma does not exist). Each of the ten actions is thoroughly explained in the Buddhist philosophical literature (including Kalu Rinpoche 1995; Khandro Rinpoche 2003, and Patrul Rinpoche 1998).

4.2.3 The Truth of the Cessation of Suffering

The Third Truth elaborates on the goal that all sentient beings aspire to achieve—the cessation of suffering. It is important to highlight this part of the Buddhist philosophy, to dispel possible misconceptions of Buddhism as offering a sad or pessimistic perspective. On the contrary, in the context of their public teachings, Tibetan masters often stress "the preciousness of human existence." They affirm that attaining a human form of existence is extremely precious, even though most people take it for granted.

While some people may take great pride in human life and are convinced of being somehow superior to all other forms of existence, they often fail to find happiness and peace. Rarely do they reflect upon the fact that they are in a unique situation, in which they must develop all their potential. As a result of this, they often waste a lifetime that could be of tremendous benefit to themselves and others. Khandro Rinpoche (2003) writes: "In the Buddhist tradition attaining a human life is said to occur as rarely as a blind turtle who, surfacing in a vast ocean once every hundred years, manages to put his head through a wooden yoke floating in all directions on the surface of the water. A more contemporary analogy is the likelihood that a pea dropped from an airplane will be caught on the head of a pin held by someone on the ground" (p. 1).

According to the Buddhist philosophy, the root of all suffering is basic ignorance. Obscured by this ignorance, one engages in all kinds of actions of body, speech and mind that produce confusion and unhappiness. Having received proper instructions, one is given a choice of whether one wants to remain ignorant, or put effort into spiritual practice, liberate oneself and others from suffering, and attain Enlightenment. The reason why suffering is so often reflected upon is to stimulate the practitioner towards engaging in spiritual actions, avoiding harmful actions, and coping with everyday problems more effectively. Gampopa (1995) teaches: "Reflecting upon death and impermanence, inspire yourself to spiritual practice" (p. 29). He further explains:

> "It is useless to care to perform protective rituals for this illusory body since it will most certainly perish—no matter how much trouble you take.
>
> It is useless to crave material things and be stingy with them, since the day you die you leave poor and empty-handed—no matter how much trouble you take.
>
> It is useless to build castles and mansions since the day you die you leave alone and even your corpse will be thrown out—no matter how much trouble you take.
>
> It is useless to thoughtfully bequeath things to your children and descendants since they have no power to help you at the moment of death, not even for one instant—no matter how much trouble you take.
>
> It is useless to affectionately care for friends and relatives since the day you die you leave alone and friendless—no matter how much trouble you take.
>
> It is useless to have possessions that will surely be squandered when given to children and descendants since they are all impermanent—no matter how much wealth you may have.
>
> It is useless to have property, dominion, and enterprises since the day you die you proceed aimlessly without fixed abode or dwelling—no matter how much trouble you take.
>
> . . . . It is useless not to practice after training your mind in leaving and reflection since there is then nothing to apply at the moment of death—no matter how much Dharma you understand" (pp. 45–46).

Having properly understood the truth of suffering and its causes, impermanence and the futility of the worldly things that most people try to grasp, one is encouraged to seek freedom—Enlightenment—in which all kinds of suffering have ceased to exist. Lotsawa Kawa Peltseg (1992) explains that cessation relates to "the abandonment of afflictive emotions such as desire and hatred as well as of non-virtuous actions such as killing" (p. 53). This results in *peace* (a state free from suffering), *excellence* (freedom from future rebirths within the three realms and no experience of suffering), and *renunciation* (having realized that the three realms resemble a prison, one goes to the blissful abode which is beyond sorrow).

According to Buddhist teachings, there is no way to liberate oneself from suffering other than by engaging oneself in spiritual actions and meditation, following the instructions of the Dharma. As presented by Gampopa (1995), mere listening is useless unless the proper methods are applied. A renowned scholar and meditation master, Lama Mipham (1973b) expressed this in a poetic way, using the following metaphor:

> "When a man is parched by thirst
> The thought of water brings no relief—
> Only drinking can quench his thirst:
> So information differs from experience.
> The exhausting search for information
> For mere objective knowledge
> Becomes needless with meditative experience
> Which quickly leads to equanimity." (p. 106)

Tarthang Tulku Rinpoche (1973b) explains the importance of gaining meditation experience as being superior to mere theoretical understanding of the nature of mind:

> "The necessary study which teaches skill in self-expression, metaphysical postulation, logic and other arts and sciences precedes practice. It is customary to look at a map before starting out on a journey. However, to believe that the knowledge which is gained from the map is the terrain itself is to mistake the concept for the reality. No mere intellectual certainty is valuable when faced with the naked reality of the depths of mind. Like accumulated wealth at the moment of death or the gift of snow in the tropics, theoretical knowledge has no relevance out of its own sphere. The spontaneous expression of the view perceived in profound equanimity, which is the acceptance of whatever may arise without addition or subtraction, replaces the preconceptions of dogma and philosophical dicta" (p. 106).

4.2.4 The Truth of the Path[19]

The Fourth Truth refers to The Eightfold Path that leads to the state of liberation from suffering and the attainment of complete Enlightenment. It involves right understanding, right aspiration, right speech, right action, right livelihood, right effort, right mindfulness, and right concentration. The Fourth Truth has been divided into the three ways of practice: 1. morality, or good conduct, 2. mental development, and 3. wisdom (Santina 1997). Dilgo Khyentse Rinpoche (2002) explains the preciousness of the teachings:

> "Our lives have no outcome other than death, as rivers have no end other than the ocean. Therefore, nothing is more precious than a spiritual teaching that can aid us at the moment of death. . . .The illusory possessions an ordinary person leaves behind, his land and wealth, are completely useless at the hour of death. The Buddhas and the spiritual masters bequeath the living expression of their wisdom in the form of teachings, providing those who wish to enter the way of liberation with a constant source of inspiration. Such teachings, inseparable from those great beings themselves, allow anyone who takes them to heart to attain their level of realization" (p. 18).

Gampopa (1995) also emphasizes how exceptional it is to be born as a human being, come across Dharma, arouse interest in it, and practice the path. He explains: "Like returning empty-handed from an island of precious gems, it is meaningless to ignore the sacred Dharma after having obtained a human body" (p. 35).

4.3. COPING WITH SUFFERING

Mercer and Ager (2005) report that the coping mechanisms used by Tibetan refugees seem significantly influenced by the Buddhist philosophical background. Buddhist teachings offer a number of methods or techniques that make it possible to bear one's suffering more effectively. Tsering Gellek (2001) writes of the common emotional responses of Tibetan refugees: "How refugees cope with the traumas of departure and arrival in foreign lands is likely to reflect not only basic features of human survival but more subtle and particular aspects of cultural and religious practices" (pp. 2–3). Khenpo Donyo (cited in Bokar Rinpoche and Khenpo Donyo 1994) explains: "Physical suffering can be relieved by medical remedies, but there is no relief for inner turmoil. Understanding how the law of karma functions places us in a relatively comfortable situation in the face of suffering and joy. Struck by suffering, we endure it without revolt, knowing it is the result of our karma. We, ourselves, have created the seed in our past lives. We are responsible for it. This attitude, in itself, diminishes suffering" (pp. 64–65).

4.3.1 Taking Refuge

Tibetan Buddhism offers a variety of practices that help believers cope with suffering. The most essential one is the Taking of (or Going for) Refuge, which is the most common practice in all schools of Buddhism. Patrul Rinpoche (1998) says that it opens the gateway to all teachings and practices. Taking refuge means adopting a certain mental attitude, while subduing oneself to the Three Jewels (Buddha, Dharma, and Sangha). Additionally, prostrations are often offered in front of an object that represents the Three Jewels (for example, an altar, a painting or statue of Buddha, or a lama). Taking refuge may express different types of motivation on the part of the practitioner:

1. Some may be motivated by fear of being reborn in the three lower realms, and so they take refuge with the hope of being reborn in the upper realms; this is called the refuge of lesser beings.
2. Others, being aware that suffering is inevitable in samsara, no matter whether one is born in the lower or upper realms, take refuge in the Three Jewels with the aspiration of attaining the level of nirvana, a state that is free from sufferings; this is called the refuge of middle beings;
3. The refuge of great beings—feeling loving kindness and compassion, one aspires to attain Enlightenment, to establish all beings in the state of perfect Buddhahood (Patrul Rinpoche 1998).

There is a popular prayer by Atisia, which can be translated as follows: "From now on, until I reach Enlightenment, I take refuge in Buddha, Dharma, and Sangha. Through the merit of practicing generosity and other perfections (*paramitas*), may I attain Enlightenment, for the benefit of all sentient beings."

There are detailed explanations of how one should understand the objects of refuge—Buddha, Dharma and Sangha. Jamgon Kongtrul Rinpoche (2003) explains: "In making this commitment to strive toward Buddhahood and become like these enlightened beings, the aspirant becomes a Buddhist and gains their protection from the vicissitudes of samsara" (p. 53).

4.3.2 Calm-Abiding Meditation

Another highly popular practice is calm-abiding meditation, or *shine*[20] in Tibetan. The aim of this meditation is to let the mind rest in a calm state. To achieve this, the practitioner may concentrate on an object of meditation—for example, one's breath, a statue or painting of Buddha, a burning candle. This kind of meditation shields the mind from distractions, and from the creation of afflicting emotions (Duff 2003). It can be used to lessen both physical and mental suffering.

4.3.3 *Tong len*

In times of adversity, in addition to contemplating impermanence and the law of karma, Tibetans commonly use the practice of *tong len.* The meaning of this particular meditation is "taking suffering and giving happiness." Kalu Rinpoche (1995) explains this practice:

> "We should think of the ocean of suffering, not only of the suffering we experience now but also of the suffering imprinted in our karmic potential, which will actualize in the future. Then we imagine that all the suffering, faults, and veils covering the mind of all beings take the form of a black light that we breathe in by the right nostril. It dissolves into the emptiness of the heart. We imagine that all beings are liberated from this suffering that we just took within ourselves. Then, we imagine all the qualities, all happiness and joys we have taking the form of a white light that we breath out by the left nostril. This light envelops all beings and they become perfectly happy. Our practice continues for a certain number of breathing cycles during this visualisation" (p. 72).

Even though some Tibetans may not meditate, they still adopt the view used in this practice, which subsequently helps them cope with their own suffering by creating meaning (in other words, it makes their own suffering meaningful). The practice of *tong len* helps the practitioner develop a positive mental attitude. Faced with misfortune or pain, Tibetans may think like this: "Being touched by this experience of suffering I can understand other people better. There are so many beings who suffer. May, through my suffering, the suffering of all sentient beings be purified." Shantideva (1979) used a metaphor to explain the necessity of changing one's perception instead of fighting against all phenomena that cause one suffer: If the road is covered with rocks and thorns, you can either pave the entire road with leather, or you can take leather and place it on the soles of your own feet. According to Buddhist teachings, the development of loving kindness, compassion, and wisdom is the remedy—the leather protecting oneself and others from being harmed.

4.3.4 Purification and Two Accumulations

Because suffering is thought to be inseparable from life in *samsara* (cyclic existence), only attaining liberation frees one from suffering. Therefore, all practices of Dharma are aimed at achieving Buddhahood. Kalu Rinpoche (1997) explains: "All Dharma practices can be categorized as purification and accumulation, that is, the purification of the veils that obscure the mind and the practice of the two accumulations of merit and wisdom. This process can be illustrated with the following image. Veiled or obscured, mind is like a sky darkened by clouds that cover its infinite vastness and brightness. The two accumulations are like the wind that dissipates these clouds, revealing the immensity and clarity of pure mind" (p. 141).

What becomes purified is one's negative karma, which is believed to be responsible for all misfortune or illnesses an individual suffers. Jamgon Kongtrul Rinpoche (2003) describes this process: "The impurities to be removed include the accumulated influences of all the unwholesome thoughts, words and deeds he [the practitioner] has perpetrated throughout his samsaric career, as well as their cause: ignorance or bewilderment" (p. 79). To achieve that goal, the Four Powers should be used, namely: 1. the power to renounce and regret the previous misdeeds as vigorously as if one had swallowed poison, 2. the power to refuse to repeat a harmful deed, 3. the power to rely on Taking Refuge and engendering Bodhicitta (the Enlightened Attitude), in other words, developing loving kindness and compassion for the benefit of all beings, and 4. the power to carry out all types of remedial wholesome actions to purify harmful ones (Jamgon Kongtrul Rinpoche 2003). A practice of Vajrasattva and repetition of his Hundred-syllable mantra is often used as a means of purification.

The term "Two Accumulations" refers to: 1. Accumulation of merits, and 2. Accumulation of Wisdom. Kalu Rinpoche (1997) describes the first type as "all benevolent and beneficial activities done for others as well as ourselves. These are actions that generate positive karma. . . . For the accumulation of merit, the act itself is important, but the underlying motivation is even more important; any act motivated by love and compassion is therefore a source of great benefit" (p. 141). The Accumulation of Wisdom is based on the first type of accumulation. Kalu Rinpoche (1997) writes: "Wisdom is direct experience of reality beyond dualistic illusions. These two accumulations—positive deeds, or merit, and wisdom—are complementary and give rise to each other sequentially; the first being right action, or beneficial activities, and the second, the nondual experience of pristine awareness, which develops in meditation practice" (p. 141). An example of practicing generosity can be used to illustrate this: giving is itself a positive action and can be an antidote to the stinginess associated with attachment. But if one offers something with the understanding that the giver, gift, and recipient are ultimately empty in their nature (have no true reality), wisdom is developed.

Kalu Rinpoche (1997) demonstrates a variety of actions that can be performed to accumulate merits:

> "Knowing and calling to mind the qualities of the Three Jewels, we can make different kinds of offerings with great faith. Traditionally, we make symbolic offerings: pure water, flowers, incense, light (butter lamps, candles, and so forth), perfumed water, delicious and aromatic foods, and beautiful sounds and melodies. We can also offer the Sangha food, clothes, lodging, other material goods or necessities, or different ornaments for temples. A secondary category of offerings, those produced by the mind, can include everything that has existed forever, divine or human lands with earth, mountains, rivers, oceans, all bodies of water, meadows, prairies, forests, fruits, fertile fields, homes, foods, clothing, silk, brocade, jewels, all goods or possessions, young men and women, domestic animals, deer, pets, birds, and wild animals. In fact, we can make mental offerings by imagining magnificent objects, beautiful sounds, exquisite fragrances, delicious flavours, gentle touches, every object of knowledge pleasing to the mind, as well as the various actual or symbolic offerings such as the eight auspicious symbols, the seven royal attributes of temporal power, the eight auspicious substances, and so on. Imagining that all these offerings extend throughout space, we present them to the Three Jewels and the Three Roots . . . if we make offerings to them with faith and respect, we can complete our own accumulation of merit and achieve the accumulation of wisdom" (pp. 143–144).

Wisdom is also accumulated through the practice of meditation and by contemplating the teachings. As will be shown in the analysis of the qualitative data gathered in this study, Tibetans strive to accumulate these spiritual merits day by day.

4.4 DHARMA IN EVERYDAY LIFE

It has already been mentioned that many Tibetans, especially the elderly, are zealous Dharma practitioners. Their involvement with spiritual practice is marked by maintaining affiliations with local monasteries and engaging in specific actions.

Affiliation with monasteries

As in the days of the early Tibetan warlords, a peculiar "patron-client dyad" has been established in exile between lay Tibetans and their spiritual leaders. Tenzin Gellek (2001) describes the monastic and patronage systems, in which lay patrons (sponsors, often chosen from among the disciples) would provide money, and the institution (monastery, teachers) would take care of the spiritual needs of the former. Such mutually satisfying relationships are visible in everyday life: lay practitioners visit monasteries and ask lamas to perform prayers, enact rituals, or give advice, all in exchange for donations. Apart from yogis, lay Tibetans are not skilled in the monastic arts and their spiritual practice is usually limited to listening to the teachings, repeating mantras, circumambulating holy places, and taking part in pilgrimages. In exchange for more advanced spiritual counsel, lay people give all kinds of offerings, usually in the form of cash.

Involvement with spiritual practice

Many Tibetans, especially the elderly ones, maintain affiliations with local monasteries. Jacobson (2002) presents an example of woman in her seventies: "She pursued a number of typical lay religious practices, and after fleeing to India had reconnected herself with some of the same religious hierarchs—then also in exile—whom her family had venerated in their homeland. This testified to the strength of her faith, in which she was typical of Tibetan refugees of her generation" (p. 267). Jacobson (2002) also refers to the practice of circumambulating holy places: "The clockwise circumambulation of temples, monasteries, sacred monuments and mountains is a common lay practice, and is generally combined with the repetition of mantra or prayers which are counted on one's rosary (when the practitioner is not engaged in gossiping with the usual fellow-circumambulator" (p. 275).

Kolas (2004) points out that Tibet's popular custom of religious pilgrimage has a significant social function: "Journeys to ritual sites are occasions that people like to talk about, and there is an evident social dimension to these journeys. On such journeys people like to dress up in their best festive clothes and travel together with their friends or relatives. Even on shorter trips they often take the time to include a picnic along the way. Visits to sacred sites are thus 'popular' in every sense of the word" (p. 136). Back in Tibet, villagers often met together to perform a special ritual for mountain deities.[21] According to the author, such group events created a sense of community, confirming and strengthening family ties and ties between the households that make up village communities. Another type of religious activity involved hanging prayer flags and performing the *sang* ritual. The Tibetans would:

> "replace the old prayer flags on the rooftop flagpoles (local Tibetan: *gyantsen bugye*) with new ones. On the first, third and fifth days of the New Year the men in each household also put up prayer flags in the five colors (red, white, blue, yellow and green) fastened to bamboo poles (ritual arrows known as *rtse sheng*). These are planted in a hilltop cairn (*rtse phung*, where *rtse* means peak, and *phung* means heap), in connection with offerings for the mountain deity (*ridag*).

Starting as early as December different types of prayer flags (*bugye*) can be bought at make-shift stalls outside the market, where they are sold by village women who want to make an extra income. If the villagers have not had a chance to go to the forest to cut them, bamboo poles can also be bought in the market. When the *rtse sheng* is put up in the cairn, this is an act of offering in itself, but is also accompanied by other offerings, including *sang* offerings as well as offerings of *tsampa*, barley grain and barley wine, which is thrown into the air. After the offerings to the *ri dbag* are completed similar offerings are made at the cairn of the village *klu* (spirit of the underworld). Offerings of *sang* are also made at religious structures such as temples and chörten (the Tibetan version of the Indian '*stupa*'; Chinese: *baita*)" (Kolas 2004, p. 112).

4.5 RELIGIOUS INSTITUTIONS IN EXILE

Having settled down in exile, Tibetans faced a number of new challenges. They had to adapt to a new environment and culture, one that often created much distress and tension. For many of them, religion became their source of strength and ethnic identity: They could affirm their ethnic background through religion. Thargyal (cited in Von Somm 1998) claims that "*Chos* [Dharma] is considered as the only source of Tibetan identity, culture and otherness" (p. 342). Below is a short description of the institution of His Holiness the Dalai Lama, as well as the role of the monastic institutions.

The Institution of the Dalai Lama

The role and influence of the Dalai Lama is emphasized by many scholars. Tsering Gellek (2001) points out that it is erroneous to think that his leadership and authority has been a "seamless continuum of power from within Tibet to exile," because originally regional and feudal powers remained independent from Lhasa. The influence of the Dalai Lama grew significantly in exile, where his leadership has provided institutional structure and continuity for the Tibetan community. The Dalai Lama seems to have a significant symbolic meaning to all Tibetans. He embodies all the traditional values Tibetans wish to maintain. At the same time, he accepts changes and encourages Tibetans to be pragmatic and reasonable. Whether or not they agree with his policy of nonviolence, to most Tibetans he is a most important and respected figure.

Monasteries

Religious institutions in exile are under the leadership of the Dalai Lama and the Department of Religion and Culture (an organ of the Tibetan Government-in-exile), which was established in 1960. The department has jurisdiction over cultural institutes (such as the Library of Tibetan Works and Archives, the Tibetan Institute of Performing Arts, the Norbulingka Institute in Dharamsala, Tibet House in Delhi, the Central Institute of Higher Tibetan Studies in Varanasi) and all monasteries and nunneries. The Department of Religion and Culture (online)[22] reports that there are more than 200 Tibetan monasteries and nunneries in India, Nepal and Bhutan with a population of more than 20,000 monks and nuns, and more than 700 Tibetan Buddhist centers abroad.

Tsering Gellek (2001) stresses the importance of the Tibetan Buddhist framework and re-establishment of the monastic and patronage systems in the creation of a successful community—one that is committed to education and health, relative gender equality, promotion of democratic principles, and human rights. He points out that these institutions have played a significant role in creating social and political networks within and outside of the Tibetan communities, facilitating community support and growth. Tsering Gellek (2001) writes: "The role of monasteries in Tibet, while formally purely religious centers of learning and training, informally provided Tibet with coalesced forms of political and economic power. Networks between monasteries naturally developed over time, as Lamas and monks would travel across Tibet to receive teachings from other great masters or to engage in philosophical debates. These social and political networks would later provide a critical form of cohesion for the exile community" (p. 5).

The patronage system has been successfully recreated in exile. Monasteries send monks and lamas to different centers worldwide in order to maintain relationships with the disciples, and to give teachings and transmissions.[23] In exchange, teachers receive donations, which they share with the monastery. Similarly, monks and lamas receive gifts (usually in currency) for their services—for example, performing rituals in private homes. Tsering Gellek (2001) views the success of the Tibetan community in exile as being owed, in large part, to the monastic institutions. He writes:

> "It has been primarily through these institutions that the dissemination of Tibetan culture has been possible. The re-emergence of monasteries in exile has thus ensured a cultural and political continuity for Tibetans. Paradoxically, however, these traditional institutions have often been at the source of significant social and economic change in the community. The Tibetan monastic system, through its dependence upon a patronage system, has helped create a complex network of social capital in Tibetan refugee communities. Despite the lack of rigorous empirical studies on this subject, anecdotal evidence suggests not only the potency of these institutions in creating internal social and political networks but also in creating networks between monasteries and foreign Buddhist centers,

> the majority located in the West. The concept of social capital helps elucidate the importance of monasteries to the Tibetan community in exile because it serves as a powerful explanatory variable of the importance of networks and trust in establishing sustainable communities. It also helps account for how a 'traditional' institution—with its established networks and channels—may be used (at times) for progressive purposes (e.g., computer archiving of texts, community treatment of tuberculosis, and women's literacy)" (p. 8).

A system of social and economic networks has been established between the monasteries in exile in their own communities, as well as cross-communally. Many of these monasteries co-operate with religious institutions in Western countries, in which Dharma centers have also been founded. Tsering Gellek (2001) reports: "The institutional support that is provided for these monasteries, while ranging from small local donations to the (rare) large multi-million dollar donations, signifies the wide spectrum of public support" (p. 9).

NOTES

1. When the texts of Buddhism were translated into Tibetan, they were translated into two main collections: "The Translated Buddha-word" (Tib. *bka' 'gyur*) and "The Translated Treatises" (Tib. *bstan 'gyur*). The first one consists of the teachings of sutra and tantra, translated mainly from the Indian texts of the time. In Tibet, there are a few different editions and therefore, it exists as either 104 or 108 volumes. The second collection consist of about 218 volumes of texts of translations (mainly from Indian texts) of the subjects of knowledge and of treatises; these are commentaries on the intent of Buddha's words in the sutras and tantras (Duff 2003).

2. Tib. *lha tho tho ri gnyan bstan*

3. Tib. *srong btsan sgam po*

5. Tib. *chosrgya mespon namsuml*

6. Tib. *gLang dar ma*

7. Tib. *yon bdag*

8. Tib. *yon mchod*

9. "Tulku" (Tib. *sprul sku*) was the title given to individuals who were officially recognized as reincarnations of a previous great being (Duff 2003).

10. The Tibetan Centre for Human Rights and Democracy has its official website: http://www.tchrd.org/

11. Tib. *'phags-pa'i-bden-pa-bzhi*

12. Tib. *sangs rgyas*

13. Tib. *sdug-bsngal-gyi-bden-pa*

14. Tib. *kun 'byung gi bden pa*

15. Tib. *gog pa'i bden pa*

16. *Bodhisattva*: the term that refers to individuals who are motivated by the wish to benefit all sentient beings and lead them to the state of buddhahood.

17. Tib. *las-gyu-'bras*
18. Sanskrit *klesia*, Tib. *nyon-mons-pa*
19. Tib. *lam gyi bden pa*
20. Sanskrit *shamata*, Tib. *zhi gnas*
21. Tib. *ri bdag or gzhi bdag*
22. CTA: Department of Religion and Culture. [On-line] Available at: http://www.tibet.net/religion/eng
23. Sanskrit *abisheka*—refers to tantric rituals in which the disciple is guided through an initiation process and receives a blessing (or an "inspiration") of a particular deity. Receiving the transmission is essential in order to engage oneself in a practice of meditation on that deity.

Chapter Five

The Traditional Tibetan System of Medicine in Tibet and in Exile

5.1 Health-Related Problems among the Tibetan Diaspora
5.2 Professional Healthcare in Tibet and in Exile
5.3 History of the Traditional Tibetan System of Medicine
5.4 Fundamental Concepts of Tibetan Medicine
5.5 Diagnosis in Tibetan Medicine
5.6 Treatment in Tibetan Medicine
5.7 Tibetan Medicine and Demonology
5.8 Tibetan Medicine and Astrology

The aim of this chapter is to present some aspects of the traditional Tibetan system of medicine, in order to get a better understanding of the qualitative data gathered in this study. A short description of health problems that Tibetans frequently suffer is followed by a general history of the Tibetan medicinal system, its fundamental concepts (including the idiom of disease), its diagnostic methods, the kinds of treatment offered, and prerequisites for becoming a Tibetan doctor.

5.1 HEALTH-RELATED PROBLEMS AMONG THE TIBETAN DIASPORA

Tibetans living in India report a number of problems that have a direct or indirect impact on their physical and mental functioning. These include changes in the sociocultural environment, in the climate, and in their nutrition, as well as the poor and unsanitary living conditions they must endure. As a result of the move to India, Tibetans have had to modify their diet from non-vegetarian food (including meat and eggs) to simple vegetarian food, with occasional consumption of vegetables. Pathak (2003) describes how, due to economic reasons, Tibetans have adopted Indian tea (which is usually taken with milk) instead of the traditional Tibetan butter tea. Some Tibetans, however, cannot even afford to buy milk. For economic reasons, many Tibetans choose to live together in cramped quarters, such as small, rented rooms. According to Pathak (2003), in 94 percent of the Tibetan households in the area he studied, from one to five family members would share this type of limited space together. Open air defecation was often practiced by Tibetans, who only bathed occasionally, and washed clothes in a river that was inconveniently distant from their settlement. Pathak also reported that the water supply in the study area was limited, and came from a single source (2003).

In the aftermath of these adaptive difficulties, many Tibetans developed severe health problems. Pathak (2004) noted: "A negative response of migration is manifested in their contemporary living condition and hygiene. . . . The main bulk of population suffer from gastrointestinal problems. Higher incidence of tuberculosis was also observed due to change of climatic condition, hygiene and nutritional status" (p. 87). He also maintained that these sociocultural changes contribute to the emergence of new ailments, which, according to Tibetans, did not exist in Tibet.

According to the Department of Health[1] (2002–2003), the most commonly reported disorders are respiratory infections, then diarrhea and dysentery, followed by skin and infectious diseases, and finally, trauma and infection. Health Department data from 1999 reveals the following causes of death by percentage:

Cancer: 13.7 percent
Cardiovascular disease: 12.9 percent
Tuberculosis: 9.5 percent
Old age: 8.4 percent
Liver disorder: 8 percent
Peptic ulcer: 6.5 percent
Asthma: 4.9 percent
Accidental death: 4.9 percent
Malaria: 4.6 percent
Epilepsy: 3.4 percent
Renal failure: 3.4 percent
Diabetes: 1.9 percent
Mental disorders: 1.5 percent
Other: 16.3 percent

5.2 PROFESSIONAL HEALTHCARE IN TIBET AND IN EXILE

Before the Chinese invasion, there were no allopathic doctors in Tibet; biomedicine was only introduced afterwards. The new authorities had little respect for traditional Tibetan medicine, and senior staff at the new hospitals were generally Chinese rather than Tibetan. Gradually, some Tibetans were trained in biomedicine. At the same time, as soon as the Chinese realized the benefits of traditional Tibetan medicine, they began to support it—while excluding its Buddhist content.

Following the invasion and the Dalai Lama's flight to India, the Tibetans re-established many of their traditional institutions in exile. These included a Tibetan Government-in-Exile, and along with many of its departments. Of these, the Department of Health (DoH) manages Tibet's medical institutions. It runs forty-four health clinics, nine primary healthcare centers, one mobile clinic, and seven hospitals in the Tibetan communities in India and Nepal.

The Department of Health is responsible for maintaining healthcare programs, administering health education campaigns, and providing basic healthcare for Tibetans as well as Indians in Tibetan settlements and villages. Health promotion in the Tibetan community has focused on the expansion of health awareness as it pertains to disease prevention, personal hygiene, and healthier lifestyles. One of the aims of the DoH was the promotion of an integrated approach to treatment, in which allopathic Primary Health Care (PHC) was combined with the traditional system of Tibetan medicine. Today, these two systems of medicine run parallel to each other, and a referral process exists between them.

The Department of Health reports: "In the two decades of its existence, the DoH has been able to establish Health Centers in almost every Tibetan refugee settlement in India and Nepal. At least one Community Health Worker (CHW) attends to the preventive and curative healthcare needs through the centers as well as providing health promotion in the community. Gradually, the services they provide have expanded from immunization and TB control to antenatal care, family planning and HIV/AIDS education among others. . . . *Men-Tsee-Khang*, the traditional Tibetan medical system, has 43 branch clinics in India and Nepal" (CTA, online).[2]

In 1993 the Department of Health initiated a program that addressed the needs of torture victims. In 1996, this was officially established as the Tibetan Torture Survivor Program (Sadutsang 2002). As a result of the introduction of fees-for-services, the DoH has come close to sustaining the non-tuberculosis, general drug supply in nearly all its hospitals and health centers. A cost-sharing system has been created, in which hospitals generate a quarter of the annual recurring budget and DoH provides the rest.

Because Tibetan traditional medicine cannot meet all health needs, the Tibetan and biomedical systems have been integrated. A number of institutions now offer treatment according to the Western allopathic model, as well as the traditional Tibetan system of medicine in exile. Practitioners in both systems consult with patients in joint clinics, while social workers, medical consultants, and project administrators meet patients in person or online. Buddhist philosophy is often used in an allopathic context, as a means of effective coping: for example, in the Torture Survivors Program. Patients are provided with Buddhist teachings and instructions relevant to the their problems, while religious coping skills and self-transformation processes take place between the monk-teachers and their patients.

5.3 HISTORY OF THE TRADITIONAL TIBETAN SYSTEM OF MEDICINE

Accounts vary as to how the traditional Tibetan system of medicine was established. Clifford (1994) reports that this medical tradition was imported from India, together with Buddhism, in about the seventh century A.D. Pasang Yonten (1989), however, stresses that there was a natural evolution of the indigenous healing methods in Tibet, in which people developed the art of healing severed blood vessels with molten butter and boils with residual barley from *chang* (beer). Lobsang Tsultrim Tsona and Tenzin Dakpa (1981) report that a variety of folk methods were used by Tibetans: residual barley on swollen body parts, drinking hot water for indigestion, and using melted butter for bleeding. Those therapies arose from practical experience and gradually formed the basis for the Tibetan art of healing.

Tsering Dhondup (2003) states that the medical tradition in written form is suspected to have appeared in the pre-Buddhist era of *Shang shung* as part of the Bön tradition, a set of shamanistic and animistic practices. At this time, a medical system known as "The Western System of Tibetan Medicine" was promoted. According to Pasang Yonten (1989) there are certain similarities between the Galen(ic) system of medicine and the Tibetan or Bön medical system, due to the fact that Tibet had established trade connections via the silk route with its western neighbors, including Greece and Rome. Similarities between the two traditions include their theories of the elements, of the three humours, and various individual treatments, as for rheumatism. Pasang Yonten (1989) writes: "The different medical systems in Asia, the Indian Ayurvedic system, the Siddhi system, the Chinese system, the Muslim or Unani system, the Greek system and the Tibetan systems were clearly closely related. Whilst they all had minor differences in terms of practice and in social and religious bias, they all seem similar as water poured into water. Due to the influences of the individual cultures and religions in their practice they came to be known as different systems" (p. 34).

Tsering Dhondup (2003) points out that during the time of the 28th king of Tibet (*Lha Tho To Ri Nyentsen*), the Tibetan indigenous art of healing was also influenced by the Indian Ayurveda. At that time, two Indian physicians (*Bi ji ga ze* and *Bi lha ga ze*) came and successfully practiced medicine in Tibet. The king was inspired by their continual successes in medical practice and requested them to stay. He also offered his daughter *Yi ki rol cha* in marriage. She later gave birth to *Thung kyi thor chog*—the first known physician in the Yuthog lineage, who mastered the arts of pulse reading, pharmacology, moxibustion,[3] blood letting, and the dressing and treatment of wounds. After *Thung kyi thor chog* there was a succession lineage of doctors who practiced medicine, preserved the teachings, and passed them on to the new generations.

In general, the teachings of the traditional Tibetan system of medicine are attributed to Buddha Shakya Muni, whose teachings were written in a medical text, "Immaculate Lineage".[4] This text has been associated with the first turning of the Wheel of Dharma[5] at Sarnath, near Varanasi. Buddha Shakya Muni also taught "One hundred thousand verses of Healing"[6] on *Jagoe Phungpo'I Ri* (Vulture's Peak) and "The Tantra of Bare Vision"[7] at Beta Groves. There is also another important text, taught during the third turning of the wheel of Dharma, which became known as the "Supreme Golden Rays Sutra".[8] It contains a chapter called "The Ways of Completely Curing Diseases".[9]

The main text, which elaborates on the art of healing, is called: "The Secret Quintessential Instructions on the Eight Branches of the Ambrosia Essence Tantra"[10] or in the abridged version: "The Four Tantras" (*rGyud-bZhi*). It consists of four Tantra texts, which are the "Root Tantra," "Explanatory Tantra," "Oral Transmission," and "Last Tantra." The "Root Tantra" contains the essence of the other three (Tsering Dhondup 2003). It was probably written down in the fourth century A.D. and then translated by Vairochana and the Pandit Chandradeva into Tibetan. It was composed in a question-and-answer format between two emanations of the Medicine Buddha: Rishi Master *Rig-pa i-Ye-Shes* (Vidyajnana) and his disciple Rishi *Yid-las skyes* (Manasija) (Dolkar Khangkar 1998). This medical text elaborates on eight branches of medicine: 1. *Lus* (the physical body, including embryology, anatomy, physiology, pathology, pharmacology); 2. *Byis pa* (pediatrics); 3. *Mo nad* (gynecology, female diseases); 4. *gDon* (disorders caused by evil spirits); 5. *mTshon* (wounds inflicted by trauma); 6. *Dug* (toxicology); 7. *Rgas* (rejuvenation) and 8. *Ro tsa* (aphrodisiacs). The ninety-two chapters of the third of the Four Tantras ("Quintessential Tantra") offer systematic explanations of each of these branches of medicine. This text includes seventy chapters on *lus*, three chapters on *Byis pa*, *Mo nad*, and *Dug*, five chapters on *gDon* and *mTshon,* one chapter on *Rgas-pa,* and two chapters on *Ro-tsa* (Lobsang Tsultrim Tsona and Tenzin Dakpa 1981).

5.4. FUNDAMENTAL CONCEPTS OF TIBETAN MEDICINE

Tibetan medicine is classified as a holistic system, which means that practitioners look beyond the physical symptoms—however serious they are—to seek the root[11] cause of the problem. Symptoms are regarded as mere reflections of deeper imbalances within the body, namely the imbalances of the three humours. According to Tibetan Medicine, trying to cure the symptoms does not address the real problem, but only suppresses the disease. Tenzin Choedrak (1995) explains: "Tibetan Medicine is a science, art and philosophy that consists of a holistic approach to health. It is a science because its principles are laid down in a systematic and logical framework based on an understanding of our body and its relationship to our environment. It is an art because it uses various diagnostic techniques to identify various problems and diverse therapeutic measures to maintain proper and optimal health. It is a philosophy because it embraces the key Buddhist principles of altruism, karma and ethics" (pp. 26–27).

Five Elements

According to Tibetan Buddhism and the traditional Tibetan system of medicine, all material phenomena (animate or inanimate) contain relative proportions of five cosmo-physical elements as their material basis, namely: earth (*sa*), water (*chu*), fire (*me*), wind (*rLung*), and space (*nam-mkha*). A specific type of influence is ascribed to each element: *sa* exerts a greater influence over the formation of muscle cells, bones, the nose, and the sense of smell; *chu* is responsible for the formation of blood, body fluids, the tongue, and the sense of taste; *me* is responsible for body temperature, complexion, the eyes, and the sense of sight; *rLung* is responsible for breathing, the skin, and the sense of touch; and *nam-mkha* is responsible for body cavities, the ears, and the sense of hearing (Tenzin Choedrak 1995; Lobsang Tsultrim Tsona and Tenzin Dakpa 1981).

Lobsang Rapgay (2001) explains: "Anatomically, the body is constituted of the five *hByung-was* (elements) which are also the substratum of all animate and inanimate phenomena. A phenomenon or object acquires its particular characteristics chiefly due to the predominant combination of specific sets of *hByung-was* in a structural unit. . . . Generally, the predominant *hByung-was* constituent is 50 percent and the remaining portion of the structural unit or atom is made up of the other *hByung-was* in equal parts" (p. 1). The four elements of earth, air, fire, and water represent the qualities of density, motility, temperature, and cohesion (Tarthang Tulku Rinpoche 1973a).

The Three Humours (nepas)

Whereas cells and tissues are recognized as structural units of the five elements (*byung ba*), there are also three *nepas,* which are identified with cells, tissues, and organs of the body and their functions. They are the living units of the body that ensure all bodily activities and maintain harmony between the forces of heat and fluidity. The five elements interact with these three basic principal energies in the human body (Lobsang Wangyal 1995). Tenzin Choedrak (1995) explains that they are the principle energy systems that mediate all physiological and biological processes. The three *nepas* may be identified with the three elements of air, fire, and water, but they are different in function than each of these elements. Lobsang Rapgay (2001) explains that the elements are not living units as such. The *nepas* on the other hand are living units and cease to exist at the death of the body.

The three principal humours in the body are *rLung*, *mKhris-pa*, and *Bad-kan.* The Wind (*rlung*) manifests the nature of the Air element. It is characterized by the qualities rough, light, cold, subtle, hard, and mobile, and is responsible for the physical and mental activities, respiration, expulsion of urine, development of the fetus, menstruation, spitting, burping, speech, and giving clarity to the sense organs. It also sustains life by means of acting as a medium between mind and body. The Bile (*mkhris pa*) is of the fire nature, and provides some of the heating functions of the body. It is characterized by the qualities oily, sharp, hot, light, fetid, purgative, and fluid, and is responsible for hunger, thirst, digestion, assimilation, promoting bodily heat, giving lustre to the body complexion, and providing courage and determination. Duff (2003) explains that *mkhris pa* is a term denoting "jaundice" (hepatitis), which is connected with the "bile" constituent. The Phlegm (*bad kan*) is cold in nature. It is characterized by the qualities oily, cool, heavy, blunt, firm, and sticky. It is responsible for firmness of the body, stability of the mind, inducing sleep, connecting the joints of the body, generating tolerance, and lubricating the body (Lobsang Tsultrim Tsona and Tenzin Dakpa 1981; Pema Dorjee 2002).

The Idiom of Disease

Lobsang Rapgay (1981) explains that the meaning of the term *napas* is "defect," and that pathologically it connotes morbidity. He writes: "rLung, mKhripa and bad.gan are called nepas because their abnormal increase, decrease or disturbance cause pathogenicity of the seven physical constituents[12]—the basic structural units of the body and the three excretory matters" (p. 1). Disease is thus understood in terms of imbalance of the three humours. Tsering Dhondup (2003) says that the three humours should have a normal level or quantity within the body system: "With the influence of causes (mental factors such as attachment, hatred and delusion) and the four main contributing factors (change of time factors, attack by evil spirits, wrong diet and unhealthy lifestyle), the levels of these humours will increase, decrease or vitiate (be disturbed) in dependence (Tsering Dhondup 2003, pp. 7–8)

Clifford (1984) enumerates a number of causes of disease, which have been classified as: 1. Long term cause: spiritual factors, the karma from past lives; and 2. Short term cause: factors in the present life, such as seasonal changes, evil spirits, poison and habits or behaviors.

Karmic diseases.[13] Even though everything is determined by one's karma according to the Buddhist philosophy, the diseases classified as karmic are those that cannot be cured by regular medicines. They are of purely spiritual cause: negative karma from present and past lives. The remedy should thus also be spiritual—for example, specific spiritual practices such as prostrations before objects representing the Three Jewels, or the performing of some ritual.

Diseases caused by evil spirits.[14] These types of diseases are believed to be inflicted by evil forces, and are also treated with religious medicines and rituals. A combination of herbal medicines and other treatments (e.g., medicine oil, massage, mantra pills) can be used. Clifford (1984) says that according to Tibetan tradition, evil spirits are claimed to be one of the main causes of insanity and psychiatric disturbances.

Immediate diseases.[15] Diseases of this type appear and disappear quickly. They could be described by the Western designation, "self-terminating illnesses," which do not require special medical treatment.

Life diseases.[16] Diseases in this category require medical attention. Otherwise, they may result in deterioration and death. They are caused by humoural imbalances, inappropriate diet, irregular and destructive behavior (lack of sleep, unvirtuous living, intoxication), as well as environmental and psychological factors (Clifford 1984).

The two categories of the causes of disease are described by Yeshi Dhonden (1977) as distant and near causes. The near causes are connected with the three humours: "Undisturbed wind, bile and phlegm are the causes of illness and when they are disturbed and in disequilibrium, they are of the nature of illness" (Yeshi Dhonden 1977, p. 67). The distant causes, on the other hand, are further divided into general and specific. The former are explained in terms of ignorance: "There is but one cause of all illnesses, and this is said to be ignorance due to not understanding the meaning of identitylessness . . . even when all creatures live and act with joy, because they have ignorance, it is impossible for them to be free of illness" (Yeshi Dhonden 1977, p. 66). The three mental poisons—desire, hatred, and confusion, which are the specific causes of disease—arise due to ignorance. This leads to the production of *rLung, mKhris-pa*, and *Bad-kan.*

Pema Dorjee (2002) explains that each humour is related to one of the three mental poisons: *rLung* is generated by desire, *mKhris-pa* by anger, and *Bad-kan* by obscuration or closed-mindedness. Thus, many of the diseases that are hot in nature are attributed to *mKhris-pa* (and anger). Tsering Dhondup (2003) also identifies three main causes of disease: 1. attachment to beautiful objects; 2. revulsion/anger towards ugly things; and 3. delusion (inability to understand the merits and demerits of right and wrong actions). When the three humours are disturbed and in disequilibrium, illness may result (Yeshi Dhonden 1977).

According to the Tibetan system of medicine, it is imperative to maintain a balanced lifestyle. Diet and behavior are regarded as important contributing factors in the creation of disease, and similarly, in maintaining equilibrium in the body. Patients are encouraged to abandon extreme tendencies, which may include always eating either hot or cold foods, extreme exercise, excessive lethargy, untimely eating, overeating, or increased mental stress, because all of these behaviors lead to imbalance. Tenzin Namdul (2000) comments: "The Tibetan art of healing has always placed a great emphasis on diet and behaviour regimen throughout the classical text (*rGyud-gzhi*). Since our body is directly or indirectly related with the environment and delicate state of dynamic equilibrium, it is very important to embrace proper diet, wholesome lifestyle and act nimbly with respect to the changes in season, for any minor problems of such could wreck the whole system" (p. 72).

Proper Attitude

Dorje Reptan Neshar (2003) points out that in Tibetan medicine, the attitude of the doctor towards the patients and their treatment regimen is crucial. He explains: "Tibetan Medicine considers the right approach to the patient and their treatment as a very important factor rather than the treatment itself. The doctor–patient relationship is considered to be the gateway of the successful healing. Doctors are viewed as that of medicine Buddha: with infinite compassion and dedication to patient care; his instructions as Buddha's own teaching: with unmistakable truth and rewarding, and medicines as deathless nectar: revitalizing and life giving. Doctors too view their patients as precious human beings, who should be treated with equal devotion given to his or her own beloved mother" (2003, online).

5.5 DIAGNOSIS IN TIBETAN MEDICINE

Tibetan medicine uses several basic techniques to diagnose a patient. Pema Dorjee (2008) lists three of÷ these: visual examination, palpation, and questioning. He stresses the importance of combining these methods to avoid misinterpreting the symptoms. In the same way one can confuse smoke with steam, the doctor can similarly make an error in diagnosis: "The physician must clearly distinguish between the different types of presenting symptoms, before reaching the conclusion that they are an indication of a particular disease. All the symptoms are an indication of an unbalanced humour, or energy, but we need to treat the unbalanced humour, and not the symptom" (Pema Dorjee 2008). The purpose of diagnosis is not only identifying a specific disease, but also the process of disturbances in the body energies before they are fully manifested. The physician aims at identifying which of the three principal energies are imbalanced (Lobsang Wangyal 1995). Below is a description of the typical diagnostic methods.

Visual Diagnosis

Visual observation involves checking the complexion, and the color and texture of the blood, as well as the nails, sputum, and feces. The condition of the tongue and urine are also crucial in making a visual diagnosis. From the moment the patient enters the doctor's (or *amchee's*) office, he or she is observed closely. By observing the patient's behavior, the doctor may note apathy, anxiety, or other affect that influences the patient's health.

Diagnosing from the Tongue

Lhawang at al. (1995) says that the tongue of a healthy person should be red, soft, wet, and flexible. When it is red, dry, and rough, or covered by a thick, pale yellow coating of phelgm, a Tibetan physician may diagnose a *rLung* disorder. In cases of phlegm (*Bad-kan*) disorders, the tongue will be covered by a pale, thick coating of phlegm, and will have a and dull, moist texture.

Diagnosing from the Urine

Patients are advised to bring a urine sample when they arrive for a consultation. This should be collected at dawn, so that the color will not be influenced by digestion. Before collecting the sample, patients are advised to have a sound and sufficient sleep, refrain from mental and emotional stress, and avoid drinking too much tea, buttermilk, or wine, which may affect the color of the sample. The doctor will test its color, steam and sediment. When the urine sample looks like water and produces large bubbles when stirred, this indicates a *rLung* disorder. A bile disorder (*mKhris pa*) is indicated by urine that is reddish yellow in color, malodorous, and produces much steam. Phlegm (*bad kan*) disorders can be diagnosed from whitish urine with little odor or steam (Lobsang Tsultrim Tsona and Tenzin Dakpa 1981). Lobsang Tsultrim Tsona and Tenzin Dakpa (1981) also describe how urine can be examined to determine whether the patient is influenced by evil spirits. If this is the case, urine is considered a mirror that reflects their shadow.

Diagnosing by Touch

This kind of diagnosis includes pulse reading, as well as observing the abnormalities in skin texture and temperature. Certain conditions of the skin suggest imbalances in the body. Lhawang at al. (1995, p. 49) explains: "Symptoms of cold chills, excessive sweating, oily skin, eruptions, etc., warn us to prevent further deterioration. Similarly, dark circles under the eyes, premature lines on the face, irritation of an itch on any part of the skin, dry surface skin, etc., indicate chronic disease or toxicity in the blood system that has accumulated inside the body over many years and is finally compelled to come forth by the general disease state."

In pulse reading, the physician examines the general beat of the radial artery: its strength, speed, nature, depth, and firmness. The pulse can be characterized as strong, weak, superficial, sunken, fast, slow, taut, or loose (Dolkar Khangkar 1998). Using pulse diagnosis, the doctor can determine whether the humours are in balance. The condition of the inner organs can also be examined by palpation. There is also a certain type of pulse that indicates disease inflicted by evil spirits.

Diagnosing by Interview

This involves interviewing the patient in order to gather information about contributory factors, such as diet and other life behaviors. The physician acquires a better, complete clinical picture of the patient by getting to know the patient's economic conditions, profession, social status, and family background. The physician also analyzes the patient's voice, including its tone and texture (Dolkar Khangkar 1998; Tsering Dhondup 2003; Clifford 1994; Lobsang Tsultrim Tsona and Tenzin Dakpa 1981).

5.6 TREATMENT IN TIBETAN MEDICINE

Treatment methods in the traditional Tibetan system of medicine include the following: 1. adjustment of one's diet; 2. changing of one's lifestyle and unhealthy behaviors; 3. application of medicines; 4. techniques of accessory therapy (e.g., moxibustion, golden needle, silver/brass/golden hammer) (Tsering Dhondup 2003). It is emphasized that behaviors and diet are crucial to maintaining health and even more important in treating diseases. According to Tibetan doctors, adopting an unhealthy diet and a demanding lifestyle will inevitably lead to disease (Pema Dorjee 2008).

Dolkar Khangkar (1998) writes about classification of diseases and their treatment:

> "All diseases may be classified as dependent diseases caused by past karma, imaginary diseases caused by demons, absolute diseases of this life, and ostensible diseases. These are respectively held to be untreatable, treatable by ritual means, treatable only by medication, and without need of treatment because they heal spontaneously. There are four kinds of diseases which can be cured by medicine and these will depend on internal medication, diet and behaviour and external therapies. The most fundamental and favored type of treatment in Tibetan medicine is modification of behavioural and dietary patterns. This is the most gentle manner of therapy and always first to be relied upon" (p. 43).

Other methods (such as herbal pills or the more invasive ones) are advised when changing diet and behaviors is not enough to cure a disease. Lobsang Tsultrim Tsona and Tenzin Dakpa (1981) state: "The first line of healthcare in Tibetan medicine involves prevention—maintenance of a proper diet and observance of a wholesome lifestyle. If these two approaches fail to bring about positive results, medicines are prescribed. The various forms of medicines include decoctions, powders, pills, syrup, and butters. Generally, the Tibetan physician starts with a mild medicine and then gradually increases its potency. The other therapeutic techniques that follow medication include gentle and drastic eliminative therapies, with surgery being utilized only as a last resort" (p. 49).

Diet and Behaviors

Dietary changes may involve the intake of certain foods, such as dairy products, oils, fermented barley beer, porridge with butter, certain kinds of meat, or light alcoholic drinks. Either food therapy or drink therapy may be prescribed. "Lifestyle therapy" may involve staying in a restful, dark room, staying in warm areas, and enjoying the company of good friends (in cases of *rlung* disorders); staying in cool areas (e.g., under the shade of trees, or by a river), relaxing, and avoiding physical disturbances (in cases of *mkhrispa* disorders); and finally, in cases of *badkan* diseases, staying in warm or dry areas, taking mild exercise, and wearing warm clothing (Tsering Dhondup 2003).

Application of Medicines

Medications applied in the traditional Tibetan system of medicine are produced from all kinds of substances: wood, roots, flowers, fruits, bark, sap, precious and semi-precious stones (e.g., coral, turquoise, pearl), salts, minerals, and some animal extracts (Lobsang Dolma Khangkar 1986). Dorje Reptan Neshar (2003) explains: "The therapeutic effect of medicines is mainly determined by their inherent taste, potency and qualities. They are combined and prepared in keeping with their taste and potency so as to ensure total and quality health of the patient without unwelcome side effects" (p. 2). Tibetan astrology is also involved in the process of medicine production—including the astrological aspects of the time when the medicine is made. Dorje Reptan Neshar (2003) adds: "Astro-calculations are also made before giving some minor surgeries and accessory therapies, and also to ascertain the nature of the disease and its prognostication" (p. 2).

The Medical Tantra explains that there are two types of therapy: 1. through tastes and inherent qualities, and 2. through combinations. In the former case, certain tastes and qualities of medicines are attributed to each of the three humours (*rlung, mkrispa,* and *badkan*) and used for treatment. Tastes are often characterized by comparison: sweet tastes like molasses or grapes; sour tastes like matured *chang gyen* or pomegranates; salty tastes like sodium chloride; bitter tastes like *Herpetospermum pedunculosum;* astringent taste like white sandalwood; hot tastes like *Piper nigrum Linn*, and so on. Qualities of medicine may describe oiliness, heaviness, smoothness (e.g., sharp like rock salt, smooth like *Rubus idaepsis Focke*), density (e.g., liquid like *Cassia fistula Linn*), and so on (Tsering Dhondup 2003).

Norbu Chophel (1983) discusses the administration of Tibetan herbs:

> "The general instructions given for taking most Tibetan medicines are that you should crush and eat them at least half-an-hour before or after meals, and that you should not take any alcohol before completing the entire course of medicine. But there are certain medicines called 'Precious Pills' for which you must memorize a whole list of instructions. Tibetans still in Tibet, and older generation Tibetans in exile, know these instructions by heart. Most of these medicines cure not just one illness, but several. And if you don't have any illness for it to cure, it simply improves your health. These medicines are also taken as a last re-

> sort cure, akin to terramycin of the allopathic system, which is taken as a last resort, before operation. These instructions that you are given in taking those 'Precious Pills' are that you should abstain from meat, liquor, eggs, raw fruits and vegetables at least one week before and after taking the medicine. You are also advised against sexual intercourse when you are taking these medicines. Except for the last precaution, all the other instructions are acceptable to anybody as having biological reasons, but there are instructions and precautions to be followed, including the one mentioned above regarding abstinence from sexual indulgence, that cannot be understood as having any relation either to the medicine or to the human body. . . . The superstition-based instructions given are that you should crush the pill under the cover of darkness (no light whatsoever should fall on it) in a clean and unbroken cup with water added to dissolve it. It is then to be covered with a clean silver cup-cover to protect it from light and dust. These instructions are for auspiciousness and an important part of the entire instructions given in taking such medicine. The pill must be taken early the next morning at dawn between 3 and 5 a.m. after reciting the special prayer dedicated to the Medicine Buddha. After taking the medicine you should go back to a very warm sleep" (p. 32).

Accessory Therapy

A number of more invasive methods used in the traditional Tibetan system of medicine are included in this category. Dummer (1988) enumerates six types of Accessory Therapy:

1. *Acupuncture and moxibustion* ("*metsa*," application of fire). A technique called "the golden needle" could also be classified as this type of therapy. One of my respondents (a Tibetan doctor from New Delhi) showed me a derivative technique, which she called a "friction stick." For this type of therapy, she rubbed a special piece of wood brought from Bhutan against a wooden plank. The end of the stick became hot and she applied it to special points on the patient's skin.
2. *Hydrotherapy*: This includes fractioning of the body with cold water, or medicinal baths (for example, bathing in hot springs, or in snow water or the waterfalls from clay-slate rocks).
3. *Humoural therapy*: This includes venesection (blood-letting), cupping, cauterization with hot irons, and the application of a golden or silver hammer.
4. *Forced elimination methods*: Cleansing procedures, such as enemas or emetics, are used as a form of treatment in and of themselves, or to prepare the patient for the administration of medicine.
5. *Pyretic treatment*: These are heat treatments, using hot stones and sandpacks. Other authors describe hot and cold fomentations, such as applying heated salts wrapped in cloth to the patient's stomach.

6. *Massage*: Therapeutic massage is performed with healing oils and ointments.

This is not a comprehensive list, and there may be other types of therapies not listed here. In the past, surgery was performed by traditional Tibetan doctors. A special medical *thanka* in the Men-Tsee-Khang Museum shows the medical instruments used by traditional Tibetan doctors in times past. Nowadays, Tibetan doctors do not practice surgery, and if patients have such a need they are referred to an allopathic hospital. (Clifford 1984; Dolkar Khangkar 1998; Tsering Dhondup 2003; Lobsang Tsultrim Tsona and Tenzin Dakpa 1981).

Spiritual Methods

Spiritual methods can also be used to accelerate treatment. Bokar Rinpoche (1996) explains that the practice of the calm-abiding meditation (*shine*)[17] and the superior vision meditation[18] have a healing effect:

> "Practicing mental calming dispels illnesses of wind. The illnesses of phlegm and bile are eliminated by practicing superior vision. Hot and cold illnesses are both gradually eliminated by mental calming and superior vision. Furthermore, we examine the essence of all illnesses, their form, origin, location, and disappearance. Visualization of sending and taking is emphasized. Illness being unborn, it is the Absolute Body (*dharmakaya*), being without location, it is the Body of Enlightenment (*sambhogakaya*), being without cessation, it is the Body of Emanation (*nirmanakaya*); its nature being emptiness, it is the Body of Essence Itself (*svabhavikakaya*). Integrating illness to practice as the play of the four Bodies, we see our mind" (p. 43).

Rinpoche refers to the empty nature of all phenomena. Being composed of inter-dependent factors, disease as such does not exist; being like space, it has no reality. From the *vajrayana*[19] perspective, disease is perceived as a mere ornament for a yogi (Lhalungpa 1997). Buddhist practitioners are thus encouraged to use their physical or mental suffering as an object of their meditation. Bokar Rinpoche (1996) also recommends a very popular "sending and taking meditation," also called *tong len* (described in the previous chapter). Thrangu Rinpoche (2002) explains this practice as sending all of one's happiness and all the causes of happiness to all beings and taking in all their suffering, along with all the causes of suffering (the negative actions and disturbing emotions). The practitioner imagines that these negativities dissolve into emptiness in one's heart.

5.7 TIBETAN MEDICINE AND DEMONOLOGY

Ordinary Tibetans tend to believe in evil spirits, ghosts, or demons (the personification of malignant forces) as if they were living entities. They often maintain that these spirits can cause diseases. In such cases, spiritual methods are advised as a solution, and a special ritual like an exorcism may be performed. An interesting illustration of these beliefs is a story related by the mother of the Dalai Lama (Diki Tsering 2000):

> "As a village folk we believed in ghosts and superstition. Most of us had encountered ghosts firsthand. There was a ghost called a *kyirong* that could emerge in a variety of forms: as a boy, a girl, or a furry cat. I encountered this ghost numerous times, and it caused me great suffering and fear on four occasions. Once, I was gravely ill, the *kyirong* appeared to me in the form of a little girl. She brought me a large bowl of Chinese tea and struck me lightly on the head. I had been lying in bed, and the moment she struck me I woke up, because of the loud sound, though I felt no pain. She then invited me to drink the Chinese tea, which I refused. When I tried to rise from my bed, I noticed that the bowl contained blood. With that she slipped to the door, laughing all the while, and disappeared. . . .
>
> "*Kyirong* was really a nasty character. If he did not like you, he would turn your house upside down and take all your furniture and cooking utensils out into the garden. In the kitchen he would upset everything in sight. Huge sacks full of peas and flour would be upturned, and havoc would ensue. This ghost could hear and understand whatever we said to him. He answered in giggles and laughter. He stole anything to eat, but he never stole money.
>
> "On one occasion my daughter and I were having tea, and I told her to fetch me the leftover roast mutton. When she went to the larder, the mutton had disappeared, the *kyirong* had taken it. Sometimes when we made dumplings, the top layers of the steamer would be full, but the lower layers would be empty. . . .
>
> "The deaths of four of my children were due to this ghost. After the birth of my son Norbu, I had two sons who both died. (Norbu was her second child, born in 1922.) Ten days after the birth of one son, he fell ill with a severe eye infection. His eyes swelled up, and he could not open them even for his feeding. At night, when I was resting beside him, I heard heavy footsteps echoing on the ceiling. The footsteps descended to the window, and the door unlatched itself, and the *kyirong* came and stood beside me. Out of fear I quickly lit a few oil lamps. I took my newborn infant and placed him on my lap, thinking that the ghost would not be able to harm the child if I had him in my grasp. The lamps gradually flickered lower and lower, until I was left in the dark and could no longer see anything. I lost all sense of reality and time. After a while I heard the sound of a child crying in the distance.

> Opening my eyes, I realized to my horror that my child was 10 feet away, on the floor, crying. The lamps were once more lit, and I was still sitting upright. I was not aware of how my child had got to the floor.
>
> "For about fourteen days after that, my son was severely ill, his eyes swollen out of proportion. He cried constantly, and nothing I could do comforted him. In the mornings I noticed bloody scratch marks in and around his eyes, and there were bloodstains on his cheeks. Three weeks later his crying ceased, but he seemed lifeless. When he could finally open his eyes, to my horror his eyes had turned from brown to blue. He had become blind.
>
> "Sometime later this ghost came to us again, this time in the form of an old man. After his visit my son's eyes became swollen again. My eldest daughter's eyes were also affected and swollen. She then grew a growth in her eye, which remained with her until her death. This time my son's illness was fatal. He was just over a year old when he died. Soon after that I gave birth to another baby. . . . He was bright and lively . . . very active, always around my skirts, begging for sweets. Unfortunately the *kyirong* struck this little son of ours. He suddenly developed diarrhea, for unknown reasons. He was sick for one night and died immediately. He was eighteen months of age.
>
> "On the night he died my husband's aunt dreamed that a stranger visited us, and on his departure he was carrying away our little boy on his back. She understood immediately that some unfortunate incident had taken place. The *kyirong* was the most frightening experience of my life" (pp. 49–54).

The Third Tantra of *rGyud-bZhi* includes five chapters that describe diseases caused by spirits and demons.[20] Tibetans believe that mental illness may be attributed to certain of these demons, for example, elemental spirits, madness demons, amnesia demons, demonic rulers of planets, and serpent-spirit demons (*nagas*). Yet Clifford (1994) maintains that the term demon is merely symbolic for Tibetans: "It represents a wide range of forces and emotions which are normally beyond conscious control and all of which prevent well-being and spiritual development" (p. 148). In the Buddhist literature, there are references to "demons" such as laziness, lust, bad companions, dualistic thinking, hypersensitivity, increased emotionality, attachment to wealth, sectarianism, spiritual pride, and clinging to tranquility (Clifford 1994).

From the *vajrayana* point of view: "What appears as a demon is an effect of the magic display of the mind. Looking at the mind as being itself the four Bodies, we eliminate demons in the same way through integrating the four Bodies as the path" (Bokar Rinpoche 1996).

To understand why rituals are performed to appease evil spirits who inflict harm on a given patient, it is helpful to review the concepts of relative (or conventional) and ultimate truth. Whereas unenlightened beings experience phenomena such as spirits, demons, and diseases as real (or truly existent), from the perspective of an enlightened being they are merely an illusion, being empty in nature.

In one of his teachings, the yogi Milarepa described the illusory nature of all phenomena and the ultimate truth: "Thunder, lightning, and clouds appear from the sky and merge back into the sky. Rainbow, mists, and fog appear from the air and merge back into the air. Honey, fruit, and crops arise from the earth and merge back into the earth. Forests, flowers, and leaves arise from the hillside and merge back into the hillside. Rivers, foam, and waves arise from the ocean and merge back into the ocean. Latencies, clinging, and attachment arise from the ground consciousness and merge back into the ground consciousness" (Thrangu Rinpoche 2001, p. 29). This also applies to disease and its causes:

> "The appearance of demons, the belief, and the concept of demons, arise from yoga and merge back into yoga. The appearances, belief, and concepts of demons may arise on the *conventional level* or relative level and from the practice of yoga they merge back into it. Obstacles and obscuring spirits are just manifestations of the mind. If one doesn't realize that they are empty, one will believe them to be demons. If one does realize that they are empty, there is a natural liberation from demons" (Thrangu Rinpoche 2001, pp. 30–31).

5.8 TIBETAN MEDICINE AND ASTROLOGY

Tibetan Astrology plays an important role in the daily lives of Tibetans, one that is also expressed in Tibetan medicine. The two disciplines share the understanding that everything is made up of five elements: Wood, Fire, Earth, Metal, and Water, which make up the elemental basis of life. According to the Kalachakra Tantra,[21] these five elements compose the body, foods, and medicines. Thus, the production and prescription of medicine should only be available to those who have acquired knowledge of astrological and astronomical principles (Dagthon 1998).

Jhampa Kalsang (1998) explains that an astrologer is often consulted about important life events, for example, the birth of a child, the time of marriage, health problems resistant to treatment, starting a new life in a new place, initiating an important project, or an impending death. When a child is born in a Tibetan family, parents will often order a birth chart or horoscope to see the potential future of their offspring, and to predict their lifespan, economic standard of living, or health conditions. Sometimes, parents will inquire as to whether or not the child should follow a monastic life, and so will plan the child's education accordingly.

In the event of unfavorable predictions, the astrologer may recommend an antidote to prevent mishaps. This can be in the form of a special prayer, or instructions to give alms to the poor. If the child's life is endangered, the Tibetan parents make an effort to save a life, usually of an animal such as a goat or sheep that is about to be slaughtered, or a fish that has been caught. Astrologers are also responsible for producing special amulets, which may be generic or specially tailored to an individual. In some cases, the services of the astrologers complement those of the doctors. When a disease is thought to have been caused by evil spirits or negative karma, Tibetans may visit an astrologer, a lama, or both, and ask them to prescribe an antidote.

Because they are familiar with demonology, Tibetan astrologers can determine which spirit has afflicted the sick person, the type of disease resulting from that spirit, and the prayer that should be performed to appease the spirit. There are eight main categories of spirits and appropriate protector deities, as well as prayers that are prescribed as remedies for illnesses. The astro-practitioners also advise patients as to which doctor or system of medicine (allopathic, Ayurvedic, or Tibetan) is the most suitable for them.

In the event of death, the astrologer makes death calculations to determine whether there is any life remaining in the body. Following decease, they will also determine when the body should be moved from the room or house. Tibetans believe that this will help them avoid bad spirits when transporting the body to the cremation ground. The astrologer fixes a favorable time and day according to the conjunctions of the planets and constellations. He or she can also indicate who can or cannot touch the body, and which prayers should be offered by the family. At least four monks are usually invited to the home of the dead person to perform special rituals. The holy texts are read and prayers are chanted for 49 days, and repeated one year after the death. Astrologers are also responsible for preparing almanacs and calendars.

Summary: The Traditional Tibetan System of Medicine

In summary, the traditional Tibetan system of medicine has a very long history, although there are conflicting opinions regarding its origins. Important points include the following:

The fundamental concepts often referred to are the five elements (earth, water, fire, wind, and space) and the three humours (wind, bile, and phlegm), believed to constitute the body and be responsible for its balance.

According to this medicinal system, different etiologies of diseases may relate to the imbalance of the three humours, as well as karma and the influence of evil spirits.

Dietary and sleep behaviors play an important role in traditional Tibetan medicine.

Diagnostic methods include visual diagnosis, and diagnoses from the tongue, urine, and pulse, as well as patient interviews.

Treatment may involve introducing changes to one's diet and behaviors (for example, sleep habits), the application of herbal medicines, or accessory therapies (which may include acupuncture, moxibustion, hydrotherapy, humoural therapy, forced elimination methods, pyretic treatment, or massage).

Meditation practices are also used as an aspect of treatment.

Demonology is an important component of the traditional Tibetan system of medicine, and it is often referred to in cases of disease resistant to treatment.

Astrology is also used as a helpful tool for decision-making (e.g., when to prepare medicines or how to deal with misfortunes).

All of the concepts described here are expressed in the narratives of the Tibetan respondents I interviewed for the present study. For example, patients frequently referred to a simplified version of the humoural theory to conceptualize the symptoms they experienced. This implies that the traditional Tibetan system of medicine is an important variable affecting the explanatory models held by Tibetans.

NOTES

1. The Tibetan Department of Health is part of the Government in Exile.
2. Central Tibetan Administration (CTA), Department of Health: Achievements. Source: http://www.tibet.net/health/eng/achieve
3. Moxibustion refers to applying moxa, which usually contains mugwort, to warm, and thus stimulate, certain acupuncture points.
4. Sanskrit *Vimalagotra,* Tib. *dri med rigs*
5. "Turnings of the Wheel of Dharma" refers to a sequential scheme of the teachings given by Buddha (from simple teachings to more complex).
6. Tib. *gso dpyad 'bum pa*
7. Tib. *gcer mthong rig pa'i rgyud*
8. Tib. *gser 'od dam pa'i mdo*
9. Tib. *nad thams cad zhi bar byed pa'i rgyud*
10. Sanskrit: *Amrta Hrdya Anga Asta Guhya Upadesa Tantra*, Tib. *bdud rtsi snying po yan lag bfgyad pa gsang ba man ngag gi rgyud*:)
11. Tib. *rCTAs*
12. The seven physical constituents are: nutritive essence, blood, flesh, fats, bones, marrow and regenerative fluids (Tsering Dhondup 2003).
13. Tib. *gzhan dbang sngon nad*
14. Tib. *kun brtags gdon nad*
15. Tib. *ltar snang 'phral nad*
16. Tib. *yongs grub tshe nad*

17. ib. *zhi gnas*

18 . Tib. *lhag mthong*

19. Vajrayna Buddhism (Tib. *rdo rje theg pa*), also known as Tantric Buddhism, Tantrayana, Mantrayana, or Diamond Vehicle, refers to the most elaborate teachings that were expounded upon by Buddha and become associated with the "Third Turning of the Wheel of Dharma." It includes advanced practices, most of which can only be transmitted by a skilled spiritual teacher. These teachings must have been received directly from one's own guru, passed on from master to disciple in an unbroken linage. As such, vajrayana is sometimes referred to as the "oral transmission path."

20. Tib. *gdon*

21. This is one of the two most important texts in Tibetan Medicine. The other one is called "The Four Root Tantras of Medicine" (*rGyud bZhi*).

Chapter Six

Empirical Research

6.1 The Sample
6.2 The Research Context
6.3 Methodology and Method
    6.3.1 Qualitative Methods
    6.3.2 Grounded Theory
        6.3.2.1 Methods of Data Collection
        6.3.2.2 Qualitative Data Analysis
        6.3.2.3 Coding Qualitative Data
6.4 Procedures for Data Collection
6.5 Planning the Research Process

The initial purpose of this research was to analyze the idiom of health and disease among the Tibetan diaspora in India, along with their illness behaviors and help-seeking pathways. In undertaking this study, I decided to remain open to all sources of data and new information, and never automatically reject things that might seem irrelevant at first glance. I also resisted the temptation to eliminate data that seemed ambiguous, or that contradicted the impressions of Tibet I had already formed in my mind. As time went on, this approach proved to be very rewarding, as it enabled me to obtain better understanding and more insights regarding my Tibetan interview subjects and the issues analyzed. It also helped me produce a multi-dimensional description of the core category that was soon identified in the process of research. In the following section, I will discuss a number of variables that affect Tibetans' health behaviors.

6.1 THE SAMPLE

In the process of acquiring my data, I identified thirty-five primary respondents, of which twenty-seven were men and eight were women. Eight of the respondents can be classified as professional health-care providers (Tibetan doctors, called *amchees,* a counsellor, and a senior nurse), and two as non-professional health-care providers (offering herbal treatments or massage services).

Table 6.1. The Sample

Name	*Age*	*Sex*	*Occupation*	*Place of Residence*
Bhumsang	23	M	student	Dharamsala
Chemey	28	F	office worker	Dharamsala
Chokey	21	F	student	Dehradun
Dawa	30	M	office worker	Dharamsala
Dolkar	50	F	senior nurse	Dharamsala
Dolma	39	F	counsellor	Dharamsala
Dorjee	31	M	*amchee*	Dharamsala
Gonpo	33	M	Photo-journalist	Dharamsala
Jamyang	28	M	monk	Sera Monastery
Jane	58	F	herbalist	USA, Kathmandu
Jigme	40	M	*amchee*/monk	Dharamsala
Jinpa	28	M	civil servant	Bangalore
Karma	40	M	businessman	Dharamsala
Kunzang	25	M	unemployed	Kathmandu
Lobsang	26	M	office worker	Dharamsala
Mary	28	F	American researcher	USA, Dharamsala
Ngawang	31	M	artist	Dharamsala
Norbu	40	M	*amchee*	Silliguri
Nyima	27	M	student	Dharamsala
Özer	54	M	restaurant owner	Dharamsala
Pasang	50	F	*amchee*	Dharamsala
Phuntsok	40	M	former monk, office worker	Kathmandu
Rabten	40	M	interpreter	USA
Rinchen	31	M	monk, lama	Sonada
Sangay	22	M	"street boy," dancer	Dharamsala
Sherab	17	M	student	Lhadakh
Sonam	27	M	Internet café worker	Dharamsala
Tashi	30	M	office worker	Dharamsala
Tenpa	40	M	*amchee*/monk	Dharamsala
Tenwang	~50	M	government official	Dharamsala
Tenzin	28	M	salesman	New Delhi
Thubten	34	M	monk, school teacher	Sera Monastery
Tsewang	30	M	monastery school teacher	Sonada
Wangchuk	28	M	masseur	Dharamsala
Yeshi	50	F	*amchee*	New Delhi

Whereas most of the respondents lived in Dharamsala, there were two informants from the Tibetan Camp in Manjnu-Ka-Tilla (New Delhi), one from Dehradun, two from Sonada, one from Silliguri, three from southern India (Sera Monastery, Bangalore), one from Lhadakh, and three from Kathmandu. Two were of American origin (one has lived in Asia for 30 years and presently resides in Kathmandu; another one had performed research on refuge trauma in Dharamsala for over a year). There was also one Tibetan who was born in Tibet and had emigrated to America about 15 years earlier. Only ten of the Tibetan respondents were born in exile; the others had escaped from Tibet. Table 6.1 below presents the informants' age, gender, occupation, and place of residence. To protect their identities, I have given them fictitious names.

6.2 THE RESEARCH CONTEXT

I conducted most of my research in Tibetan refugee camps located in Northern India, namely, in Dharamsala, Majnu-Ka-Tilla, and Silliguri.

Dharamsala (or Dharmsāla), which literally means "Rest House," is a town located in the Kangra district of the state of Himachal Pradesh (Northern India). Its average elevation is around 9 miles (ca. 1457 metres), and in the past, it was a popular hill station for the British Army. Its role as a military post came to an end in 1905, when a massive earthquake killed an estimated 40,000 people at the site. The British Army's summer headquarters were then moved to Shimla (Simla). After the Dalai Lama escaped from Tibet in 1959, the Indian Prime Minister, Jawaharlal Nehru, gave him Dharamsala as a residence. Since then, the town has absorbed massive influxes of Tibetans. Most of them now reside in Upper Dharamsala, which is also known as McLeod Ganj. Upper Dharamsala is situated around 5.6 miles (ca. 9 kilometers) up the hill from Lower Dharamsala, which is a commercial center mainly populated by Indians. The Tibetans have established schools, temples, and medical institutions in and around Upper Dharamsala, which is surrounded by rich forests of pine and deodar. Not only does it attract people interested in Tibetan Buddhism and culture, but also those keen on trekking. The temperature ranges from 32 °F to 58.1 °F (0 °C − 14.5 °C) in December and January, and from 71.6 °F to 100.4 °F (22 °C − 38 °C) during the summer.

Majnu-Ka-Tilla (Manjutilla), the Tibetan colony in Delhi, is a major transit hub for Tibetan people traveling within India and abroad. The entire settlement resembles one large street, densely crowded with pedestrians during the daytime, and lined with numerous guesthouses, restaurants, Tibetan shops, and small stalls selling jewelry and other handicrafts. Tourists who wish to visit Dharamsala can avail themselves of the daily buses that run from Majnu-Ka-Tilla to the mountain settlement.

Silliguri is a densely populated and lively town in northeast India. It serves as a point of departure for visits to Darjeeling, Kalimpong, Mirik, Sonada, Gangtok (Sikkim), and the North-East states. Silliguri is also an important trade center for north-east and eastern Nepal. The Tibetans have established a few monasteries and temples there, along with a branch clinic of the Tibetan Medical and Astro Institute (Men-Tsee-Khang). While I was staying in Silliguri, I gathered qualitative data in the clinic and at the monastery of His Eminence Kalu Rinpoche. Using Silliguri as a base, I traveled to each of the places mentioned above.

In Tibet, people normally identify themselves with the particular region they come from. Jacobson (2002) maintains that: "familial and regional loyalties are virtually always stronger than national loyalties" (p. 266). In exile, identification with a particular ethnic group could be expressed by the dialect spoken, the traditional garments worn, the involvement in typical religious practices, the customs maintained, and the traditional cuisine and type of residence found within the Tibetan refugee community.

Although the Tibetan community in India presents itself as a rather homogeneous group with a strong allegiance to the authority of its leader, Misra (2003) says that historically, "Tibetan diasporic nationalism has witnessed an abundance of intrigue, in-fighting and violent conflicts. The desire for separation on the part of various sectarian groups was very potent during the early years of their exile. . . . Although all sects within the Tibetan Buddhist pantheon owe their allegiance to the Dalai Lama, some nonetheless enjoyed both limited temporal and spiritual autonomy in the past" (p. 190).

6.3 METHODOLOGY AND METHOD

In this section, I will present the methods I used in the present study. There are several reasons why qualitative research methodology is recognized as an effective tool in cross-cultural research. First of all, it may be more efficient when the aim of the research is to get a better understanding of certain phenomena and provide descriptions of them. Secondly, it is often difficult to adopt Western quantitative research tools in different contexts. For example, Crescenzi et al. (2002), who also did their research on a sample of Tibetans, noted that the Tibetans lacked an appropriate vocabulary to communicate their mental reactions. The authors translated and adapted one of the psychiatric measurement tools to create the Tibetan Hopkins Symptom Schedule-25, and wanted to study mental disorders of refugees with a history of trauma.

Apparently, a number of difficulties emerged: "We found that illiterate patients of our program could not fully comprehend written Tibetan language when the items were read to them, because the language used in written Tibetan tends to differ from spoken Tibetan. Also, wide variations between Tibetan dialects resulted in communication difficulties. Moreover, translations of words involving direct expression of emotion were poorly understood because Tibetans typically communicate without such words." (p. 370).

Another argument is given by Bhui (1999) and refers to research in cross-cultural psychiatry. The author maintains that using Western systems to comprehend and measure phenomena in other contexts may prove inappropriate: "The use of dimensional measures aims to identify symptoms which are commonly presented in all cultures, and then to signify comparative levels of severity across cultural groups. The danger with such methodologies is that items that are uniquely symptoms of a common mental disorder, specific to one culture, are not necessarily of utility in comparisons with other cultures. It might be argued that psychiatry is culturally bound itself, and that any instrument developed in accord with psychiatric nosology is established on certain premises that include Euro-American conceptualizations of illness, distress and its alleviation" (p. 142). This is one of the reasons why using standard tools may fail.

Furthermore, in planning this research, I was not able to make any assumptions about what I might find, and so the best solution was to adapt the open, inductive approach that is characteristic of grounded theory (thoroughly described later in this chapter). Glaser (2004) claims, that grounded theory is a methodology distinct from Qualitative Data Analysis. In this section I will present the methods I used for collecting, administering, and analyzing the data, according to the grounded theory approach.

6.3.1 Qualitative Methods

As cited in Ritchie and Lewis (2003), Denzin and Lincoln define qualitative research: "Qualitative research is a situated activity that locates the observer in the world. It consists of a set of interpretive, material practices that makes the world visible. These practices . . . turn the world into a series of representations including field notes, interviews, conversations, photographs, recordings and memos to the self. At this level, qualitative research involves an interpretive, naturalistic approach to the world. This means that qualitative researchers study things in their natural settings, attempting to make sense of, or to interpret, phenomena in terms of the meaning people bring to them" (pp. 2–3).

The aim of qualitative research, then, is to provide an in-depth and interpreted understanding of the social world. In order to achieve this, the researcher investigates various areas of the lives and experiences of the subjects, including their social and material circumstances, personal perspectives, and life histories. In this type of research, it is quality, not quantity that is important, and for this reason, small samples are usually selected on the basis of predetermined criteria. Data collection involves close contact between the researcher and the target group. It is interactive and leaves space for all kinds of issues to be explored. The information gathered is usually extensive, and the analysis is descriptive, often multi-dimensional. The output result focuses on the interpretation of social meaning (Ritchie and Lewis 2003).

The great advantage of the qualitative method is that because the researchers do not limit themselves to a pre-defined set of questions or data collection methods, they may be able to discover important topics that might not have been apparent at the beginning. Even though some general questions may be formulated, and choices made regarding the collection method, these can be modified during the course of the research (World Health Organization 1994). Myers (1997) supports this assessment: "Qualitative research methods are designed to help researchers understand people and the social and cultural contexts within which they live . . . the goal of understanding a phenomenon from the point of view of the participants and its particular social and institutional context is largely lost when textual data are quantified."

Miles and Huberman (1994) have enumerated the features of qualitative research: It is conducted through an intensive, prolonged contact within a "field" setting or life situation, one that reflects the everyday life of the studied target. It aims at obtaining a holistic (integrated) overview of the context; data is gathered "from the inside" by means of deep attentiveness, empathetic understanding, suspension of any preconceptions about the research topics; and the isolation and review of certain themes. It is important for the researcher to "explicate the ways people in particular settings come to understand, account for, take action, and otherwise manage their day-to-day situations" (p. 7). Analysis of the gathered material is done with words, which are specially organized to enable contrasting, comparing, analyzing, and the finding of patterns.

Qualitative Research has been proved to be an especially effective tool in the following situations: when the subject matter was unfamiliar to the researcher; when concepts and variables were unknown or definitions unclear; when in-depth understanding was required; when meaning rather than frequencies was sought; and where flexibility was required, so that the discovery of the unexpected could take place (WHO 1994). The same source notes that: "ideally, researchers who intend to conduct qualitative field research should also have experience or training in a field relevant to the topic to be studied" (p. 9).

Miles and Huberman (1994) describe three main approaches to qualitative data analysis: interpretivism, social anthropology, and collaborative social research. Of these, the second approach—social anthropology—was most relevant to my study. Social anthropology involves extended contact with the studied community, participating in and observing day-to-day events, focusing on the individual's perspectives, and interpreting their world. With this approach, there is little structure and extensive use of recorded material, such as audio and video recordings. Other data sources include diaries, photographs, and personal artifacts. Researchers who follow this approach are particularly interested in the behavioral regularities used in everyday situations—language use, artifacts, rituals, and relationships—and aim at finding patterns or rules that express these regularities. In other words, the goal is to "uncover and explicate the ways in which people in particular (work) settings come to understand, account for, take action and otherwise manage their day-to-day situation" (Van Maanen, cited in Miles and Huberman 1994, p. 8).

Strauss and Corbin (1990) note that qualitative research may vary according to type (grounded theory, ethnography, the phenomenological approach, life histories, conversational analysis); purpose (clarification and illustration of the quantitative findings, building research instruments, developing policy, evaluating programs, providing information for commercial purposes, guiding practitioners' practices, scientific research); and approach (as to how much data analysis should be involved, varying from the mere presentation of data and allowing the informants to "speak for themselves," to accurate descriptions by the researcher). Another important aspect is connected with building theory, which implies having to interpret data, conceptualizing and relating the concepts to create a "theoretical rendition of reality (a reality that cannot actually be known, but is always interpreted)" (Strauss and Corbin 1990, p. 22).

6.3.2 Grounded Theory

According to Strauss and Corbin (1990), grounded theory (GT) is a research method in which a systematic set of procedures is used "to develop an inductively derived grounded theory about a phenomenon. The research findings constitute a theoretical formulation of the reality under investigation, rather than consisting of a set of numbers, or a group of loosely related themes" (p. 24). The generated theory should be grounded—that is, it should derive from data—and it should be conceptually dense and well integrated. The researcher generates analytical theories and their dimensions, and identifies relationships between them. One of the important prerequisites for a GT researcher is to develop "theoretical sensitivity," indicating "an awareness of the subtleties of meaning of data" (Strauss and Corbin 1990, p. 41). Grounded theory also stresses the personal qualities of the researcher, such as the ability to induce conclusions from important information.

Grounded theory was first developed by two sociologists at the University of California, Barney Glaser and Anselm Strauss. They described the new approach in their book, "The Discovery of Grounded Theory." Subsequently, they refined the methodology and published their findings in a number of individually authored articles and books. Afterwards, the authors of the method started to disagree about theoretical and practical issues, and each of them would develop his own approach (Babchuk 1996). For the most part, in the present study I have followed the description and methodological research instructions presented by Strauss and Corbin (1990).

Data Collection

Researchers who follow the GT approach can use a variety of data sources. The technical literature is a rich source of background information. This may include readings on theory, individual research studies, government publications, and biographies, all of which may "sensitize"[1] the researcher. Another important source is the researcher's own professional experience and background knowledge, which can enrich understanding of the phenomena being investigated. It should be noted, however, that being an expert in a field can also become an obstacle: "it can block you from seeing things that have become routine or 'obvious'" (Strauss and Corbin 1990, p. 42).

Primary and Secondary Data

Material gathered during research becomes data, which will be specially administered, reflected upon, and presented. Two different sources of data can be distinguished in qualitative research: primary and secondary. The first type refers to material collected by the researcher from the interviewees, plus his or her own field notes. The secondary data are collected by someone else (Ashwin-Hirst 2001). Myers (1997) explains that the primary sources "are data which are unpublished and which the researcher has gathered from the people or organization directly. Secondary sources refer to any materials (books, articles etc.) which have been previously published" (online). Both types of data can be in written form (for example, books, journals, company documentation, reports, newspaper articles, faxes, letters, e-mail messages, memos, etc.), or non-written form (videos, charts, diagrams, photos). It is up to the researcher whether or not to augment his or her original data with secondary sources (Ashwin-Hirst 2001; Myers 1997).

Using the Technical Literature in GT

The technical literature in grounded theory can be used to stimulate theoretical sensitivity. While it is a good idea to have few preconceptions when entering the field, some issues frequently turn up in the literature and seem to be of significance. This knowledge of extant writings and theories can influence the way in which the researcher examines the data and what is given special significance: sometimes in a prejudicial manner. Glaser (2004) states that extensive reading prior to research could unduly influence the pre-conceptualization of that research. It can also "cloud the researcher's ability to remain open to the emergence of a completely new core category that has not figured prominently in the research to date, thereby thwarting the theoretical sensitivity" (p. 12).

On the other hand, for some researchers, a review of the literature may provide an opportunity to extend or enrich an existing theory. It can also be mined for secondary sources of data. Descriptive materials concerning events, actions, settings, and quoted materials in research publications can also be treated as data and analyzed along with the original data. Additionally, when discrepancies are discovered between one's own research and the findings presented in the technical literature, it should stimulate the researcher to go back to the field data and find out why such discrepancies occurred. Presenting one's theory, the researcher can relate original concepts to appropriate themes in the writings of others, while differences may also be disclosed (Strauss and Corbin 1990).

Using Non-Technical Literature in GT

Although this type of literature is rarely used in quantitative studies, it can be very valuable in GT research. The non-technical literature refers to sources including letters, biographies, diaries, reports, videotapes, and newspapers. These can supplement standard sources such as interviews and personal observations. Strauss and Corbin (1990) suggest that these should always be cross-checked against the primary data, due to the difficulty of authenticating them.

6.3.2.1 Methods of Data Collection

Qualitative research utilizes a number of methods to gather data. According to WHO (1994), interviews and observational methods may vary based on the degree to which they are structured. Grounded theory encompasses specific procedures for data collection that are classified as theoretical sampling. Glaser (2004) explains that this is "the process of data collection for generating theory whereby the analyst jointly collects, codes and analyzes the data and decides which data to collect next and where to find them, in order to develop the theory as it emerges" (online). Theoretical sampling is an interactive process. The researcher picks an initial sample, and after having analyzed the data, may proceed to choose further samples. The key criteria used for selection are theoretical purpose and theoretical relevance. The aim of theoretical sampling is to refine the categories and theories that emerge. This process is continued until "data saturation" is achieved, meaning the point at which no new insights are obtained (Ritchie and Lewis 2003). During the research process, the researcher may identify a number of gaps in the theory, and is subsequently "guided as to the next sources of data collection and interview style" (Glaser 2004).

The Interviews

In the field of cultural anthropology, unstructured interviews are commonly used to collect data. Generally, the researcher knows beforehand what kinds of questions he or she would like to ask. There is, however, no structured set of questions, as is typical of structured interviews. In structured interviews, all the respondents are exposed to the same questions, in the same order. If the unstructured interview style is adopted, the researcher can use a topic list for reference. If completely new topics emerge, the researcher will often come up with new questions and discard the original ones.

The strength of the unstructured interview is that it enables the researcher to be responsive to individual differences and situational characteristics. It is very helpful at the stage of building initial rapport with the interviewees, and it enables the researcher to conduct interviews in an informal setting. In a semi-structured interview, the researcher may use a list of questions that need to be covered, but he or she remains flexible and adapts the order and wording of the questions according to the situation. In semi-structured interviews. new topics are also accepted, but they are merely a supplement to the main topic of interest (WHO 1994).

Observation

Like the interviews, personal observations can be structured (recording only the behaviors present on a pre-defined observation list), or unstructured (observing behaviors in their holistic contexts to discover unknown aspects of a problem) (WHO 1994). Ritchie and Lewis (2003) note that this method "offers the opportunity to record and analyze behaviour and interactions as they occur, although not as a member of the study population. This allows events, actions and experiences and so on, to be 'seen' through the eyes of the researcher, often without any construction on the part of those involved" (p. 35). Using observation as a tool to collect data, the researcher will register signs or indicators of behavior.

WHO (1994) also describes a situation in which "the investigator becomes, to a greater or lesser extent, an active, functioning member of the culture under study . . . [and] participates in any activities appropriate for a person of the status which is assumed, observes what others do, and in general attempts to see through the eyes of a member of the culture rather that through those of an outsider" (p. 28). This technique is called "participant observation," and combines interviews with more unstructured data-gathering methods, such as everyday conversations and casual observations.

The strength of this method is that the interviewees come to feel increasingly comfortable with the researcher's presence. It also stimulates the investigator's intuitive understanding of the situations and the collected material. Thus, it can be very useful in new contexts, where the researcher has little or no background knowledge or experience. On the other hand, it often requires speaking the local language and possessing observational skills so as to notice small but important details of life situations, as well as a good memory for recording them later. There is also a potential trap: "Sometimes the researchers become so familiar with the culture that it becomes more and more difficult to notice things that should be considered different or important" (WHO 1994, p. 29).

Field Notes

Field notes have been a common "method of data collection in ethnographic research, and particularly in observation form the primary data" (Ritchie and Lewis 2003, p. 132). Field notes are descriptions of what the researcher experienced (saw, heard, felt, smelled, thought about, imagined, etc.) during field observation or in the course of an interview. Glaser (2004) refers to field notes in GT as non-threatening and selective in nature, and as providing description, not conceptualization. Field notes should be written down immediately, following interviews or observations.

Validity and Generalizability

The issue of validity and generalizability is often discussed in the context of qualitative research methodology. WHO (1994, p. 54) explains: "validity refers to the extent to which a particular method of measurement (i.e. interviews or observations) actually represents that which it claims to measure."

Strauss and Corbin (1990) claimed that if grounded theory is carried out appropriately it meets the canons for doing "good" science: significance, theory-observation, compatibility, generalizability, reproducibility, precision, rigor, and verification. Haig[2] clarifies, however, that "these methodological notions are not to be understood in a positivist sense. The general goal of grounded theory research is to construct theories in order to understand phenomena. A good grounded theory is one that is: 1) inductively derived from data, 2) subjected to theoretical elaboration, and 3) judged adequate to its domain with respect to a number of evaluative criteria."

WHO suggests that to increase the validity of qualitative data, researchers can triangulate data collection methods—for example, use a variety of interviewing techniques and respondents instead of a single source. An example of using multiple data collection could be a combination of individual and group interviews or interviews and observations. Subsequently, "confidence in the validity of findings is increased when there is agreement among the different methods and types of respondents about a particular issue" (WHO 1994, p. 54). The representativeness, on the other hand, can be increased by conducting research in a number of different sites and in the larger population (WHO 1994).

Recording and Transcribing the Material

GT does not require tape recording interviews. Field notes are sometimes preferable (Glaser 2004). If an interview is taped, the researcher can either use the tape itself for reference, or produce a transcript. In qualitative research, transcripts can vary from the selective to the minutely detailed. In some cases, the material is transcribed verbatim. Strauss and Corbin (1990, p. 30) advise transcribing "as much as is needed" and encourage the researcher to be selective (i.e., there is no need to transcribe the entire tape word for word). The authors do suggest transcribing the first few interviews of taped field notes entirely before progressing to the next set of interviews or field observations, because "this early coding gives guidance to the next field observations and/or interviews" (Strauss and Corbin 1990, p. 30).

Before proceeding to analysis, the raw data (the scribbled field notes, the dictated tapes, and the direct tape recordings) must be appropriately processed, that is, converted into "write-ups." While field notes are sketchy, fairly illegible and contain private abbreviations, a "write-up" is "an intelligible product for any reader" (Miles and Huberman 1994).

6.3.2.2 Qualitative Data Analysis

In most instances, analysis of the qualitative data begins at an early stage of the research. Ritchie and Lewis (2003, p. 199) explain: "the pathways to forming ideas to pursue, phenomena to capture, theories to test begins right at the start of a research process." While some researchers use up considerable time and energy in collecting data, so that they may analyze it later, this "rules out the possibility of collecting new data to fill in gaps, or to test new hypotheses that emerge during analysis" (Miles and Huberman 1994, p. 50). This is why the authors encourage performing analysis of the data from the earliest stages of the data-collection process, as it is obtained in the field. It then becomes a continuous, lively enterprise.

The various levels and types of data analysis include ethnographic accounts—descriptive narratives that portray the lifeways of particular individuals, groups, or organizations. Other types of analyses include life histories, narrative analysis, content analysis, conversation analysis, and discourse analysis, which focuses on how knowledge is produced within a particular discourse, such as medicine. Grounded theory is yet another category, one that "involves the generation of analytical categories and their dimensions, and the identification of relationships between them. The process of data collection and conceptualisation continues until categories and relationships are 'saturated,' that is new data do not add to the developing theory" (Rinchie and Lesis 2003, p. 201).

Most of these approaches focus on the use of language, or on understanding the views and culture of the sample being studied. While grounded theory focuses on theory building Bryman (cited in Rinchie and Lewis 2003) points out that "theory building may be part of both language-based and descriptive or interpretative approaches" (p. 201).

Data Management

Miles and Huberman (1994) stress the importance of efficiently managing the qualitative data from the earliest stage of the research, as this will influence the entire process of analysis. By its nature, the data will be quite extensive, and may include hundreds of pages of field notes and interview transcripts. As a way of managing this data, researchers may produce a one-page Contact Summary Form. This form can include information about the main issues or themes touched on in the interview, a summary of the information received from the informant, any comments that seem important or new, and any remaining questions the researcher would like to ask. Memos are also used to record important information that relates to the process of analysis and building up a theory. Computer software can be an important aid in managing qualitative data.

Computer-Aided Qualitative Data Analysis

The last ten years have witnessed phenomenal development of new computer software for qualitative data analysis. Miles and Huberman (1994) state that three-quarters of the researchers they interviewed reported using computer technology to enter data, perform coding, retrieve information, make displays, and build concepts. PC technology lets researchers "reduce analysis time, cut out much drudgery, make procedures more systematic and explicit, ensure completeness and refinement, and permit flexibility and revision in analysis procedures" (p. 44). Because of the "richness" of qualitative data (which usually makes it cumbersome to analyze), the software facilitates data handling and supports its analysis. Using the appropriate software, researchers can do the coding more quickly and efficiently. Theoretical associations and links can also be created within the data (Fielding 1994; Miles and Huberman 1994).

There are different types of data-analysis tools, including text retrievers, code-and-retrieve packages, and theory-building software. In addition, word processors are essential for transcribing and editing field notes, preparing files for coding and analysis, and writing reports (Miles and Huberman 1994). In data analysis, the researcher codifies the text by providing it with appropriate labels. In this way, the data is sorted into categories by marking codes. The text retrievers "recover the data pertaining to each category on the basis of keywords that appear in the data" (Fielding 1994). This software finds all the instances of words, phrases, and combinations of these, and helps in operations, such as marking or sorting the text into new files, hyperlinking memos, and making annotations to the original data. The code-and-retrieve software is used to divide text into segments (chunks), attach codes to them, and then retrieve and display the chunks with codes. As Fielding (1994) explains, "they take over the kinds of marking up, cutting, sorting, reorganizing and collecting tasks that qualitative researchers have traditionally done with scissors, paper and sellotape." The theory builders usually include code-and-retrieve capabilities, but also help in finding relationships between categories and data. They can be used to develop higher-order classifications and categories, and formulate propositions or assertions, implying a conceptual structure that fits the data (Miles and Huberman 1994). Examples of such software include ATLAS, or NUDIST and its newer version, QSR N6, which I used for qualitative data management in my research.

6.3.2.3 Coding Qualitative Data

The heart of grounded theory is the coding process. Three kinds of coding can be identified: open coding, axial coding, and selective coding. GT starts with a research situation, in which the researcher gathers data and tries to distinguish certain phenomena. He or or she may initiate the process by formulating questions, such as: What is happening here? Who are the actors? How do they manage their roles? Data can be recorded as field notes or in the form of interview transcripts. The researcher will then name or label distinguishable phenomena (coding) and move on to gather more samples, trying to see if similar phenomena will occur in them. Strauss and Corbin (1990) note that the "data collection and data analysis are tightly interwoven processes, and must occur alternately because the analysis directs the sampling of data" (p. 59).

Open Coding

Strauss and Corbin (1990) define open coding as "part of analysis that pertains specifically to the naming and categorizing of phenomena through close examination of data" (p. 62). It is connected with conceptualizing the data "by breaking apart an observation, a sentence, a paragraph, and giving each discrete incident, idea, or event, a name, something that stands for or represents a phenomenon" (Strauss and Corbin 1990, p. 63). Open coding can thus be done through a line-by-line analysis (involving a detailed examination of single phrases or sometimes words), by sentence or by paragraph. Glaser (2004) points out that this process "allows the analyst to see the direction in which to take the study by theoretical sampling before he/she has become selective and focused on a particular problem. The researcher begins to see the kind of categories that can handle the data theoretically."

The next step in open coding is categorizing, Having identified particular phenomena in the data, the researcher groups concepts around them, to reduce the number of units. A conceptual name is given to a phenomenon, which is represented by a category. In some instances, an "in vivo" coding is practiced, in which words and phrases said directly by informants are used as a code. Categories are also made in terms of their properties and dimensions. Strauss and Corbin (1990) explain that "properties are the characteristics or attributes of a category" and "dimensions represent locations of a property along a continuum" (p. 69). The properties become dimensionalized. While each category can have a number of properties, "each property varies over a dimensional continuum" (Strauss and Corbin 1990, p. 70). Let us take an example of a category named "somatic disease." Within this category we might identify dimensions, such as: "severity" or "duration." These dimensional continua will then include properties, such as "acute" or "mild" to describe the severity of the symptoms, and "brief" and "chronic" to denote their duration.

Axial Coding

This type of coding, phenomena are specified in terms of the conditions that give rise to them; the context (set of properties) in which they are embedded;

the action or interactional strategies by which they are handled, and the consequences of those strategies. Axial coding is explained as "a set of procedures whereby data are put back together in new ways after open coding, by making connections between categories. This is done by utilizing a coding paradigm involving conditions, context, action/interactional strategies and consequences" (Strauss and Corbin 1990, p. 96). This process leads to the creation of subcategories, which are then linked to a category in a set of relationships "denoting causal conditions, phenomenon, context, intervening conditions, action/interactional strategies, and consequences" (Strauss and Corbin 1990, p. 99). The use of this model makes grounded theory analysis dense and precise.

Selective Coding—Building Theory

Selective coding refers to integrating the categories to form a grounded theory. While it does not differ much from axial coding, it is done at a higher, more abstract level of analysis. Strauss and Corbin (1990, p. 116) define this type of coding as "the process of selecting the core category, systematically relating it to other categories, validating those relationships, and filling in categories that need further refinement and development." Glaser (2004) explains that the goal of selective coding is "to delimit coding to only those variables that relate to the core variable in sufficiently significant ways as to produce a parsimonious theory."

Selective coding is a complex process, which involves: 1. explicating the "story line," 2. relating subsidiary categories around the core category by means of a paradigm, 3. relating categories at the dimensional level, and 4. validating those relationships against data. It is not necessarily a sequential process, because the researcher can move back and forth among these four stages. The story line is the core category or the conceptualization of the story, or "a descriptive narrative about the central phenomenon of the study" (Strauss and Corbin 1990, p. 116). The previously mentioned paradigm of conditions, context, strategies, and consequences is used to relate secondary categories to the core category: "A (conditions) leads to B (phenomenon), which leads to C (context), which leads to D (action/interaction, including strategies), which then leads to E (consequences)" (Strauss and Corbin 1990, pp. 124–125). However, the methodologists remind us that these relationships may be more than causal, due to the existence of intervening sets of conditions. According to Strauss and Corbin (1990), in the course of the study, the researcher will identify differences in context, and group the categories along the dimensional ranges of their properties in accordance with discovered patterns. Data will then be related at both the broad conceptual level and at the property and dimensional levels for each major category. To complete the process, the researcher's task is to validate the emergent theory against the data. The result of this coding is "a picture of reality that is conceptual, comprehensible, and above all grounded" (Strauss and Corbin 1990, p. 117).

After performing a continual comparison of data, a theory may emerge. Dick (2005) notes: "what most differentiates grounded theory from much other research is that it is explicitly emergent. It does not test a hypothesis. It sets out to find what theory accounts for the research situation as it is" (online). That is why grounded theory is said to be grounded in data, as it gradually develops and interpretations are accumulated.

6.4 PROCEDURES FOR DATA COLLECTION

I gathered most of the data for this research via in-depth interviewing. These interviews were conducted on a one-on-one basis with the respondents, in their homes, in health clinics, or in casual settings such as restaurants. Most of the respondents spoke English at an intermediate or upper-intermediate level. There were also a few interviewees whose language proficiency was low. In such cases, I contracted with a Tibetan interpreter to translate the conversations.

The interviews were open in structure, which let me build a good rapport with the respondent, and also allowed unexpected topics and issues to arise. I also had a list of predetermined questions in mind. While most of the interviews were digitally recorded, in cases where tape recording was not possible, the transcripts were made from notes. Recorded interviews were transcribed verbatim. These textual files were managed by QSR N6 (a newer version of NUDIST; see above), a computer software for administration of qualitative data. This program tended to accelerate the analysis procedures, including the data coding, retrieval and display. Using QSR N6, the free coding and axial coding could be done efficiently.

My field notes were an additional source of information: Having observed various situations, I made a descriptive narrative that was coded according to the GT methodology. I also made field notes based on an analysis of photographs of Tibetans, which were taken in various situations of daily life. Then I wrote up descriptions of the selected photographs on three levels: 1. the perception level (what can be seen in the picture; who are the actors; how do they behave, etc.), 2. the interpretative level (what is the meaning of their behavior? what do they want to express?), and 3. the meta-conceptual level (how can the identified phenomena be understood in terms of research questions?). These conceptual descriptions resembled memos, which are popular in qualitative research. I also acquired material from personal communications via e-mail, Internet chats, leaflets, biographies, and posters. These valuable sources of information were coded separately.

6.5 PLANNING THE RESEARCH PROCESS

As is characteristic of qualitative research methodology, this study was a sequential process and involved several stages: theoretical sampling, followed by open, axial, and selective coding. After having created a grounded theory of illness behaviors of Tibetans in exile, I validated my theory against new data obtained during the follow-up stage. I then analyzed the literature, to gain additional insight into some issues touched upon in the study: migration, acculturation, and the unique problems faced by political refugees. Finally, I wrote up an analysis of the qualitative data, together with a discussion based on my findings and the information gleaned from the technical literature. These subsequent phases are included in Chapter Eight, "Discussion and Conclusions."

Theoretical Sampling and Coding

Theoretical sampling refers to the phase of my field work in which I was collecting numerous kinds of data. This involved interviewing selected informants, making field notes, taking pictures, and gathering other sources of information. During this phase, I followed two main principles: 1. that data can be found everywhere, and 2. that all data may be valuable. Apart from data collection, theoretical sampling also involved open and axial coding. I also used specialized computer software for administrating the qualitative data, to manage the interview transcripts, and to make annotations and memos. Open coding was based on identifying meaningful chunks of texts and labelling them as free nodes. A listing of free nodes can be seen in Table 6.2.

At a later stage, I classified free nodes into groups and labeled them with conceptual names; these groups often included sub-groups. An example of tree nodes is shown in Table 6.3.

At a later stage, I analyzed the relationships between various nodes to identify patterns and associations. Another stage of analysis involved axial coding, a conceptual process that involved specifying phenomena in terms of conditions, context, actions, and consequences. An example of axial coding could be a case in which the severity of the illness stimulates the patient to react ("I was so desperate when I could not get rid of those symptoms, even though I took allopathic medicine") and the patient is involved with the culture of origin ("My girlfriend is very religious and she believes in traditional ways"). The patient is likely to seek advice and help from lamas ("So I went to Rin-

Table 6.2. A Few Examples of Free Nodes Generated in QSR N6 During the Open Coding Phase.

(F 1)	//Free Nodes/RESEARCH DIARY
(F 48)	//Free Nodes/referral
(F 15)	//Free Nodes/born in exile
(F 3)	//Free Nodes/absorbed in practice
(F 26)	//Free Nodes/death
(F 23)	//Free Nodes/feeling emotionally weak
(F 35)	//Free Nodes/professional services in Tibet
(F 39)	//Free Nodes/sponsorships
(F 51)	//Free Nodes/helping dead people
(F 47)	//Free Nodes/hygiene
(F 29)	//Free Nodes/immunization
(F 17)	//Free Nodes/involvement with the culture of origin
(F 21)	//Free Nodes/length of the medical consultation
(F 13)	//Free Nodes/medicine is cheap
(F 30)	//Free Nodes/memories from Tibet
(F 18)	//Free Nodes/paying for treatment
(F 4)	//Free Nodes/possession
(F 6)	//Free Nodes/rapport with a lama
(F 8)	//Free Nodes/Reasons for Leaving Tibet
(F 32)	//Free Nodes/reflectivity
(F 14)	//Free Nodes/remoteness
(F 11)	//Free Nodes/remorse
(F 56)	//Free Nodes/responsibility
(F 10)	//Free Nodes/shared knowledge on medicine
(F 16)	//Free Nodes/stereotypes
(F 9)	//Free Nodes/taboo
(F 5)	//Free Nodes/trance healers
(F 44)	//Free Nodes/unhealthy behaviors

poche, who said I should take some spiritual actions and gave me some holy pills"), and as a result of this, he may cope with the situation more effectively ("I felt more peaceful and my health got better after some time"). Exceptions to such patterns were sought and different intervening variables were analyzed, to create a multidimensional description of the phenomena.

The final stage of analysis involved selective coding, in which I created my grounded theory by selecting the core category and relating it to other categories (a process similar to axial coding but conducted on a more abstract level). I then validated the relationships between categories against my field data.

Follow-Up Phase

During this stage, the grounded theory I had created was validated against the new data. On returning to Poland, I established communication via e-mail or

Table 6.3. A Few Examples of Tree Nodes Generated in QSR N6 During the Axial Coding Phase.

(3)	/disease
(3 2)	/disease/symptoms
(3 2 1)	/disease/symptoms/severity
(3 2 1 1)	/disease/symptoms/severity/acute
(3 2 1 2)	/disease/symptoms/severity/mild
(3 2 2)	/disease/symptoms/duration
(3 2 2 1)	/disease/symptoms/duration/brief
(3 2 2 2)	/disease/symptoms/duration/chronic
(3 3)	/disease/attitudes
(3 3 2)	/disease/attitudes/affective
(3 3 2 1)	/disease/attitudes/affective/angry
(3 3 2 2)	/disease/attitudes/affective/sad
(3 3 2 3)	/disease/attitudes/affective/crying
(3 3 2 4)	/disease/attitudes/affective/hope
(3 3 2 5)	/disease/attitudes/affective/anxious
(3 3 3)	/disease/attitudes/behavioral
(3 3 3 1)	/disease/attitudes/behavioral/coping strategies
(3 3 3 1 1)	/disease/attitudes/behavioral/coping strategies/karma
(3 3 3 1 2)	/disease/attitudes/behavioral/coping strategies/prayer
(3 3 3 1 3)	/disease/attitudes/behavioral/coping strategies/prayer flags
(3 3 3 1 4)	/disease/attitudes/behavioral/coping strategies/pilgrimage
(3 3 3 1 5)	/disease/attitudes/behavioral/coping strategies/kora*
(3 3 3 4)	/disease/attitudes/behavioral/seeking help
(3 3 3 4 1)	/disease/attitudes/behavioral/seeking help/from family and friends
(3 3 3 4 2)	/disease/attitudes/behavioral/seeking help/from health professionals
(3 3 3 4 3)	/disease/attitudes/behavioral/seeking help/from lamas
(3 3 3 4 3 1)	/disease/attitudes/behavioral/seeking help/from lamas/blessing
(3 3 3 4 3 2)	/disease/attitudes/behavioral/seeking help/from lamas/divination
(3 3 3 4 3 2)	/disease/attitudes/behavioral/seeking help/from lamas/ritual

*"*Kora*" refers to circumambulating holy places

chat with a select number of the Tibetans living in India. Several of them responded and I could check, whether my theory could be applied to describe illness behavior of informants I had not met before.

Study of Technical Literature

Once I completed the qualitative data analysis, I engaged myself in studying literature on the interdependencies between culture, religion, and health. I then compared the findings of my own research with studies performed in other cultural contexts. I was able to identify a number of regularities among the studies, which are presented in the "Discussion" section of Chapter Eight.

The next chapter, Chapter Seven, "Presenting and Analyzing the Qualitative Data," presents a sequential analysis of the material, including how certain hypotheses were developed and tested towards my final conclusions.

NOTES

1. This refers to the "theoretical sensitivity" mentioned later.
2. Haig, B.D. (2008). *Grounded Theory as Scientific Method.* University of Canterbury. Source: http://www.ed.uiuc.edu/EPS/PES-Yearbook/95_docs/haig.html

Chapter Seven

Presenting and Analyzing the Qualitative Data

7.1 Support and Treatment Methods
7.1.1 The Traditional Tibetan System of Medicine
7.1.2 Paramedical Solutions
7.1.3 Western Allopathic Medicine
7.2 Factors Affecting Illness Behavior
7.2.1 Age Factor
7.2.2 Severity of Symptoms and Duration of Treatment
7.2.3 Economic Effects Factor
7.2.4 Treatment Availability Factor
7.2.5 Idiom of Disease
7.2.6 Views on Treatment Methods
7.2.7 Three Levels of Acculturation
7.2.8 Educational Background
7.3 Grounded Theory of Illness Behavior

The field work I performed among the Tibetan diaspora in the Indian mountain settlement of Dharamsala provided me with data for a multidimensional understanding of individual responses to illness among members of this community. I described my exact procedures for data collection and analysis in Chapter Six, "Empirical Research." The core category—namely, illness behavior—was identified during the research process. As I analyzed the qualitative material, which was based on interviews and field notes, certain patterns emerged, along with a number of influencing variables. I was able to formulate and test various hypotheses during this stage of the analysis. A description of these hypotheses follows a discussion of the available treatment methods. To illustrate the material, this section also contains highlights of the interviews with my respondents. These interviews have been transcribed verbatim.

7.1 SUPPORT AND TREATMENT METHODS

The available support and treatment methods were classified into three categories. The first category was the traditional Tibetan system of medicine. A second category, "Paramedical solutions," included alternative or complementary treatment methods, as well as spiritual support and psychological counseling. The third category, Western allopathic medicine, refers to the biomedical model described in Chapter Two, "Health and Illness Behaviors." Both the Tibetan and Western medicinal models were represented by health professionals, all of whom were educated in their respective approach, and who offered their services through public institutions or private clinics.

7.1.1 The Traditional Tibetan System of Medicine

In Tibet, up until the Chinese invasion, the traditional Tibetan system of medicine was the prevailing medical system. In addition to certain shamanistic practices, it was the only form of health treatment available to Tibetans. Most of the doctors lived in the city of Lhasa, and nomads from the plateau usually had to travel for a couple of days to consult a health professional. Due to the severe environmental conditions of Tibet, with its snow-covered mountain ranges, it was difficult to transport a sick person to a far-off physician. Such a trip was often exhausting for the patient. A Tibetan doctor recalled:

> Dorjee, male, age 31: "In Tibet patients went directly to Tibetan doctors because there were no other medicines like allopathy or Ayurvedic. When they have problem, disease, when they want to consult a doctor, they would go on a horse-ride to receive a doctor. In the past in Tibet, we don't have vehicles to travel. We don't have bike, we don't have car. We really have to take the patient—a day's journey, three-days journey on horse, to see the doctor. It was very tiring for the patient."

Another doctor reported that after the Chinese invasion, practicing Tibetan medicine was initially banned and the officially accepted allopathic treatment was only available in largely populated towns:

> Norbu, male, age 40: "Actually, when I was in Tibet we had hard time; we don't have much facilities. There were no doctors around, no injections. When I was child, we don't have any Tibetan medicine. They [Chinese] banned everything—all kind of traditional knowledge, especially Tibetan medicine, also. In

> my area . . . there just one monk in the monastery but the old monasteries were closed. But the doctor who was in the monastery, he wear lay clothes . . . then stay in the village, try [practicing Tibetan medicine] sometime . . . not allow the government to know, they go somewhere secretly and take some medicine—gather some plants, then they give the pills. They didn't told the people."

The delivery of healthcare for Tibetans in exile is much better, however. The traditional Tibetan system of medicine has been preserved, promoted, and developed, due to the establishment of the Tibetan Medical and Astro Institute (TMAI or Men-tsee-khang), under the auspices of the Dalai Lama and the Tibetan Government-in-Exile (Department of Medicine). TMAI is based in Dharamsala and runs branch clinics in most Tibetan settlements across India. (Additional information about TMAI appears in the Appendix under "Medical Institutions").

TMAI is the major institution providing medical services based on the traditional Tibetan system of medicine. Apart from TMAI, there are a few private clinics run by independent *amchees,* doctors qualified in the Tibetan medical arts. In Dharamsala, there are two such clinics: Dr. Yeshi Dhonden's Clinic and the Dr. Lobsang Dolma Khangsar Memorial Clinic, both of which offer diagnosis and treatment according to the Tibetan model.

The diagnostic methods used in the traditional Tibetan system of medicine include visual diagnosis (patient's general appearance, examination of the tongue and urine), pulse reading, and patient interviews. Treatment methods include modification of dietary habits and behaviors, application of medicines (mostly herbal), and accessory therapies (acupuncture, moxibustion, hydrotherapy, humoural therapy, forced elimination, pyretic treatment, and massage). These diagnostic and treatment methods are described in Chapter Three, "The Traditional Tibetan System of Medicine in Tibet and in Exile."

7.1.2 Paramedical Solutions

The paramedical category includes a number of treatment methods that are offered by non-medical, non-professional caregivers. The methods may be divided into four sub-categories:

Home Methods

This sub-category refers to the folk healing methods that Tibetans sometimes use. These methods have been transmitted from one generation to another, and include manual therapy (such as providing massage treatment and setting dislocated joints), or using herbs and other substances believed to have a healing effect (for example, drinking hot water, or inhaling different kinds of smoke).

Shamanistic Practices and "Tantric Power"

This sub-category refers to rituals performed by faith healers or yogis. Some of these practices derive from the Bön tradition; others are connected with the Buddhist path of *vajrayana* and usually involve a sophisticated use of ritual language (for example, the chanting of mantras) and symbolic actions (ritual dance, hand signs or *mudras*). These methods may involve the use of ritual objects: for example, a bell and a *dorje*, a *driggu* (curved knife), *phurba* (ritual dagger) or symbolic offerings. This sub-category also includes elaborate Buddhist rituals for appeasing deities, or relieving the patient from the influence of malignant forces (exorcism). The "tantric power" referred to in these rituals is the transmission of blessings from lamas or yogis, who are believed to impart objects or medicines with their spiritual energy. I was able to observe such practices in a number of monasteries, where the holy men produced pills known as "lama medicine" during lengthy rituals.

Spiritual Methods and Counseling

This sub-category refers to specific religious practices performed by Tibetans to cope with their health problems. These rites may include repeating prayers and mantras, performing prostrations, or making offerings. Sacred offerings may include lighting butter lamps, hanging prayer flags, or donating money to lamas, monks, and monasteries. Circumambulating holy places (*kora*), taking part in pilgrimages, and visiting monasteries are other acts of faith offered to accumulate positive karma and enhance healing. The spiritual-methods category also includes seeking support and divination from lamas, who usually recommend the actions listed above.

Other Forms of Healing

This sub-category refers to a variety of alternative methods that have been brought to the larger settlements from other cultures, and are promoted there. They include various styles of massage, such as Shiatsu, Reflexology, Acupressure, Cranio-sacral massage, Reiki, Pranic Healing, and Tsampa technique. Services and training in the art of the Indian Ayurveda are also provided by a number ayurvedic centers and schools.

7.1.3 Western Allopathic Medicine

Both Tibetan and Indian doctors provide Western allopathic medical services to Tibetans living in exile, through a number of allopathic hospitals and private clinics in the settlements. In Dharamsala, where I performed most of my research, Western medical services are provided by Delek Hospital and

Tibetan Children's Village Hospital. Delek Hospital has a surgical department, a maternity ward, an outpatient clinic, a laboratory, and a pharmacy. A special unit is dedicated to eradication of tuberculosis, while a mobile team provides basic community health services, and an eye-care clinic.

The hospital is managed by Tibetans in exile, sometimes assisted by volunteer doctors and dentists from Western countries. The hospital provides training for Tibetan healthcare providers who work in the more distant settlements; it also offers low-cost or no-cost health services to the needy. The Tibetan Children's Village Hospital is another important source of Western medical services for Tibetans. Inpatient services, including minor surgery, consultations with specialists, emergency treatment, laboratory tests, and diagnostic procedures are among the services provided by both hospitals.

In the Tibetan settlements, minor medical procedures (such as injections) are performed by nurses working at hospitals or schools. Allopathic medicines are available through hospital or school dispensaries and small private pharmacies.

Psychological counseling, a sub-category of Western allopathic medicine, is also available. Both counseling and social support that focuses on mental health and well-being are provided through the Mental Health Clinic at Delek Hospital. Other services provided by the Department of Health include the Tibetan Torture Survivor Program, and the Kunphen[1] Center for Substance Dependence, HIV/AIDS, and HRD, which provides counseling services and health education.

The three types of treatment modalities available to Tibetans—the traditional Tibetan system of medicine, paramedical solutions, and Western allopathic medicine—were registered as coexistent solutions in the respondents' statements. Community support was also identified as an important variable affecting help-seeking behavior.

7.2 FACTORS AFFECTING ILLNESS BEHAVIOR

In this section, I will present and analyze the various factors affecting Tibetans' individual responses to health problems, along with the relationships between these separate factors. The factors to be discussed are: age, severity of symptoms, duration of treatment, availability of treatment, economic effects, idiom of disease, views on treatment methods, acculturation level, and educational background.

7.2.1 Age Factor

In this section, I will analyze the individual response to disease according to the age of the patients. This was found to be one of the key variables affecting illness- and help-seeking behaviors and pathways. In the course of my analysis, a number of patterns emerged, and I will describe them here, paying particular attention to religious methods of coping with illness.

The first hypothesis tested was based on observation that individual reactions to disease differed according to the age of the patients. The Tibetan population was classified into two categories, namely: "the young generation" and "the older generation." There is, however, a degree of arbitrariness and generalization in this classification, as it is difficult to set precise age boundaries for each group.

Statements referring to each group were made according to the respondent's own age perspective. This means that the interview subjects made statements relating to the respondent's own peer group (for example, when a 20-year-old man talked about the young generation), as well as to other age groups (when a doctor in his forties talked about the youth). When referring to the young or older generation, respondents used other modifiers[2] alternately: "The young generation, the young, the youth, youngsters, teenagers, young men/people/Tibetans, students, younger generation, the new generation, boys and girls." The older generation was variously referred to as the "the old, elderly, grandmas/grandpas, old men/people/Tibetans, older generation, older ones, old age people."

Twenty-nine respondents in their teens, twenties, thirties, or forties identified with the young generation. They referred to the older generation as another group of people who were much more advanced in age (for example, when they talked about their parents and grandparents). Five respondents who were approximately age fifty talked about "the Youth," meaning those who were much younger. While they did not really identify themselves with "the older generation," they reported sharing some similar beliefs, as well as attitudes regarding a number of social issues. Although I did not interview any respondents in their late sixties or older, twenty-four respondents of different ages (including nine who were regarded as local authorities) talked about the differences between both generations. Another generalization could be made that the modifier "the older generation" mostly referred to individuals who were born in Tibet, and then escaped as refugees following the Chinese invasion.

Patterns Relating to the Age Factor

Having observed certain regularities in relation to the age factor, I focused on how they affected help-seeking pathways: specifically, decision-making between available treatment options). These seven patterns were as follows:

- Pattern 1: The older generation reveal a greater tendency to ignore the symptoms of disease.

- Pattern 2: Whereas the older generation favor treatment based on the traditional Tibetan system of medicine and home methods, the young generation prefer Western allopathic medicine to obtain quick relief.
- Pattern 3: The older generation reveal a greater tendency to use spiritual strategies to enhance the recovery process or cope with the situation more efficiently. Religious coping is also reported by the young generation, but the younger the subjects are, the less frequently they use this coping strategy.
- Pattern 4: The older generation reveal a greater tendency to use shamanistic methods and "tantric power" to deal with difficult situations; these strategies are much less frequent among the young generation.
- Pattern 5: Neither the young nor the older generation reveal much interest in paramedical forms of healing.
- Pattern 6: None of the respondents report the choice of psychological counseling.
- Pattern 7: Representatives of both generations report seeking support from the community (family and friends).

Pattern 1: The older generation reveal a greater tendency to ignore the symptoms of disease. A number of interviewees (especially doctors) reported a general tendency in the Tibetan community to neglect health issues, to pay little attention to the symptoms of disease, and to avoid looking for treatment. This behavior was more strongly attributed to the older generation, however, and in some cases, this strategy led to death.

> Dorjee, male, age 31: "Sometimes Tibetans ignore disease. The old ones. The old one try to really suppress it and that is very dangerous. In Tibet, if you go back, let's say 50 years ago, you are very macho if you do not express your illness or pain. So, some who are like over fifty, sixty, they still have that kind of feeling. If you cry, you are not macho. So, when they are sick, they try to suppress and ignore. When it gets worse, then it is really difficult to cure. That happens."

> Norbu, male, age 40: "Old age people, they are a little bit uneducated. For example, if they suffer from stomach-ache, like that . . . they think: 'Slowly and slowly it will heal automatically without any medicine.' They neglect and it grows more severe. Then, they go to the doctor's place."

> Tsewang, male, age 30: "I think most Tibetan neglect their health and this is the biggest problem in Tibet. They just suffer, just wait and then it is too late. My uncle for example had a problem with his leg. He had a strong pain and could not walk for many years. He was lying in bed and did not want to see the doctor. After a long time he was once visited by a doctor when he got worse but the doctor said it was too late and my uncle died."

I then made an analysis of whether the young generation would report a similar strategy. Examples of ignoring symptoms of disease were found in this group as well.

> Jigme, male, age 40: "In Tibetan society, lot of people they neglect their problem. They have small pain—they don't care. Same with the disease. They do not care it. They just neglect."

The next step in the analysis was based upon the question: In what circumstances would Tibetans NOT ignore their symptoms; that is, when would they seek professional help and treatment. The reaction to disease was analyzed according to the severity of the symptoms.

Pattern 2: Whereas the older generation favor treatment based on the traditional Tibetan system of medicine and home methods, the young generation prefer Western allopathic medicine to obtain quick relief. I asked most respondents about their preferences in relation to particular treatment models and methods. I also asked them what kinds of methods their friends and family would use, and in what circumstances. Frequently, they reported that the older generation favored the traditional forms of healing: consulting *amchees*, taking Tibetan herbal medicine, and using accessory therapies such as massage.

> Dolkar, female, age 50: "In TCV we have both allopathic and Tibetan traditional medicine, you know. The doctor [*amchee*] comes twice a month and most of the older people prefer to take the Tibetan medicine, not allopathic.

> Dorjee, male, age 31: "When they are getting old, or become chronic, then they of course want take medicine and of course come to Tibetan medicine. So they take medicine for long time."

> Norbu, male, age 40: "Mostly, at Tibetan settlement, all aged people used to come . . . because young people, those who are spending in school, they have their own clinic, dispensary. Western. And old age, they used to come here."

Respondents also reported that the older generation often favored using home methods—even before consulting a health practitioner. Respondents reported a number of such methods, such as manual therapy, drinking hot water for digestion problems, inhaling special kinds of smoke or steam, and using herbs (either collected on their own or obtained from a Tibetan doctor).

> Tenpa, male, age 40: "They have their own techniques. Like passed for generations. Physical methods for dislocated joints. These people help others. They have their own techniques . . . family heritage. Their father and grandfather and

grand grandfather—like that. It is not sure the grand grandfather was a doctor. For the generation of five levels they might pass that. Sometimes, when people have very acute pain in the stomach, or the small intestine, then they use this special folk method . . . hair of goat—they burn it and then smell the smoke. Yeah. This is a kind of folk method of curing such kind of acute pain."

Gonpo, male, age 33: "If someone had fever we would boil hot water and let the person inhale the steam. Sometimes we would use some herbs. I take hot water before going to bed and so that it would keep me warm from inside the body."

Yeshi, male, age 50: "Actually, there are many home methods but in Tibet we mostly used plants. Because we lived in the mountain. Around there are many, many plants. We say: 'Oh, this plant is good for headache!' Normally, when people have headache they think, this is good for headache."

Rabten, male, age 40: "In Tibet most Tibetans saved those things [medicines] from doctor. Because this is like a powder—this herb medicine, so you can keep it for years and years. And because it is powder, it doesn't get bad. It not a liquid [writes down Tibetan names] *norbu dyn thang*—this are the basic medicine Tibetan use for cold, for getting sick, fever, so this is the commonest thing that we use—*thang*. *Thang* is always powder. Nowadays, you can get powder as well as pills. So, based on this, sometimes this comes like seven [different herbs mixed together]—which called *norbu dyn thang*. Then, there is twenty five—*thang chien nye nga*. It means twenty five different herbs [are included in the *thang* powder]. We always have this at our family, mostly. Each time a person get sick, we boil *norbu dyn thang* or *thang chen nye nga* and give them before they go to sleep. Often, when you get a good night sleep with that, it heals you. Because they are given so often, most family knows which one [should be applied in a particular situation] . . . because *thang chen nye nga* [has an] acting benefit for all type of sickness. So [for] any sickness, they try to give you that. So everybody says: 'I'm not well today, headache'—they take *thang chen nye nga*, they have something . . . stomach-ache and they take *thang chen nye nga*. So, it is something that is helping all sort of things. And when they get real things like . . . three or four days of sickness and seems that these things are not helping, we do consult doctors. . . . The common methods beside *thang* is . . . *men drub*. We have like . . . blessing pills. Actually, these blessing pills have little taste of . . . like a citron. So, this is really blessing and it is like a black powder stuff. All lamas—especially *kagyu* and *nyigmas* used to make all the *puja* . . . months of *puja* and they make *men drub* and this is something . . . before they make *puja,* they always put on altar. And if you get sick, Tibetans first take actually those blessing. Often, they will try this. Than, second stage is like . . . *thang*. The third is going to doctor."

Sherab, male, age 17: "Truly speaking, by the previous karma I never been sick now, except some cold. But I don't consider it a sick. I got injured on my feet jumping on nails, but that time I put some snuff and some spider web to stop the blood. This what I did till now."

The younger generation reported a greater tendency to use Western allopathic medicine, and in some cases, showed a marked aversion to the traditional Tibetan system of medicine and its treatment methods. Most reported a desire to obtain quick results, which they believed were only available through allopathic medicine.

> Jigme, male, age 40: "Especially the younger generation. They just . . . they have a headache, they want to stop the pain and they go to allopathy."

> Ngawang, male, age 31: "Some people go to a Tibetan doctor, some to the Indian. The older people prefer traditional Tibetan medicine. The young people want quick relief. They prefer to go to a pharmacy and buy painkiller or get an injection at hospital."

> Sherab, male, age 17: "It wasn't my intention to go the *amchee* for consultation because I am not used to go to them. When I have a health problem, usually I prefer to take Western medicine, even though I know it is side effects. But I don't care of that but I care for fast recover, in which, Western medicine is good for."

I then analyzed why the younger generation were reluctant to use the traditional Tibetan system of medicine and its treatment methods. Many young people preferred to get quick relief so that they would not miss too much school or work. Secondly, some expressed their reluctance to use the traditional Tibetan methods, because they required diligence on the part of patients. The administration of Tibetan herbs, for instance, involves preparing hot water to drink with medicine three times a day. In some cases, performing special "rituals" is required, as in the case of *rinchen rilbus* (taking holy pills at night to keep them away from sunlight). Especially for minor ailments, Western medicine is much easier to administer.

> Thubten, male, age 34: "Younger generation are very busy. They don't have much time to make the water hot every three times a day. You need to take a Tibetan medicine very long time and it takes very long time cure also. It is very hard to eat. You have to eat it after or before half hours of breakfast, lunch, and dinner with hot water."

> Sangay, male, age 22: "Well, I'm gonna choice that [western allopathy], if I had a big pain . . . but some other people . . . I don't know exactly what they are gonna choice. I'm sure that some of my friends take that [Tibetan] medicine, but some is not. They would like to use Tibetan medicine, a lot. They say: 'Oh, this very . . . I need to keep clean.' I don't really like to use Tibetan medicine. Really, I will tell you truth! There is so lot of. I eat every day, every day. After every meal. It is so difficult I can eat that all. So, I usually take the [Western] medicine. I don't like to take [medicine] every day. If I had some problem, the

> doctor gives me this much [Tibetan] medicine for a month. I never take it. For example . . . I never . . . I don't like to use all these medicine."

> Sherab, male, age 17: "With the Tibetan pills you also need to be careful, diligent. I mean you should take them regularly. Sometimes you receive three or four different [kinds of] pills and you take the first ones half an hour before breakfast, then the other ones half an hour after lunch and then supper. If you are busy, you forget sometimes."

A few respondents complained that the herbal remedies were hard to crush and swallow and had a bad taste:

> Chokey, female, age 21: "Till now I can't take Tibetan medicine because it's not tasty. I think because of taste . . . not so good taste. You know, one of our school mate . . . she have a very serious problem, so she take a Tibetan medicine. One day I taste it."

> Kunzang, male, age 25: "I was given Tibetan medicine twice and gave up my treatment after one or two weeks. The doctor said I should take three different kinds of medicine, three times a day (before or after a meal). I didn't like the bitter taste of the pills, which I should chew! The doctor said I should take them for six days and then a *rinchen rilbu* on day seven. The taste was terrible! Then my regular pills for six days and so on . . . for a couple of months. I was not sure when to take them because I didn't have regular meals quite often. On the second occasion I received some *thang* [powdered herbs] for my stomach. I did not want to eat anything, then. I mean, no hunger. I got many bags [sachets] with a sour powder. Every time I took it I really choked. I didn't like the taste."

There were also statements about young people who exhibited fear of the invasive methods used in the traditional Tibetan system of medicine (for example, acupuncture, moxibustion, and the "golden hammer"):

> Norbu, male, age 40: "They are afraid. Lot of old patients, they really like moxibustion very much. They say: 'Can you do moxibustion for me? I have pain!' They are also afraid of some methods, but especially the younger generation. Actually, moxibustion is more painful than the golden hammer. You know, we have special plants to make this moxa. Then we put it on the skin, on the point, then burn it. It goes directly to skin. After finish, it goes 'puff.' It goes burn. It make sound 'pah.' We think, the sound . . . if we've got big sound, then it is good. It will be very healthy, good result. But many young people fear that."

Irregularities in Pattern Two were also reported: there were older patients who sought professional support from the clinics that provided services based on Western allopathic medicine, as well as representatives of the younger generation who consulted the Tibetan *amchees* at Men-tsee-khang and used the Tibetan herbal pills. The Tibetan doctors frequently reported patients who combined both types of treatment methods. A few doctors reported cases in which Tibetans replaced the allopathic treatment with the traditional Tibetan system of medicine if the Western method failed to cure the disease or caused side effects.

> Tenpa, male, age 40: "The young generation go to allopathy, but of course after one or two or three times, they come to Tibetan [clinic]. The old age people, first they take Tibetan medicine. They don't before . . . like Western medicine take."

> Tsewang, male, age 30: "When I was at school I had TB. I first went to the school nurse and she sent me to a doctor. So, I went straight to the Western medicine practitioner. They did some tests, X-rays. I was then taking injections for two months and some other medicine for six months. After that I suffered from a terrible stomach-ache which was side effect of the medicine. That is why I consulted a Tibetan doctor. He checked my urine only and gave me pills. After a few days the pain disappeared. If stomach-ache, most of my friends would advise me to go to a Tibetan doctor even though it may take more time to cure the disease. If you have a eyesight problem for instance, it may take sometimes a year or two to cure it."

The choice of the traditional Tibetan system of medicine by the older people was often justified by their adherence to tradition. Young people, on the other hand, preferred Western allopathic treatment, which many respondents characterized as modern. Additional questions pleaded for answers, for example: In what circumstances do young and old Tibetans combine both treatment options? Is there any referral of patients between the two systems? I also analyzed irregular behaviors, and subsequently identified other important variables that affected the choice of treatment. These were the economic status of the patient, the idiom of disease presented by the patient (beliefs and understanding of the nature of disease), patient's health awareness, and knowledge of the treatment methods available to them.

Pattern 3: The older generation reveal a greater tendency to use spiritual strategies to enhance the recovery process or cope with the situation more efficiently. Religious coping is also reported by the young generation but the younger the subjects are, the less frequently they use this coping strategy.

The spiritual methods described in Pattern 3 involve spiritual counseling offered by lamas and a variety of spiritual methods to cope with disease. For the older generation, tradition and customs strongly influence treatment choices. When the older people experience health problems or need to make important decisions, they are very likely to visit a lama and ask for a prediction/divination *(mo)*. The divination-seeker asks a particular question, and the lama uses two dice with the six syllables of Mañjushri[3] mantra written on them. Often the dice are replaced by a *mala,* or rosary, and the lama will count the beads in a special way to make the prediction. Although this strategy was especially ascribed to the older people, I found examples of such strategies among the representatives of the young generation (in their twenties, thirties, and forties) who also had an experience of seeking divination from lamas.

> Chemey, female, age 28: "When someone is ill, we go to lama. Make offering to lama. Mostly people go for *mo* to see: the Western doctor is good or Tibetan. If I have to go for certain operation, we consult *mo* also."

> Norbu, male, age 40: "Some people who are very religious-minded and some people who have strong faith in such kind of lama and they might have been following such kind of tuition for a long period and they have also experiences of consulting lamas, they will choose to consult lama when they have a problem. Say, there are lot of patients who, first consult . . . when they have a problem, first consult a lama to ask for . . . which kind of system is better for them. OK? And then, after knowing . . . if the lama says, that: 'OK, for you it is best to get treatment from a Tibetan medical doctor,' then he will have another question. Next question is always: 'Which doctor to choose?' He might have some doctors that he likes to consult. So, he might have names: three, four names, or five, whatever. And out of these five, then again, the lama might tell according to divination [using a mala] or dice throwing or whatever: 'OK, this name of a doctor is good for you.' Then, he will consult. Whereas now, at the present, I think . . . I think it is not so common. I think it is not so much being followed as in the past, I think so. So, this is maybe influenced by the Western communities or in our different environment or community."

> Dolkar, female, age 50: "Well . . . older people, I think, they take little bit longer to come to hospital. Because in that case, the cultural belief, you know, take place an important role. Because first, they have to decide, whether to go to a Tibetan doctor or to the Indian doctor. And if you decide Tibetan doctor, then to which one? Because there are choices. And sometimes they have to decide, whether to go to outside—private one, or to a local like us, or to Delek. That depends. I told you. Tibetans have a way of seeking divination, you know. You know *mo*? So, that belief and practice, still exist. They will go to lama and lama will say whether to go to Western or Tibetan and then, whether to Delek, TCV, or to the other—zonal hospital. They will see, which place is more suitable."

She further points out that this strategy often delays diagnosis and treatment:

> Dolkar, female, age 50: "With the cultural beliefs. It's a big hindrance sometimes. Because you cannot diagnose earlier and treat in time. Suppose, if you come early, you can detect, do all necessary test and you can find the diagnosis, get the treatment. Otherwise, you keep deciding which place is more suitable,

which doctor is more suitable. Then, the symptoms will get more serious and you need more expensive treatment and even more expensive tests, isn't it?"

One respondent also reported that apart from lamas, there are cases of lay practitioners offering similar services in the community:

Chemey, female, age 28: "Mostly lamas also doing *mo* because lamas have to do so many mantras, early morning for this *mo*. I've heard that it is very difficult to do *mo*. But lay people . . . there are also some lay people who are doing *[mo]* also. Those who are religious, who do so many *pujas*. They have this skill, that it really goes right. There is one old man, who has been spending his whole life doing *pujas* in every houses. He is reading out a script. He is lay but he spend all his life in everybody's house. I also invite him once in a year for two days. He is really busy. We have to book him two months in advance and . . . he is a little bit dumb also but he has been spending all his life . . . and you will very surprised to see him. He takes that thick script, big *puja*—he is finishing in one day. Now, in small, small cases my mother goes to him also, to do *mo*. His *mo* comes true also. The most important thing is the belief, you know. But in some cases, it goes true."

Another question appeared in the analysis, namely: In what circumstances do young individuals use spiritual counseling, and what variables influence this? I produced a hypothesis, which assumed that seeking spiritual counseling depended on feelings of powerlessness and apprehension, as well as the level of involvement with the culture of origin. Powerlessness and apprehension refers to a state in which the individual experiences a situation as being beyond his or her control. High involvement with the culture of origin, on the other hand, implies better religious socialization and higher familiarity with traditional coping strategies, such as religious coping. The more religious young people are, the higher the probability that they will seek spiritual counseling.

The hypothesis that refers to the state of powerlessness and apprehension has been confirmed by a number of respondents, who said they turned to lamas when they could not find any other solution to a problem. One young respondent reported that he would normally never seek spiritual counseling, but at one point of life he felt so desperate that he agreed to use this strategy. In this, he was encouraged by his girlfriend, whom he described as being a religious person.

Lobsang, male, age 26: "After the doctors, desperately I went to see rinpoche who advised me to do some *pujas* and after done that really helped me a lot, but not fully. I went to the lama because my girlfriend wanted me to. I also thought it might be useful because I also experienced some feelings that I never used to have, such as fear and aggressiveness."

Data from my field observations and interviews also confirmed that people who were more involved with the culture of origin (that is, who lived with their relatives or friends who performed Buddhist practices regularly, and who maintained customs and traditions) were more likely to use this kind of coping strategy at crucial moments of their lives.

In addition to spiritual counseling, most respondents reported using other coping strategies that involved religion. These were believed to accelerate the recovery process, and help them deal with the situation emotionally. While the highest intensity of use of such strategies was reported for the older generation, these strategies were also very frequently reported by the young as well. Many of the respondents made statements referring to religious methods of coping, as a way to find meaning. These methods involved both benevolent religious reappraisal and demonic reappraisal (see RCOPE in the Appendix). In other words, a number of respondents reported a tendency to redefine their disease through religion as being benevolent and potentially beneficial. The concept of reincarnation was common, as well as the belief that it was better to suffer in the present life (and engage in spiritual actions to cope with the difficult situation) than in future lifetimes. Some respondents said they could never be sure whether more favorable conditions for spiritual practice would come again. Many believed that if they managed to endure their misfortune or health problems, simultaneously practicing kindness, compassion, generosity, and patience, their negative karma would be exhausted.

> Sonam, male, age 27: "When I listen to the teachings of His Holiness, he is always talking about love and compassion. Then, I think I would like to become a monk, have no wife, no children. I think to myself: 'Life is so short and we have such a great opportunity. I can practice now and time is running so quickly. Should I waste it on raising children, relationship or the practice?' Only practice. I believe in heaven—*dewachen zhing khang* [The Pure Land of Dewachen]. It is very important to me."

Many perceived their difficult situation as an opportunity for practice and transformation of negative attitudes into positive ones (e.g., anger into patience). Some referred to the practice of *tong len.* (See Chapter Four, "Tibetan Buddhism in Tibet and in Exile," Section 4.3.3. on *Tong-len*.) They said it helped them make the situation of suffering more meaningful and thus bearable.

> Sonam, male, age 27: "Oh, I pray and think: 'I am now sick but there are so many beings that suffer. May their suffering be purified through my suffering.' I send them good wishes. Religion also helps if you lose friends, family. We then

say to ourselves: 'I will die too. Why worry about trying to grasp earthly things?' We should think of what is helpful at the time of death. I am religious."

This strategy was commonly used by both generations. Respondents were also asked about exceptions, that is, if they knew people who would think differently. While none reported any particular cases, some admitted it might be possible among some representatives of the young generation, who lacked religious socialization and were not involved with any religion, and were thought to rely less on religion as a coping strategy. In response to disease, such people were believed to develop anger:

> Tenzin, male, age 28: "If they are not religious and get sick, then they think: 'Oh, why did this happen to me? Others are healthy and happy.' Then, they become more angry, jealous and have more hatred."

A considerable number of statements referred to redefining disease as an act of evil spirits or serpent deities (*nagas*). This strategy was reported to be especially common among the older generation. In some cases such redefinition was presented by a Tibetan doctor or a lama whom the patient consulted. Understanding pathogenesis in terms of affliction by malignant forces presented further options of using spiritual means to cope with the situation.

Many statements frequently addressed religious methods of coping to gain control. Respondents who defined themselves as religious and involved with spiritual practices often sought control through a partnership with a deity. They tried to follow the advice of doctors and lamas: to implement treatment and engage themselves in actions to purify their karma, and so accumulate merits. They were also told to simultaneously rely on the blessing of their favorite deities, such as the Green Tara,[4] the Guru Rinpoche, and others.

> Sonam, male, age 27: "When I am sick, I often think about Dharma, compassion. Every morning I recite the Praises to Tara. She is my girlfriend [laughs]. She is my main one. But the goddess is supreme; you cannot compare anyone with her. Just like Buddha—he was a man who collected merits and because of good karma . . . good practice she [Tara] went through 10 *bhumis* [stages the *bodhisattvas* go through until they attain Buddhahood] and reached Enlightenment. How can we compare ourselves with Tara? That would be stupid to think I am equal to Tara. She is superior. So, you pray and make good actions."

Many respondents reported making offerings to Dharma protector(s).[5] Protectors are the deities who protect Dharma, the practitioner and his or her spiritual practice. There are some very popular Dharma protectors, such as Mahakala[6]—a wrathful, protective form of Avalokiteshvara (the bodhisattva of love and compassion), and lesser classes of protectors—such as Dharma guards,[7] or field protectors.[8]

> Chemey, female, age 28: "Some people offer *sang*. Yeah, it is good. Upstairs here the landlord also does that every morning. This is like . . . a prayer flag. They do offering and say special prayer. That's all for good wishes. Mostly for good wishes."

A considerable number of statements reported that lamas "prescribed" certain religious actions to help sufferers cope with disease. These involved making all kinds of offerings (of butter-lamps and prayer-flags, ordering a *thangka* to be painted, or giving money to the poor), going on pilgrimage, performing certain rituals, or repeating particular prayers. If an individual was unfamiliar with a recommended practice, he or she could offer money to monks or nuns, who would visit the home of the sponsor and pray, read scriptures, or perform a *puja*. In other cases, they did the rituals for the sponsor in their own monasteries or nunneries.

> Chemey, female, age 28: "I was not well for months . . . when I was not well and feeling not happy, then I just go to a lama for prediction, for a *mo*, because I am a little bit believing in religion. So, I went for prediction and the *mo* didn't come well—in the *mo* rinpoche told me that, you know, the *mo* is little bit not good . . . He just used dice and then read *pecha* [scriptures]. So, rinpoche said that: '*Mo* is not good. If you do all these pujas it is really good,' he said. I have got long list. But these *pujas* are really big *puja,* you know, that I can't do myself, you know. Even I'm not good in doing all this *puja*. So. . . . I. . . . we offered money to the monasteries to do prayer. So I did all that. I spend about five thousand rupees. I also went to *link khor* [path around the temple] to put prayer flags, and whitewash all the *link khor*. Whitewash—it's called *kuka sul*. It is something like a *stupa,* that we have to white-wash. When you go down *link khor* there are so many stones. . . . I did all white-wash. People do like this. Whatever it is we just whitewash. Make it clean. For purification. So, people . . . mostly do that when it comes in *mo*. In *sava dawa* people do like that for their own. When I did that I purify my karma. But you know, whenever I pray, I don't pray for myself. I always think like: 'People like me, who have same sufferings, please help'—like this. Because I know, we can't pray for us, you know. And that doesn't help for me. I always pray for people like myself—[so that] they don't have suffering like me. Like this, then I feel much. . . . Like when we go around temple, pray, I always pray for *sem chen tham che* [all beings]. It is always better . . . it feels for me much more helping. I always do. So, I did all these prayer offering in a week. Whatever I can do, I have to do. But the big *pujas,* we offer it [money] to *gompas,* to see the date, good date according to hour *lobta*, you know . . . horoscope . . . they do the date."

Certain forms of religious activities were typically ascribed to the older generation—for example, sitting in meditation and turning prayer wheels while repeating mantras. Many respondents also referred to grandmas and grandpas circumambulating the temple with small prayer wheels. The young people were hardly ever observed with prayer wheels. Nevertheless, representatives of both groups (irrespective of age) were seen counting the beads of their *malas,* which might imply they repeated mantras silently. It might also have been a habitual behavior. Elderly people were also seen doing prostrations in front of the temples, while fewer young people performed this practice.

Some made statements about representatives of the older generation who performed religious actions daily, hoping to attract favorable conditions, wealth, and good health. They did not necessarily need any encouragement to engage in these activities—it was natural and customary for them. The intensity of these behaviors increased when they faced life challenges or disease. Respondents in their thirties or forties also reported using religion to cope with disease, but the intensity of these practices varied, with some using the strategies more often than others. Some reported that it was natural for them to use religious methods of coping in which they copied their parents and grandparents. Statements about the representatives of the young generation in their teens and early twenties suggest a lower frequency of using such actions. But exceptions were also found in this group, as with young respondents who frequently used religious coping behaviors.

Further Hypotheses

My analysis of the material led me to a further question: What other variables might affect levels of involvement with religious methods of coping? I then made a hypothesis that assumed there was a positive correlation between high levels of involvement with religious practices (including religious methods of coping with disease) and high levels of involvement with the culture of origin. On the other hand, low levels of involvement with religious practices would have a positive correlation with high levels of involvement in the host culture, as well as exposure to Western culture. Involvement with the culture of origin would also imply increased religious socialization.

Some individuals reported their complete surrender to the power of Buddhas, bodhisattvas, and protectors at periods of challenge or disease. I found that this was particularly true of monks, irrespective of their age. Some of them refrained from seeking help from health professionals and hoped that the higher power would guide and heal them. Many respondents believed that they could receive the blessings of the Buddhas, bodhisattvas, and protectors by praying to them directly, or through lamas and rinpoches—particularly those who were regarded as highly realized, because they are believed to channel the stream of blessings. Here is an example of a monk who had problems with his eyes:

> Jamyang, male, age 28: "I had problems with eyes. Very serious. I was afraid I become blind. I had pain and could not see well. It was worse and worse. I do not go to doctor. I prefer to ask lama advice. I went to lama and he said special *mynlam* [prayer] and puffed air into my eyes. Lama did that several days [running]. I pray and visited him every day for some time and problem disappeared. I prefer to see lama. Through blessing of the Lord Buddha I become healed."

> Sonam, male, age 28: "You know, I smoked a lot. I smoked two packages of cigarettes a day. I went to H.H. Dalai Lama, kneeled and said: 'I want to stop smoking.' He gave me his blessing and I have not smoked for months ever since. I also want to give up alcohol. I drink just a little bit from time to time with my friends. But I think it is important to socialize with friends sometimes. I have very little free time. I work most time of the day. In my free time I study."

A degree of active surrender (see RCOPE in the Appendix) is also expressed in one of the most common and fundamental Buddhist practices, namely Taking or Going for Refuge. Respondents reported that both the young and older generations, who used religious methods to cope with disease, usually searched for comfort and reassurance through the benevolence of Buddhas and bodhisattvas when they were in distress or experienced life challenges such as disease. Tibetans of all ages referred to the deities for support, strength, and guidance, while making offerings, repeating mantras, or circumambulating holy places. They believed in the presence and guidance of their protectors. Even though this strategy was less common among teenagers, they still used it at critical moments. For example, while the young people reported fewer health problems, they would visit monasteries and pray to Buddhas and bodhisattvas before important school exams.

Individual Image of the Buddha

In general, respondents perceived enlightened deities as benevolent, manifesting "the four immeasurables"—immeasurable love, immeasurable compassion, immeasurable joy, and immeasurable equanimity. Equanimity referred to sharing equally and unconditionally, with love and compassion. In other words, enlightened beings were believed to be impartial and to regard and treat all sentient beings as equal, irrespective of their behavior.

Many of those interviewed perceived Buddha as a supreme being. They said he set an example for them, representing a human (just like them) who practiced the meditation path and finally attained buddhahood. Buddha embodied a state that the faithful aspired to achieve. Yet respondents differed as to their personal image of Buddha.

Respondents reported that activities like praying, repeating mantras, and sitting in meditation helped them divert their minds from personal problems and achieve a more peaceful state. Physical actions such as performing prostrations, turning prayer wheels, and using their *mala* beads to count mantras also had a beneficial effect.

Many respondents claimed that religious methods were important to them for coping with psychological problems, such as symptoms of anxiety, depression, or emotional crisis. Not a few of the younger respondents said that religion let them experience a sense of connectedness with higher forces. It also let them connect with other Tibetans, helping them to maintain their Tibetan identity. For these young Tibetans, religious activities helped them alleviate feelings of loneliness, and of distance from family members left behind in Tibet:

> Sonam, male, age 27: "I think religion is very important. Tibetans are known for religion around the world. When His Holiness travels he always puts his hands like that [makes the praying gesture and bows down] and talks about religion. If we lose this part of our culture we will become like all the other refugees."

Representatives of both generations reported using "religious purification," if they considered their diseases and other types of suffering in terms of negative karma they had accumulated. These individuals also reported using confession as a means of purifying the mind, sometimes accompanied by a special prayer. In a number of cases, Buddhist practitioners were taking vows to strengthen their commitment. Such vows could be taken individually, by making a promise in front of a symbol representing the Three Jewels, a statue or painting of Buddha, or in front of one's teacher; or else in a group. Many *pujas* performed at monasteries included confession and taking vows as part of the ritual.

During a public teaching, one of the rinpoches explained that in order to make confession meaningful, practitioners should use the "four powers": 1. the "power of renounce" (regretting previous harmful actions or misdeeds); 2. the "power of refusing to repeat a harmful deed" (making a resolution to avoid repeating unvirtuous actions); 3. the "power of rely" (on Taking Refuge and developing *bodhicitta,* which refers to developing an Enlightened Attitude, that is, a wish to attain liberation and buddhahood for the benefit of all beings); and 4. the "power to carry out all types of remedial wholesome acts to purify harmful ones."

Most respondents related the teachings of Dharma to all aspects of life. Those aspiring to be good practitioners of Buddhism made an effort to perform virtuous actions and abandon harmful activities. The perspective of achieving Enlightenment and investing one's energy in spiritual practice helped them cope with poverty, ailments, and other sources of distress.

One of the students reported that maintaining a strong faith and thinking of His Holiness the Dalai Lama helped him cope with imprisonment in Nepal for illegal immigration. At this time, he was also experiencing health problems. When we met for the interview, I asked him a provocative question, to see what the Buddhist tradition meant for him: "What would you say if I offered you a visa, and a nice place to live in the West, where you would have a nice car, a girlfriend, and whatever else you needed—but you would have to trade that for your culture and forget about the teachings of His Holiness the Dalai Lama." His response was:

> Sangay, male, age 22: "What!? [laughs]. This is very difficult question [laughs]. Actually, I really like money, because I need it for the living, but. . . . I don't know actually [laughs]. No, I'm sure I can't do that. Really. That means I am not Tibetan. Believe nothing religion. I don't know . . . maybe some crazy people would do that. Besides, even I don't know how to give you that question. That means . . . if you're gonna say that . . . you will give me building, car, money . . . everything I want . . . Yeah?. . . . But forget my family, culture. Yeah? And His Holiness, Dharma . . . forget it? [thinks]. No! This really. I think nobody would do that. I don't think so. I don't know. I tell the truth. I like car, building, everything, but . . . His Holiness forget . . . it's a little bit difficult, you know. I'm sure I'm gonna be choice His Holiness Dalai Lama. [I asked him why.] Erm. Precious . . . human life. You know . . . His Holiness and . . . this is the spiritual leader for all the people. Almost people can die for His Holiness and Dharma. I am sure they can die. They never think about property. If you're gonna die, you can't take this building, money, to the heaven or hell. So, even if we stay here, listen to His Holiness, make more prayer, and also *pujas* . . . then we can get result. Like . . . I do this *puja* . . . I don't wanna go to hell. Like that. If I've got lot of money, building, and I don't care [about] this, 'Kill this!' [points to something as if it were a living being], OK . . . give you money . . . 'Kill this! Do that! Do that!' You know, at this life I've got lot of result, because I have money, I have car, I have building. But when I die, I can't take it to any place. And *puja,* like this, result I can take to future life."

Next, I analyzed what variables affected the intensity of using religious methods and spiritual counseling, for individuals of both generations. First of all, I observed that there was a relationship between the tendency to use spiritual counseling and religious methods and the duration of the disease. There was also a relationship between these spiritual health behaviors and the effectiveness of the treatment applied—to be discussed below.

Pattern 4: The older generation reveal a greater tendency to use shamanistic methods and "tantric power" to deal with difficult situations; these strategies were much less frequent among the young generation.

Respondents described a variety of healing methods that the medicine men and women employed, and a few reported their direct experiences with these shamans. In some cases, they characterized the healer's behavior as frightening; for instance, when he or she was making strange sounds, screaming in a trance, and dancing with a *phurba* or a *driggu* (two types of ritual knives). Jane (age 58) recalled a situation in which she visited a Tibetan medicine woman known for her shamanistic practises. The medicine woman shouted at her: "You are all demons! Evil spirits!" She then went into a trance, in which she claimed to be possessed by a certain deity. Then she started screaming at the patient, listing a number of evil actions the patient had done in her previous lifetimes. Next, she bit the patient and began spitting out blood (even though she did not harm the patient), and then danced with the *drigu.* The patient was both terrified and confused. After this session, however, her health improved.

While the use of these types of practices were ascribed to the older generation, there were also cases of young respondents who had some experiences with faith healers. One of them explained that his choice of this strategy was strongly influenced by his elderly mother, as he did not himself believe in the effectiveness of such treatment:

> Sonam, male, age 30: "When I was very much sick. Swelling . . . eye, and I couldn't get my arms like this [shows he is trying to lift them], so I have myself treated with Chinese medicine like injections, antibiotic medicine, everything. . . . I took them two weeks but it doesn't work. Then, my mother . . . my mother is very religious, very much religious. And she took me to a . . . not a doctor. Just someone very much experienced in people . . . not a doctor and not a lama. Like a yogi. You know *ngakpa*. Someone like that. Then I went him and of course, I had suspicion. I think . . . maybe, if he is really good enough to treat me, to cure, to recover this kind of disease, but . . . anyway my mother insist me to go there one day. Then he did just, you know, butter . . . mix butter which . . . is said to have the blessing of his . . . something like that. He put . . . applied butter all over my arm, and said some prayers. It was really funny, to be honest. I though: 'How can that work?' He . . . doesn't give me medicine, no any other treatment. Anyway, he said: 'OK, once you come to me, you are not allowed to take any medicine—whether Tibetan or the Chinese. OK?' 'OK.' I was worried a little bit. If I don't get medicine, I was afraid it might get worse. Anyway, I

went there for three days. Early in the morning. After three days, it's completely recovered. Even there is not any cut left. It seems like nothing happened. Three days, no medicine, no any other treatment, just like that."

Another respondent described traditional beliefs relating to unfortunate deaths, and how Tibetans coped with such situations:

Ngawang, male, age 31: "We call a lama, Rinpoche and ask him to perform special rituals. We give offerings. There are different offerings. If someone dies on Sunday, we believe it is very unfavorable. Additionally, according to the Tibetan astrology there are special bad days. The black days. Then we have to perform special rituals. Lamas would buy heads of certain animals. If someone died on such bad day three heads were needed. They would bring heads of camels from far away, from abroad, but they would never kill an animal for that purpose. If no head is available, they would use *tsampa*[9] and write on a piece of paper the name of the animal. That would symbolize the offering."

Further Questions

My analysis of Pattern 4—that the older rather than the younger generation reveal a greater tendency to use shamanistic methods and "tantric power" to deal with difficult situations—led to further questions. These included: Under what conditions might young people also use this kind of coping to deal with disease? What other factors determine such choices? I created a hypothesis that assumed a close relationship between the ways of coping with disease and the effectiveness of the treatment applied, the idiom of disease, and the degree of involvement with the culture of origin.

Pattern 5: Neither the young nor the older generation reveal much interest in paramedical forms of healing.

While the availability of a number of alternative or complementary treatment options was observed in Tibetan settlements, no respondents reported ever using such methods. Two of the young respondents had learned massage and offered it to tourists as a way of earning money. They did not have any special qualifications, however. The lack of interest in these complementary or alternative forms of treatment was explained in terms of money—these were paid services, generally addressed to Western tourists and beyond the means of most Tibetans. But the Tibetans would occasionally share these services amongst themselves:

Wangchuk, male, age 28: "Well, most of the clients are people from the West. They have money for that. Massage centers became more and more popular here. Tibetan massage. Reiki, Ayurveda. I don't know Tibetans who use that. I mean, I do not any who go to the centers but if they know massage they can help each other. I help my friend sometimes and he gives me some massage too. Not often."

Pattern 6: None of the respondents reported the choice of psychological counseling. Information on using this strategy in the Tibetan community has been provided by the counselor from Delek Hospital; however, none of the respondents themselves claimed that he or she had ever used this kind of support. Dolma (female, age 31) who worked as a counselor reported that patients of all ages, suffering from both mental and somatic disorders, sought help at Delek Hospital's Mental Health Clinic. Hospital nurses referred some of these patients to the counselor, following an initial health-screening interview. They also might be sent to counseling via the "Reception Center"—an office where new refugees registered upon arrival to Dharamsala.

Dolma, female, 31: "The nurses . . . when the patient comes they will ask: 'How do you feel? Do you have cold? Cough? Fever?' Maybe check for what reasons he is having that. If he says: 'I have nothing but I am getting headache,' first time, maybe they will give a pain-killer and next time when they come, if they find out he has some tension . . . has got tension headache, then they will ask me to look."

The most frequently reported psychological complaints were symptoms of depression, anxiety, and somatic disorders. There were also cases of Post-Traumatic Stress Disorder:

Dolma, female, age 31: "Many are anxious, stress. For example, we have many cases in Soha School. Young boys: 22, 23, 24, 25 [years old]. They are depressed because they have no family, language problem, no money. Family bonds seem very important to Tibetans. They try to cope: play basketball, they go to talk to the friends, or just . . . [try] to forget."

She also stressed the lack of health awareness in the Tibetan community, irrespective of age.

Dolma, female, age 31: "Depression very common. The problem of our Tibetan community is they are still not aware of mental disease and . . . most of them come with a somatized complaint: 'I have a headache. I have a back pain.' They never say that 'I am unhappy,' or 'I am depressed,' or 'I am anxious.' Some say they don't have emotions, just tension and headaches. When we say health problems can be connected with emotions, they say : 'No, no, no. I don't have any emotions.' Big problem in our community. Because they don't see. The emotion is there, they get this headache and back pain . . . they think this can only come from physical disease. So, when we give a training or when we go to settlement, I always give talk to our community. Like . . . any disease can come from your mental . . . or any tension, or worry, or stress, so you can get any physical problem. One thing is they are not well educated . . . like they have no idea. That disease can come from that and they are suppressing. When they worry or they are in tension, stressed or . . . how to say . . . they don't see the importance of expressing, telling people that 'I am feeling upset,' 'I am feeling unhappy.' They just keep that in themselves."

The counselor acted as a social worker as well—she visited her patients at their homes and checked whether they took their medicine.

Dolma, female, age 31: "I am not only a counselor. I am doing all the social works. Check to the patients. Schizophrenia patients. Check, whether they are taking their medicine or not. How many medicine are left. If the family is not able to buy, then I have to go to buy."

Pattern 7: Representatives of both generations report seeking support from the community. Apart from using religious methods of coping, other coping strategies were also identified in relation to disease. These involved seeking comfort and reassurance from family and friends. A few respondents reported that Tibetans generally liked to share their concerns with others, and to ask for advice (despite a tendency to maintain an image of someone who is serene, brave, and self-dependent). The influence of the support group can thus be regarded as an important factor affecting the process of choosing between available treatment solutions.

Sonam, male, age 28: "If someone has problems, we all meet. All family meets and discuss what we can do."

Norbu, male, age 40: "They would openly share about the problem with somebody and get some ideas about where the treatment could be received and which treatment could be better for oneself. Choosing a method is mainly due to the public influence and education also. So, if the public have more understanding of the particular example . . . like a diabetic, for example . . . they might have a lot of friends, Tibetan friends, Indian friends or Westerners . . . they normally tend to . . . [seek advice] Of course it is a habit to talk about problems."

Yet the same respondent also reported topics (usually related to sexuality) that were avoided, particularly by the older generation. Tibetans were less open to discussing and sharing these issues among other members of the community.

Norbu, male, age 40: "Here, in India or particularly in the Tibetan community other than AIDS, we would share. AIDS is a difficult topic and . . . different disease also. I would say . . . normally people . . . and of course since they are educated they know that it . . . they would be infected in . . . somehow, somewhere . . . so if they say they have AIDS, they will be . . . they will face a lot of problems in the community. [I asked him: "Is it because it is associated with sex?"] Sure, of course . . . of course . . . now we are going from one question to . . . somewhere else . . . erm. . . . AIDS could be infected in different ways. I have already told you that lot of Tibetans, educated youngsters are working in the exile government or offices so they have lots of education and general ideas of what this kind of disease is and how it could be infected, and how we can prevent and avoid this kind of problem. So, there is of course . . . if somebody lives together with AIDS patient, in a family or in a community, there is of course some chances. Sometimes, even if one is very careful of oneself and if someone uses the same . . . or whatever, it would infect the other person—by accident or unknowingly. So, there is always a chance of getting infected from somebody who is already infected. So therefore, AIDS is a different topic. Whereas other than AIDS we would share. Tibetans they would love to . . . I mean not that they would love to but . . . they would openly share about the problem with somebody and get some ideas about where the treatment could be received and which treatment could be better for oneself."

Some statements described individuals who isolated themselves and refrained from sharing their problems with other community members. Instead, they would use religion as a coping method—by trying to establish an intimate relationship with a deity through the practice of meditation, prayer, or mantra recitation.

Jamyang, male, age 28: "I do not like to show [my problems; smiles, looks shy]. Sometimes, I talk. My friend's father died and my other friend was to tell him. This monk cried and cried and the other monks said after some time: 'There is no need to cry, we must all die, crying will not benefit him. You should better do some prayers.' Then we performed a special ritual. We made offerings, many butter lamps. When I was ill, I prayed and meditated."

Bhumsang, male, age 23: "Sometimes, when there no money I very sad. Then go to mountains. Alone. Sometimes talk to friend. Better go to mountains alone."

Some respondents reported that the religious methods helped them find direction in life and cope with feelings of sadness, emptiness, and solitude.

7.2.2 Severity of Symptoms and Duration of Treatment

In this section, I will analyze individual responses to disease, including help-seeking behavior, according to the severity of symptoms and duration of treatment. In their statements, most respondents juxtaposed two properties in relation to disease: acute versus chronic. According to Western medical science, the term "acute disease" refers to high intensity of symptoms and short duration, whereas "chronic disease" is characterized by long duration of symptoms and often (but not necessarily) milder intensity. Many diseases are classified as chronic, even though the severity of symptoms is high (for example, many cases of cancer, respiratory problems, or heart disease). But the Tibetans' frequent use of this pair as opposites implies that the interviewees associated chronic conditions with both prolonged duration of disease, as well as milder intensity of symptoms. For this reason, the term "chronic" will refer to both of these qualities: mild and long-term.

To begin with, acute/chronic states will be placed along the same dimensional continua, that is, intensity of symptoms. Inasmuch as it refers to symptom severity, "chronic" will be replaced by the label "mild." Apart from these two main properties, other modifiers have also been distinguished: "acute conditions, severe, serious, strong, life-threatening, mild conditions, not strong, not serious, bearable." The respondents automatically classified particular complaints into one of these categories. For example, the property "acute" was ascribed to conditions including injuries, acute pains, severe lung diseases (tuberculosis, asthma), cardiac diseases (hypertension), jaundice, hepatitis, epilepsy, food poisoning, and diarrhea. The property "mild" (which replaces "chronic") referred to common colds, headaches, or minor pains.

With respect to the duration of treatment, two properties will be listed: brief and chronic. "Brief" refers to situations in which evident recovery could be obtained within a relatively short period of time. Here, recovery is understood in terms of the elimination of pathological symptoms, as in the biomedical model of medicine. "Chronic," on the other hand, will refer to cases in which recovery could not be achieved and the symptoms of disease are still present. It characterizes conditions experienced by patients over a longer period of time (for example, rheumatism, skin diseases), and requiring more time for treatment. In many cases, complete recovery is never achieved.

Patterns Referring to Severity of Symptoms and Duration of Treatment

The analysis of both factors (severity of symptoms and duration of treatment) produced patters that will be presented in this section:

- Pattern 1: When the severity of symptoms is high, Tibetans are likely to use Western allopathic medicine; whereas with mild conditions, they are likely to neglect it, use home methods to cure themselves, or seek help from a Tibetan *amchee.*

- Pattern 2: Western allopathic medicine is usually recommended for diseases of short duration, and the traditional Tibetan system of medicine for chronic diseases.
- Pattern 3: Cross-referral is often practiced by doctors, and a combination of the two treatment methods is often recommended to patients.
- Pattern 4: When recovery has not been achieved in the expected time frame, Tibetans may use para-medical solutions.

Pattern 1: When the severity of symptoms is high, Tibetans are likely to use Western allopathic medicine; whereas with mild conditions, they are likely to neglect it, use home methods to cure themselves, or seek help from a Tibetan *amchee.*

It has been reported that Tibetans tend to choose Western allopathic medicine in case of acute problems or life-threatening diseases . Many young respondents admitted that they were interested in a quick recovery, and thus frequently used modern allopathic medicines to reduce the symptoms of disease. If they suffered from intense pain, they chose a pain killer:

> Chemay, female, age 28: "We go to Western doctor if it is really serious or unbearable pains are coming, then we go. Then they have . . . it is frequent [to use a] pain-killer or injection, you know. Tibetan medicine doesn't have like . . . strong effect. For certain, certain illness, like headache, or something, then go to Western doctors. Because it is the on the spot condition that they can deal."

> Norbu, male, age 40: "If it is serious and sudden I think I might go to Delek Hospital [Western allopathic] or see any Indian doctor. . . . My parents would probably choose the traditional Tibetan medicine. They prefer the natural methods and have great faith in that medicine. If I had a very strong headache, for instance, I might first take a pain killer and then go to see the Tibetan doctors if the problem comes again."

> Dorjee, male, age 31: "If the problem is more serious or acute I think I would visit the Western medicine practitioner first. I could then see the Tibetan doctor."

> Jinpa, male, age 28: "To be very frank with you . . . I consulted [a doctor] only one time in my whole life. It was a general checkup and the doctor told me my problem correctly. That time I consulted Tibetan allopathic doctor. . . . Tibetans usually consult *Men-Tse-Khang* in small illness and chronic diseases. When there is serious and needs urgent attention, they consult allopathy, private Indian doctors."

Patients reacted differently when the symptoms were mild—that is, when the illness was not serious enough to stimulate them to seek professional treatment. In such cases, they reported a tendency to neglect the symptoms, as described in the previous section with respect to age.

Nyima, male, age 27: "When I get some headache or little fever or cough, I never used to go to doctor or even bother taking medicine. I used to think like this . . . you may call it orthodox . . . if I take less medicine by now, then when I get serious problem one day, the medicine will be more effective . . . but at the same time I never let the small problem grow old by not taking care of myself . . . I used to think positive all the time."

Other strategies for coping with mild symptoms involved the patient's own resources, such as home treatments, or paramedical solutions like "holy pills":

Chemey, female, age 28: "Some people when they have, like . . . food poisoning also, we took that religious pills. It is very good, you know. At home, you know. This is the hope medication. People take pills. Then, if it is not good or is getting worse, then we go to doctor."

Nyima, male, age 27: "I often have a cold but I don't take any medicine. I just end up [in bed] . . . till recover itself, I use hot water. Using drugs for small disease . . . is not good for health, so I don't use any one of them. . . . It is best . . . not drinking cold water and keeping yourself warm . . . if it continues more than a week . . . I use light medicine only . . . only after the checkup."

Finally, many would seek professional help from the Tibetan *amchees* if the home methods proved ineffective. They would visit Men-Tsee-Khang, or any of the private clinics, and go through the traditional diagnostic procedures, obtaining herbal pills or other therapeutic instructions.

Jigme, male, age 40: "So, here, in exile countries, people who have chronic disease, like *rLung* disorders and other chronic disorders of bile and phlegm, used to come directly to Tibetan doctors."

Chemey, female, age 28: "Tibetan people, when they have illness, suppose like jaundice, long time illness . . . *mkhris pa* [bile][10] or something happened, like *pokha* [stomach pain]—gastral, intestinal problems . . . for that, they really consult Tibetan doctor. They consider that it will purify. "

A number of respondents reported that they used Western medicines initially to cope with severe symptoms and eliminate danger. Afterwards, they would visit a Tibetan *amchee.* This shows a sequential application of various coping strategies according to the severity of the symptoms. Some respondents also expressed their resistance to Western medicines, as long as the symptoms were bearable. If they could not cope with the condition any more, they would use allopathic medicines for a short time, until they obtained full or partial recovery. Combining Tibetan and Western Medicine was frequently reported. Some replaced the Western allopathic treatment with the natural herbal remedies:

> Norbu, male, age 40: "If I take an example of myself, generally if I have a headache . . . if it's very, very severe and very severe headache and I cannot bear the pain, then I would choose to have a painkiller at the moment. I would choose a painkiller and I would consult a Western medical doctor at that period. But not for a very long duration. If I am having a headache within some intervals—within a week, within a month, then I would rather choose to take Tibetan medicine. With mild headache, personally I would not choose to have a Western medicine, because I can bear the pain. It's not something I cannot bear and the main reason why I am not choosing to take Western medicine is, we try to abstain from taking Western medicine when they have pain like this one's, because we know that this kind of medicine will effect—in other way round. Even if it helps to reduce the pain, subsides the pain, whatever, then the other way round it might harm to have problem with digestion or like that."

Exceptions to Pattern 1

Exceptions to Pattern 1 emerged in which several statements referred to individuals who suffered from acute conditions and sought help from the traditional Tibetan system of medicine, despite having Western allopathic medicine available to them. Yet such tendencies were only ascribed to the older generation, who normally expressed a very strong adherence to tradition (including traditional forms of treatment). They also exhibited more resistance to acculturation and assimilation. Subsequently, they resisted forms of treatment other than the ones with which they had been familiar.

Another exception to Pattern 1 was presented by one of the respondents, who resisted seeking any professional support when he suffered from serious liver problems. Instead, he claimed that he had decided to rely on his own powers of healing. In general, this young Tibetan (born and educated in India) presented strong tendencies towards marginalization: alteration of the original and new cultural practices to create his own unique entity.

> Gonpo, male, age 33: "I was very close to death when I got very sick with liver. I got jaundice. Jaundice is like . . . liver problem—enlarged. Maybe I was drinking too much and eating lots of fats, animal fat. So, I became very sick, but I don't believe in medicine very much. I mean, yeah, I do believe but . . . I do believe more in myself, you know, the self-healing part. I think that's more powerful. So, at one point, maybe it was the worst of that particular period, that I had to go to death stage. Liver enlarged and I was like . . . feeling bad and then . . . meditation. I meditate, then . . . not every day—I mean at that particular period. . . . So like . . . this disease doesn't go out of the sudden. It doesn't come out of the

sudden, go out of the sudden. . . . Never . . . only in accident. Disease comes slowly and goes slowly, if it does. So, it went up, and up [deteriorated]. Maybe it has to go to this extent [makes a scaling movement]. And then . . . beyond that, maybe I would have died. It stayed there and then at that particular moment I was contemplating death. I said: 'Yeah, maybe this is finally my last time and I'll die.' You know! But I was not scared because I believe in rebirth. I knew that I would come back . . . 100 percent, you know. I had strong vision in my mind, and then . . . thinking that, I was meditating on this . . . and then next moment I don't remember. It was a long, good sleep. Then from then on I started to go better, better and better, because . . . when I realized I was getting sick, then I control my food, no oil, no fried things . . . dieting . . . now I go normal. I don't drink anymore, now. I never used to smoke, anyway. I don't eat much fat. I do eat but not as what I used to. I used to . . . was eating chunks of fat, and in fact . . . I was not willing but I was invited . . . you know, so I do not want to make that person unhappy not eating that chunk, you know. So what happened was . . . it was required by this disease . . . and in that point I didn't die. I went into a nice sleep and it started to reduce, come slowly down. I didn't go to doctor. My friends did not see me for many days. They came to me and knocked on my door and say: 'Gonpo, this is not a good idea!' But . . . then I washed every day and go to the market . . . slowly, slowly. . . . I do shopping, I know what I need to eat. Then like . . . very light, boiled rice . . . like a porridge—very light. No, other things, just very light. So . . . when you have enlarged liver, it takes the space of your stomach. So, you are not so much hungry. So, I knew these things. Then I knew, when I could not eat much at a time, I need to eat several times a day. So, I used to eat six times a day. Little. . . . So, because of all these things together, it completely gone. And my friends came to my house and said: 'Gonpo, we are taking you to a doctor!' I was very unwilling. But they forced me. So, I did not want to make them unhappy, angry or sad, so I said: 'OK, fine." But if doctor gave me a prescription and they buy any medicine I was not going to eat anyway. So, I went. We went by taxi. That day it was doctor's strike day. There were no doctors. I was very lucky. I was very happy. I believe in my mind and the karma. And my karma has to be like this. The doctors went on strike."

Pattern 2: Western allopathic medicine is usually recommended for diseases of short duration, and the traditional Tibetan system of medicine for chronic diseases.

Dawa, male, age 30: "For temporary matters, if we sick, like temporary, Western medicine is quite good. But if you still sick for a long time, it is better to take Tibetan medicine. Like . . . Western medicine cure out sickness very fast, and very easily. But if long time it cannot sometimes cure the root. If you take Tibetan medicine, it takes time but you will be, like . . . completely recovered."

Pattern 3: Cross-referral is often practiced by doctors, and combination of the two treatment methods is often recommended to patients.

Tibetans are encouraged to use their common sense and choose between available treatment methods according to the nature of the symptoms. In some cases, however, doctors may suggest to the patient that he or she should use a different form of treatment where it seems more appropriate. For example, patients who suffer from severe hypertension and seek help from a Tibetan *amchee* may then be referred to a Western allopathic doctor:

> Jigme, male, age 40: "Sometime we ask. Especially for acute hepatitis, we say: 'Oh, please, you should go this . . . and you should take this medicine. You go to take Western medicine.' We refer the patient."

> Tenpa, male, age 40: "Sometimes we would advise the patient to have the Western medicine or go to a Western clinic or hospital, and just to receive the treatment from their medical, hospital or whatever. I would say . . . in the case of . . . like sometimes severe asthma. When somebody is being attacked by asthma, at the very immediate period it is very important that she should go and have the quickest means to relieve that problem. We wouldn't . . . it is wrong for the patient to wait for the Tibetan medical doctor to receive treatment. At the very immediate period he has to go to a Western medical doctor. Similarly, there are lot of other diseases when we need to have an immediate relief . . . you see, like brain . . . somebody is being having a severe . . . accident. Of course we have to go and receive immediate [help] and . . . he needs to have received emergency treatments, care, whatever. There are lot of other diseases which we can say . . . for example TB. [For] tuberculosis . . . it is best to receive Western medical treatment. Normally from my personal experience, I would say patients should receive medicine from a Western clinic. Specially for that bacteria . . . acid . . . bacillus. That bacteria needs to be removed or cleaned through that [allopathic] medication. At the same time we can also advise a lot of Tibetan medicine to heal his liver, the lungs, and also to have good sleep and to gain a lot of energy. There are a lot Tibetan medicines, which can be used complementarily."

> Dorjee, male, age 31: "We have to think about the patient, what is best for the patient. Not, what is best for one's own system, to get fame or name or whatever. So therefore, we have to tell the patient that, for instance: 'For you it is best to receive the treatment from the Western medicine . . . like a doctor or hospital. At the same time, if you take this and this kind of [Tibetan] medicine, it will help to get quicker relief and you will be relieved in a . . . I would not say shorter duration. Of course, in a better way. You can combine both.' The main thing is that we don't talk about comparative medicine but combined treatment. So, we say like . . . right now if we have work to be done, I know that if we combine—you and me together to do that job, it would be much better, than handling by yourself and myself. Similarly, there are lot of other systems of medicine. They have their own potential. So the thing is that we have to think about the patient. This is one of the main principles in Tibetan medicine, that we have to. . . . There are certain vows for the Tibetan medical to follow. Vows to be accepted as a Tibetan medical doctor. We say that we have to be very compassionate, very loving, very

caring for the patient. So, if we think only about gains, or fame, or name and whatever . . . other things that are related with our own happiness and feeling, rather not for the patient, that is wrong. It's a wrong concept."

Norbu, male, age 40: "They have this option: Tibetan medicine or allopathic Western medicine. The younger generation are very good in that [knowing how to choose]. This time not only younger people like that. Also the old age people. They used to come to Men-tsee-khang first, and then go for check—each and everything. And, if it is little bit serious, like that, we advise him to go for check to the allopath system, pathology . . . whatever they do: ultrasonography, scanning, blood check and then give, show me the report. And through the combination they [allopathy doctors] also used to go like that. What they diagnose, from our diagnose . . . if it was equalized [confirmed], then it was very easy to treat the patient. Some of the case it is very easy like that: 'I am suffering from stomach, pain over here, headache, nose running,' or just small cases. These are the things they go for option like that. Sometimes, they used to go for quick relief to the Indian doctor place [allopathy]. Those who want to take our medicine, slowly and slowly . . . but what they used to say: Tibetan medicine, after taking our medicine, it will clear up from the root. So they used to come. And for our advice. If there is any necessary, taking any other medication, then we give advice: 'Let's go further. You go for allopathy system, you go for check-up and everything, and then bring a report, whatever the doctor has given.'"

Combining Western allopathic medicine with the traditional Tibetan system of medicine is officially promoted by doctors, health institutions, and the government.

Yeshi, female, age 50: "We always have to tell the patient, that depending upon the problem of the patient, and depending upon the severity of the disease, we can advise to the patient: 'OK, you can receive first Western medicine for . . . maybe six months." OK?' Or, whenever he is much better. Then, to fully remove the disease, or fully energize or make really healthy he can receive lot of Tibetan medicine, which we say that it has minimum side effects."

His Holiness the Dalai Lama (quoted in Lobsang Tsultrim Tsona and Tenzin Dakpa 1981) states: "Tibetan medicine is far more advanced in the understanding of the nature of mind than Western medicine. In matters of understanding the physical functioning of the human body, the Tibetan medicine . . . is less advanced than the Western medicine. Without mixing the two approaches, and without saying one is better than the other, both schools should work together in order to find ways of understanding each other and thus boost the effectiveness of the two healing techniques."

Tibet's Department of Health (part of the Government-in-Exile) has issued a brochure on healthcare, in which they state: "The two systems of medicine run in parallel to each other and are used equally by the refugees; there is also a referral process between the two health care systems. [In case of mental problems:] References are made to Indian psychiatrist and follow up care is provided by the health workers."

Pattern 4: When recovery has not been achieved in the expected time frame, Tibetans may use para-medical solutions.

In many instances, respondents reported situations in which neither Western allopathic medicine nor the traditional Tibetan system of medicine could produce any positive results. In such cases, patients often experienced worrying thoughts, and attributed their problems to supernatural causes, negative karma accumulated in the past, the evil eye, or other baleful influences. As a result, many of them consulted lamas, yogis, or healers. If the lama or other respected person confirmed that the disease was "karmic," or inflicted by malignant forces such as evil spirits or *nagas*, they would also advise performing special rituals. The advice from lamas was often based on divination (*mo*). As one of the Tibetan doctors pointed out, spiritual support from a respected guide and performance of rituals played a significant psychological role:

> Tenpa, male, age 40: "Also . . . especially those people who are very chronic disease. They take allopathy and Tibetan medicine and still there is little improvement, then they go to high lama to ask him something, then they check what is wrong and what they should do. Then after, [doing] some prayer or some *puja* . . . [and] after taking medicine . . . some really good result. Also, this because of the doubt of the patient . . . I mean the patient have lot of doubt for the nature, for doctor, surroundings. If they got this kind of problem, then if they do *puja,* they think it's OK. It is really . . . actually . . . before the medicine is working but still they have doubt. If they did some prayer . . . of course the prayer will give a lot of energy. Of course, first they come to . . . take medicine, see the doctor, then take [it] for a long time medicine, then after not so good result, they go to lama and check, ask what is wrong. Lama often tells them to continue this medicine and do this and this *puja.*"

Tibetans are often encouraged to use their common sense and knowledge of symptoms to choose between available methods of treatment. But this produced another question: How do Tibetans know which method is effective for treating particular symptoms? In response to this question, I made a hypothesis, which assumed that those who were more educated could make such decisions more skillfully. I also observed that help-seeking behavior was significantly influenced by the support group (family and friends).

7.2.3 Economic Effects Factor

The economic aspect of Tibetans' lives is one of the factors influencing their help-seeking behavior. Many Tibetans in exile still find their life conditions to be challenging. Although the unemployment rate is high, they are reluctant to work for the Indians. Instead, they may engage in production and trade in the food-service business—running restaurants, or making and selling dumplings *(mo mo)*[11] through small stalls. They may produce handicrafts (woollen garments, carpets, jewellery, *thankas*), or offer services (massage, dressmaking and tailoring, teaching school, working at hospitals or clinics). Many of them are self-employed or run family businesses. Some become very effective and successful. They may own big shops, restaurants, or hotels, and have established international trade connections.

The young, school-age Tibetans, along with the elderly, have been reported poorest. In particular, those living in remote settlements often suffered from extreme poverty. Monks and nuns also represent this part of the community who have limited chances to obtain money to sustain themselves. Even though some individuals or groups of monks run small monastery shops or restaurants to earn money, most of them are dependent on the monastic institution and resources provided by their families.

Because medical treatment requires money, those who are economically underprivileged may refrain from seeking professional support as long as possible, if they are not provided with free-of-charge medical services. Most respondents considered Western allopathic medicine expensive and reported using this method only when absolutely necessary—even though it provided instant relief, as compared to the slow-working, and cheaper, Tibetan herbal remedies:

> Tenzin, male, age 28: "When they are ill, there is just more suffering and more problem with the money. There are lot patients who cannot spend money for treatment. Lot of expensive medicines. . . . Some operations or treatments . . . you have to pay a lot for the problem to be treated."

> Dolma, female, age 39: "Apart from difficulties and adaptation problems . . . we have some patients who also get depressed because of physical problems. They get physical disease and in the monastery, when they are monks, they have to pay by themself and these people don't have money and they have to study very hard, they cannot take care of their body. To go to hospital they have no money. And this don't get better."

Special insurance was granted to students, who were provided with free-of-charge medical treatment by the school nurses and doctors. They could also obtain medicine from the school dispensaries.

Sangay, male, age 22: "We have to pay [for treatment in institutions outside the school] but Transit School[12] people—they don't have to pay. They have health paper. I have it, too. For six months I don't have to pay. I can use it for six months only. When I came here I had so cough. I was thinking: 'Oh, what's happening!?' Then, I've been to Delek Hospital to make . . . x-ray . . . and gonna check everything. And doctor said: 'Everything is good. Nothing is problem. Your health is good.' Then, one time I went to this . . . Men-Tsee-Khang. You know? We've been there and even I don't need to pay it. I don't need to pay for registration. But if I didn't have this paper, I have to pay, it's a lot of money . . . I cannot go to other hospital, because I need to pay money. These two [Delek Hospital and Men-Tsee-Khang] are part of exile government, so I don't need to pay it. So, that's why I chose."

Respondents characterized the traditional Tibetan system of medicine as a relatively cheaper healthcare solution. In Men-tsee-khang, which offered traditional Tibetan medical services, patients paid about 100 Rupees for consultations. But this clinic offered discounts or free-of-charge services to those older than 65, to monks and nuns, and to students. Patients also had to pay for herbs prescribed by the Tibetan doctors. While this was economically challenging to some people, it was still cheaper in comparison to Western allopathic medicine. Thus, Tibetan Medicine was particularly appreciated by those who had less money.

Dawa, male, age 30: "There were certain times that I have taken Tibetan medicine and I found that it is cheap which was very good for everyone. I agree it has effects but is very slow."

Norbu, male, age 40: "Younger people, those who are spending [time] in school, they have their own clinic. Dispensary—like that. Western. And old age, they used to come [to Men-Tsee-Khang]. Because we used to run our Men-Tsee-Khang Clinic each and every of the branch. So they are coming and those who are above 65 age, we are distributing free medication for them. Suppose . . . those who are monks, students, they are giving consultation rate like that. For the students, it is difficult to get money, those who are monk, they can't survive, can't get a money for everything . . . like that. Those who are aged people, they can't do a work by themselves. So, for them we are giving [medicines] free or consultation on that line. And those who are affordable, we are charging [them for the] medicine. This how the charity goes like that. Mostly, at Tibetan settlement, all aged people used to come."

Sherab, male, age 17: "There is homeopathic and Tibetan [clinic] and I usually see most of the monks and older people refer Tibetan and those having good money prefer taking homeopathic."

Dolkar, female, age 50: "We have to pay for this consultation, as well as for the medicine. But I think [in Men-Tsee-Khang] they have a special budget for people who cannot afford, you know. Then . . . I think they give them free [medicine]. Especially, like for nuns, monks and older people, you know. From older people . . . they don't take money for the medicines, only for the consultation."

Considering the above, the economic effects factor can be regarded as one of the important variables influencing help-seeking behavior. Those who struggle against material problems may tend to choose treatment solutions that would not significantly reduce their budget.

7.2.4 Treatment Availability Factor

The availability of certain forms of treatment is another factor affecting help-seeking behavior. In places like Dharamsala, most of the available solutions could be accessed. I made the hypothesis that people would tend to choose the treatment solutions that are the most readily available to them, and thus, easy to utilize. In the case of school children, for example, seeking help from a school nurse or doctor can be regarded as convenient as well as affordable. So, their choice of Western allopathic medicine is easy to understand.

Sangay, male, age 22: "To be very frank to you, I consulted Tibetan Men-Tse-Khang doctor in 2003 . . . only one time in my whole life. It was a general checkup and the doctor told me my problem correctly. You know, Tibetans usually consult Men-Tse-Khang in small illness and chronic disease. When there is serious and needs urgent attention, they consult allopathy, private Indian doctors. In 1995 I also suffered TB . . . first year in college . . . that time I consulted Tibetan allopathy doctor. We have a Tibetan allopathy hospital in our settlement, so naturally we consulted that hospital and doctor present there was specialized in TB."

There are also some institutions that offer treatment through both the Western and Tibetan models of medicine—for example, the Tibetan Children's Village Hospital. On the other hand, there are schools where Tibetan Medicine is regarded as unscientific, and so no services based on this model are provided.

Thubten, male, age 34: "No lecture in Tibetan Medicine in our school. It is not scientific. It is very old tradition, practical and it may helpful to some, but it may also harm to some. Before two years back, Tibetan Medicine is ban in Switzerland, because they found something in one Tibetan particular pills—*ngul chu* [Tibetan: *dngul chu*; English: mercury]. You know Rinchen Ratna Shamphel—very powerful Tibetan medicine pill. Expensive also. There is *ngul chu*, silver water [in it] . . . that silver water is poisonous."

While ease of access increases the likelihood that the Tibetans will use a particular treatment, other important factors shape their decision-making process. One of the most crucial is the idiom of disease.

7.2.5 Idiom of Disease

My analysis of the qualitative material revealed that the idiom of disease is an important factor affecting help-seeking behavior. This category includes the local disease categories (general beliefs about the nature of diseases shared in the community) and explanatory models (notions about a particular episode of disease held by the patients and practitioners).

Respondents reported that they acquired knowledge about the nature of disease from different sources, two of which were most significant: 1. health education at school, via public talks given by doctors or nurses; and 2. from experience transmitted via the support group (family and friends), who openly shared common beliefs and superstitions about illness. A number of factors were recognized as potential causes of disease:

1. Imbalance of the three humours in the body
2. Accumulation of negative karma
3. Supernatural (malignant forces)
4. Psychological disturbances and stress
5. Biological causes

As described below, certain help-seeking behaviors were associated with a given explanatory model.

Imbalance of Humours

The concept of the three bodily humours, or *nepas,* has already been discussed in Chapter Five, Section 5.4, "Fundamental Concepts of Tibetan Medicine." Respondents often referred to them when they talked about health problems. For example, when someone suffered from symptoms of depression or anxiety, it was often associated with the disturbance of wind (*rlung*). In these cases, methods based on traditional Tibetan medicine would normally be included in the prescribed regimen. The patient might take some herbal medicines (usually kept at home) or visit a clinic, where after a diagnostic procedure, remedies or other forms of treatment would be prescribed by the *amchee.* Advice on modifying dietary habits were often given, as humoural imbalance was often attributed to improper nutrition.

> Tenpa, male, age 40: "In the society, you will find that most Tibetan people seem to have hypertension—means . . . maybe due to the diet, you know . . . because we butter tea . . . high intake of butter and oily things. It could be due to heart or whatever."

Accumulation of Negative Karma

The Tibetans also understood illness in terms of karma. According to the Buddhist philosophy, everything can be perceived as a result of good or bad imprints in one's mind. This was expressed by one of the respondents:

> Tenzin, male, age 28: "I always think about karma [laughs]. Maybe, because of my bad karma or I did that. . . . Not blaming on others. It is just superstitious that we blame. It is not good."

On the other hand, some statements referred to conditions that were specifically "karmic." The Tibetans believed that diseases in this separate category could not be cured by means of medical treatment, but only through spiritual methods.

> Phuntsok, male, age 40: "Well, if someone has been ill for a long time and nothing, no treatment could bring any relief we may think it is because of the person's karma accumulated since beginningless time or evil spirits. So, quite often the person may visit a high lama who can tell what the cause of the disease is. In many cases, where no medicine and doctor could help lama may perform a ritual or advise on sponsoring a special *puja* and then the problem may disappear, the patient may fully recover."

Understanding the causes of disease in terms of karma was also referred to as a useful coping strategy. It let the patients give meaning to the challenging situation, and create a feeling of control. They could then incorporate a number of spiritual methods into their regimen.

> Tenpa, male, age 40: "Well most of them . . . elderly Tibetan understand the law of karma. So, we know it is our karma. We have done something and so . . . we learn to accept it. But accepting does not mean ignore: 'OK, I deserve sickness.' We will try to find a method, any medicine—Tibetan medicine, Western . . . to overcome."

For many respondents, religion was characterized as an effective coping strategy. Those who could not apply it experienced emotional problems:

> Lobsang, male, age 26: "There are some people who are religious and some who are not. If they are not religious and get sick, then they think: 'Oh, why did this

happen to me? Others are healthy and happy.' Then, they become more angry, jealous and have more hatred."

Tashi, male, age 30: "We do not feel, like: 'Why me?' Or we do not get angry like at the God or something. 'Oh, why are you punishing me?' We have no feeling like that because it is our karma. So, the younger ones, especially those who are born like . . . in the West, Europe, America, they can go in the same way like Western society: blame—'Why me?' or something like that. Or maybe they think that God has punished. This is really when you don't have knowledge of the laws of karma. That happens. And also, when you believe that there is a creator. Because, when you don't believe in cause and effect, when you get sick (like a cancer), then you think: 'Why am I sick? There are millions of healthy people but I am sick. I cannot cure myself. I must be the worst person in the world and I do not deserve to live because God thinks I am that bad.' They are so angry. They have to have so strong anger, to destroy themselves. It is not out of joy they are destroying themselves. This anger comes from not understanding the laws of karma. They think, that someone has effected that sickness. So, the law of karma . . . if you believe in it, you know it is your karma, not really . . . it's your doing. And then, what remedy should I do . . . because you are also the one who cultivated, so you need to purify that. You have to work hard. So, by knowing the law of karma helps you to accept the suffering. By accepting, of course the suffering will not go away. Cancer will not go away but the intensity of suffering is less. Because your are not angry, you have accepted it. This is my karma—you know. So the intensity is lesser."

When the causes were understood as karmic, special spiritual methods had to be incorporated into the treatment. Patients usually sought support from lamas, who gave clear instructions on how to deal with the problem. These often included paramedical solutions, such as those described in Section 7.1.2.

Supernatural (Malignant Forces)

The Tibetans often understood the pathogenesis of disease in terms of influence of malignant forces, such as evil spirits, *nagas,* and ghosts. Pathak (2003) writes: "It was believed that the causation of ailment was due to the effect of supernatural intrusion or possession by ghosts on the morbid person which was responsible for the imbalance of body constituents. The tradition of various types of offerings to appease the angry deities or nature worship such as sun, moon, stars and so on was the only resort for the curing of ill-health in Tibet"(p. 46).

Ghosts are believed to be entities who failed to obtain a better rebirth, due to their attachment to worldly possessions or an unexpected death in anger. *Nagas* are serpent deities, powerful beings who are believed to take the form of frogs or snakes and inhabit forests or other wilderness lands. Some spirits may be visible to the human eye, while others are not. It is believed that when their abode is violated, they can inflict harm upon people. Violation is usually attributed to open air defecation or urinating into streams and ponds where the spirits reside. Diseases attributed to malignant spirits are thought to be resistant to medical treatment, and require alternative, spiritual methods:

> Yeshi, male, age 50: "There may be some diseases caused by evil spirits. The skin diseases most of all. . . . There are different kinds of spirits and ghosts. If someone died suddenly, unexpectedly—like in an accident for instance—he or she may become such a spirit if very much attached to the worldly possessions. They may feel they do not belong anywhere and become more and more frustrated. If they felt harmed they may be angry and wish revenge. Sometimes, we also violate the peace of certain formless beings. We may disturb their place—Tibetans often pee into rivers or streams or cut trees. If a spirit inhabits such place it may get angry. If the person's vital energy is weak then the spirit may be powerful enough to inflict harm or possess the person. I heard many examples of people who started behaving strangely. Only after a special ritual was performed they recover."

Belief in ghosts was reported as being quite common in the Tibetan community. Even young respondents shared a number of beliefs: for example, that one should not whistle in the evening as it attracted ghosts. Some, however, spoke more critically about these beliefs:

> Pasang, female, age 50: "Ghosts? No, no. We are modern but ghost we not, not, we now modern. All people say ghost, ghost, if stomach they say ghost, some evil spirit. Little old people they maybe ghost think or evil spirit." [However, I could not resist a feeling that my respondent was anxious about being ridiculed by a Western scientist. When I asked her whether she herself believed in ghosts, her response was: "Maybe 1 percent, maybe believe. Otherwise, hmm. . . ."]

Tibetan doctors claimed they could determine whether the patient was affected by a spirit. For this purpose they either used urine diagnosis or pulse testing. Certain behaviors also indicated that the patient could be possessed.

> Jigme, male, age 40: "Evil spirits are very common and I also met such patients. Pulse is very much different than in normal people. Like in our case the pulse is very . . . like . . . round but in their case it's very flat. Those cause diseases caused by evil spirits, pulse is very flat and then very flexible. So this is very much true in general in Tibetan community that diseases are caused by the evil spirits. Diseases which are caused by the evil spirits are called in Tibetan in the medical *kun brtags gdon nad*. So this disease cannot be cured by Tibetan doctors. It has to be asked for a lama, for spiritual performance. So, *kun brtags gdon*

> *nad* is not to be cured with a Tibetan doctor. The cause of disease is related with the evil spirits. So, once people, when they have such sickness caused by the evil spirits, then, they have to be . . . asked to the lamas or rinpoches or they have to be . . . do spiritual things like . . . give their life for the spiritual . . . like sometimes they also wearing different clothes as they used to wear previous time. Like sometimes they wear before yellow, sometimes totally black, sometimes even shave hair. These are such rituals for those, cause evil spirits."

Phuntsok, male, age 40: "My relative had a certain skin problem—it was some kind of rash, pimples from the palm to elbow. When she would get better, her husband would develop same symptoms and then their children. Again and again they would suffer from the skin disorder. She consulted the Tibetan doctor and took medicine with no results. Finally, she went to the Venerable Tenga Rinpoche and asked for *mo.* Rinpoche did the Dream *Mo* [divination using conscious sleep]. He then told her that she has recently got a wooden box elongated in shape and red in color. The wood which the box is made of came from a tree that belonged to a certain being, which is now angry for having his home place violated. Rinpoche advised that she should offer it to someone. First she said it was not possible because she could not recall any red wooden box but Rinpoche was very sure about it. So, she searched and searched in all her house for the box but could not find it. One day she noticed a box with incense in her shrine room. She had already forgotten about it. It was made of wood and painted red. She brought it to Rinpoche who recognized it. He said: 'Yes. It is the box I was talking about.' When she finally got rid of it the symptoms disappeared in all family members."

A number of respondents told stories about possession by spirits. Most victims were young girls:

> Tenpa, male, age 40: "One time, when I was studying here, Tibetan medical, there was one woman. She was not nun. And that time she got that disease . . . I mean not disease. This spirit came on her . . . like . . . possessed. So, then . . . Actually, I thought: 'Oh, she is doing something wrong.' She is pretending by herself, I mean. I really thought. Then, every night we went to look after her. All the students—boy students. They changed every night. Because I am a monk I thought I don't want to go there. So, few days I didn't go to visit her even though all the students have to go there. Then, one day the class teacher asked some students who didn't came to look after her to come . . . all the students one by one. Each in small groups.
>
> "So, one night I went there and on my first day like . . . I looked after her with four other students, and then out of four . . . others they rest for a while, take a sleep next to the girl who was possessed by some other spirit. So, that night . . .

like . . . suppress by someone . . . like . . . I know there was something but I did not see. Suppress . . . I couldn't stand up. Somebody suppressed on me and then I was thinking that: 'Now, I am dying.' Also I had pray a lot to free from that. I could not speak or read mantra by myself.

"But I'm imagine. All this, this, this by myself. But still not so power. So, I though I might be dying. But then, afterwards, you know . . . I really . . . I didn't though that . . . the statue of Guru Rinpoche in the main temple . . . it is very similar . . . I mean, I think it is same statue like this but very small . . . immediately I saw it in that moment . . . when I saw it like that in one moment, then I got kind of power, but still not . . . wake up. Then I got power from that image, small image of Guru Rinpoche. Then, I got power but still, I can't speak out. And then I was . . . kind of dream. But still I was, kind of fighting.

"Fighting with this [speaks very expressively]. As I was fall from the bed, and then . . . like something happening . . . like fighting with that spirit. . . . It was not a dream but like dream. Not like that we sleep and have dream. I was fell from the bed, still I was fighting with that spirit. I got like . . . his arm . . . one of spirit arm here and his feet here and pull the hand of spirit very strongly. Then I pull this and then I broke the hand—the hand of spirit. Then, I felt: 'Oh, I am sorry.' *Nying je*—[compassion]. I felt very kind . . . sympathy, that I had broken than hand. Deeply I thought: 'Oh, I am sorry, sorry.' I released this hand. My . . . like imagination, I saw an unclear picture of . . . kind of human figure but I could not see proper features. Then it get up and got out. It closed door behind him. Then I got like . . . was very much deeply believe in that spirit that she got some . . . possessed by spirit. I felt very sorry for her. Then she get better, because she went to His Holiness and His Holiness advice . . . she should go to Kamdro Rinpoche . . . there is another Nyigma Rinpoche. He is recommend. She got advice that: 'You should go to Kamdro Rinpoche' and get initiation from him and do practice. After she did, then she . . . problem gone and after she become a nun. Nicely . . . she is in Lhadak."

In his book about beliefs and superstitions, Norbu Chophel (1983, p. 27) explained such events: "Many Tibetans complain of having been 'pressed down upon' by a ghostly spirit at night in their sleep. It is not necessary that this should occur only during the night, it can also happen in the day time. A Tibetan says that he has been pressed down by a ghost at night when he had a dreamy feeling of someone exerting pressure on him and trying to strangle him. In such cases the person experiences great difficulty in breathing and struggles violently in sleep." Another respondent presented a different example of possession:

Ngawang, male, age 31: "There was a boy in my school. He behaved strange. Sometimes, he would lose his consciousness a few times during a day. Sometimes, he threw stones at his friends, called them names. It lasted for some time. After some years one lama said it was because of the evil spirits and advised him to go back to Tibet. He did not, however. No doctors could help him—neither Tibetan nor Western."

A few respondents also reported a common custom in Tibet of making offerings to all kinds of deities and family protectors. Upon arrival in exile, these activities were sometimes abandoned. It was commonly believed that unenlightened spirits could get angry if offerings rituals had been stopped, and as a result of this they manifested obstacles. One monk-respondent said that he suffered from an acute stomach problem, which his spiritual guide attributed to the effect of a powerful being called *Shug den*. The monk had established connection with that deity in Tibet, when he was unconsciously repeating the deity's mantra. Later that connection was broken and the respondent believed he was experiencing the results of it:

> Tenpa, male, age 40: "This often happens. Also for me. First time I came here [to Dharamsala] I had pain. I had stomach problem and I got very sick. Afterward, it was not so good result. Then, I went to one Rinpoche and he says: 'You should not. . . .' Actually, there is one deity in Tibet. Is known in Tibetan society. That deity has become big problem. You know . . . *shug den*. It make big problem. When he [Rinpoche] asked me: 'Did you connect with that?'—high lama asked me. Because, when I was child. Not child—like 18, 16 years [of age], a lama taught me . . . actually I didn't know what it is . . . this lama [in Tibet] told me: 'You should read this sometime.' He gave me some words. It also . . . one word was about this *shug den*."

When the problems were attributed to supernatural causes, most patients used paramedical solutions. They usually sought advice from lamas and performed (or rather sponsored) religious actions. In case of spirit possession, special rituals were usually required. In some cases, help from the yogis or faith healers was also used.

Psychological Disturbances and Stress

Some doctors referred to psychological conflicts as important components of disease and potential causes. However, none of the respondents viewed stress or other emotions in such terms. On the other hand, they did recognize disease as a stressful reaction.

> Dolkar, female, age 50: "You can have headache. We should be able to differentiate what kind of headache they have. What could be the most possible cause. Some headaches . . . you cannot fight. Even if you give analgesics, you may not get better. Like, suppose you have tension headache, I don't think medicine will help, isn't it? You'll have to change your attitude, your way of thinking."

> Norbu, male, age 40: "I would include all the different conditions, when I have a [health] problem. Sometimes, when I have work tension on some problems, or whatever. Then according to that problem, according to the hectic time schedule, very stressful, no rest, then . . . I would give the reason that it may be affected due to stress or work problem."

Tension and traumatic experiences were also recognized as potential causes for mental and somatic problems. Very often the tension would be repressed, or barely expressed. Health professionals understood the symptoms that subsequently emerged in terms of somatization.

> Dolkar, female, age 50: "Like some people have gone through, gone through Chinese repression, you know. Torture. Then you come to Dharamsala or to India and you can't speak the local language, you can't get a job. It's difficult, isn't it? It's natural that people feel stressed. Then some get sick."

> Dolma, female, age 39: "The problem of our Tibetan community is, they are still not aware of mental disease and most of them come with a somatized complaint: I have a headache, I have a back pain. They never say that: 'I am unhappy' or 'I am depressed' or 'I am anxious.' They just complain about the pain."

If the patient or the health practitioner acknowledged psychological disturbances or stress to be the key factor in pathogenesis, the patient was often referred to a counselor at the Mental Health Clinic. In some cases, a consultation was provided with an Indian psychiatrist, who prescribed Western psychiatric medicines. Patients were also encouraged to use the traditional methods of coping, which were mainly focused on religion. They often consulted lamas and performed a number of paramedical practices, at the lama's instruction.

Biological Causes

Some respondents understood the causes of mental illness from the perspective of modern Western science (for example, as being caused by a biochemical imbalance). One of the health practitioners talked about a depressive patient. She admitted that her medical allopathic training influenced her understanding of the depression, and for this reason, it differed from the explanatory model of her patient:

> Dolkar, female, age 50: "Since I am trained in the allopathic line, you know, my concept of thinking is a bit different. I think it does affect sometimes . . . brain. Patients often say *rlung*. That's very common [laughs]. Imbalance, all that. This is more in the Tibetan traditional medicine, you know. *rLung* means you get more . . . how to say in an allopathic way . . . more of temper. This is when we

have people [who are] more self-centered. Your ideas or whatever you do is not appreciated or accepted by your peers, or friends, or colleagues. Then people feel irritated, or you feel rejected, isn't it? During such times you get more upset, you may get more of what to say . . . negative emotions, isn't it? So, for such things, I think there people say: You have more *rLung*."

When respondents understood disease in terms of biological causes, they frequently referred to modern allopathic science. This was usually the case with ailments such as colds or food poisoning, or contagious diseases like tuberculosis. In these instances, modern allopathic medicine was the treatment of choice; if the disease was unrecognized, the patients might seek spiritual advice:

Lobsang, male, age 26: "Mostly, when we are sick and the sickness is obvious sometimes, like if you get a cold, you can go to hospital and get medicine and heal it. But sometimes we were ill . . . like unrecognized sickness, we ask lamas, what kind of things we should do, what is wrong. Then the lama will show you, will give advice, what kind of things you have to do."

The respondents may have failed to mention other explanatory models of disease. For example, Norbu Chophel (1983) described a number of superstitions related to health. One of these is that disease can be caused by "human mouth" (usually associated with people's envy): "If people talk much about you, whether in criticism or praise, a curse known as *mi-kha* (literally meaning 'human mouth') falls upon you and you become sick, or a similar misfortune befalls you. In the case of a child, the same belief applies even more seriously: many children die from the effects of *mi-kha*" (Norbu Chophel 1983, p. 8).

Jacobson (2002) pointed out that lay and professional understandings of medicine were distinct, even though closely related. His observations revealed that patients often used illness names and simplifications of the classical theory in their discourse. These simplifications were based on explanations provided to the patient by the *amchees*. A good example of how the patients' explanatory model affects help-seeking behavior is presented below:

Lobsang, male, age 26: "Even I had a small, like . . . spirit harm. We used to piss everywhere, you see. In a spring. We used to pee near that and sometimes my organ [penis] swells. And when I go to lama, he say: 'This is harm of *nagas* because you did something wrong.' So, they would tell me to do this prayer and I do. But also . . . I may have some . . . like, I may have slept with another woman who may have some problems. If that . . . I think, if that is cause, then I should go to a doctor. It depends . . . "

The next step in my analysis aimed at investigating factors that affected the idiom of disease: in other words, what influenced the patient's understanding of the nature of disease and its causes. I hypothesized that acculturation level and educational background (also affecting acculturation) would be among the most crucial determining factors. I also believed that the same factors would influence the patients' views on treatment methods, as described below.

7.2.6 Views on Treatment Methods

For this segment of my analysis, I asked healthcare professionals and patients for their views about treatment methods. Both groups had comparable opinions and often used similar phrases to express their attitudes. For this reason, I made the hypothesis that the attitudes of the healthcare receivers were shaped by the authorities, such as doctors, nurses, and schoolteachers. The respondents reported that public talks on health education were frequently held in the Tibetan settlements. These talks were usually given by the allopathic doctors, the *amchees,* or the nurses, who explained the causes of various diseases, as well as the available treatment methods. In some cases, Tibetans were instructed about how to assess the severity of their condition and choose a method of treatment, and advised about which treatment methods were most convenient for them.

Most respondents characterized Tibetan medicine as safe, natural, gentle, and as that which roots out the real cause of the disease and produces no side effects. On the other hand, it was characterized as working slowly. Some pointed out the fact that it required taking many pills, which they said were difficult to carry, chew, and swallow. Tibetan medicine was reported as better for diseases that were chronic and not too severe. In cases of acute health problems, severe pain, or life-threatening diseases, most Tibetans relied upon allopathic forms of treatment, which they saw as fast and effective. But many respondents were cautious about the potential side effects of allopathic medicines:

> Chokey, female, age 21: "I think that most of old people take a Tibetan medicine because I told you before Tibetan medicine it's good for health not so much acid like Western medicine because it is made of herbal. So mostly they take those medicine."

> Özer, male, age 54: "For [Tibetan] medicine I am not trained to practice but just sure medicine I eat. No side effection, not chemical, so it is good for health. My wife [takes Tibetan medicine] also."

> Chemey, female, age 28: "Tibetan medicine works slowly to purify all disease, you know."

Dorjee, male, age 31: "We enjoy Tibetan Medicine because the side effects of herbs is almost zero. Some [people] also like, Western medicine—they work fast [snaps his fingers]. Tibetans medicines are very slow, but we say that eventually, it works best."

Norbu, male, age 40: "The Western medicine is not so good. I mean it is quick and you can get the relief quickly but you cannot get rid of the cause. Tibetan medicine is much slower but it is natural and helps you balance your whole body."

Sherab, male, age 17: "All the people . . . my mother, father, grandmother, grandfather . . . they normally take Tibetan medicine. They say, generally it will work very well. But this medicine [allopathic], like Chinese medicine works really fast, but still you know, some make problem. They [older people] usually check Tibetan medicine. But the young generation, they say: 'Oh, Tibetan medicine, this is so difficult to carry them. There are so many of them.' They do not know, which to take today, which tomorrow. So, they like Chinese medicine."

Tashi, male, age 30: "The Western medicine works fast but the Tibetan will get rid of the real cause of disease."

Dolkar, female, age 50: "The Western medicine is very expensive sometimes but it work fast. It is good for emergency. They also have good diagnostic tests. Very good equipment. But sometimes there is no need to do so many tests."

Dolma, female, age 39: "Young people like Western medicine? They think it is modern."

Norbu, male, age 40: "They [Tibetans] know that this kind of medicine [allopathic] will effect . . . in other way round. Even if it helps to reduce the pain . . . subsides the pain, whatever, then the other way round it might harm to have problem with digestion or like that."

Sangay, male, age 22: "Yeah, [Western allopathy] it's fast! I heard that the Tibetan medicine effect is so slow—I heard it from the doctor. But I studied nothing on health, nothing. The doctor say: 'If you take this, the effect is so slow, but after . . . complete take out from your body.'"

Tashi, male, age 30: "If it is serious and sudden I think I might go to Delek [Western allopathic] Hospital or see any Indian doctor. But the Western medicine is not so good. I mean it is quick and you can get the relief quickly but you cannot get rid of the cause. Tibetan medicine is much slower but it is natural and helps you balance your whole body. My parents would probably choose the traditional Tibetan medicine. They prefer the natural methods and have great faith in that medicine. If I had a very strong headache, for instance, I might first take a pain killer and then go to see the Tibetan doctors if the problem comes again. If my problem is more chronic, I would go to the Tibetan doctor. Tibetan medicine works slowly but I can deal with the root of the problem. The Western medicine works quickly but they do not eliminate the cause."

Although Western allopathic medicine was reported as being better for acute conditions, one of the Tibetan *amchees* pointed out that the traditional Tibetan system of medicine could also be effective for diseases with severe symptoms.

> Tenpa, male, age 40: "People say Tibetan medicine is not very effective and would not give a quick relief. It is sometimes a wrong notion. It would not apply to all the medicine. There are some medicine which helps treat disease in immediate period. Whereas most medicine, they will take longer duration. It depends upon the medicine itself also."

Respondents often reported that Tibetans chose a particular method of treatment based upon their knowledge of the disease, and their views on the methods of treatment. In the process of decision-making, Tibetans used their common sense and knowledge:

> Tenpa, male, age 40: "Sometimes we would say Western medicine is very good in treating some particular kind of disease, whereas similarly Tibetan medicine has some potential in treating other kind of diseases. So, when these people or staff, or community knows about the effectiveness and potential of these different kinds of system they will choose with the right system, for the right disease."

According to my field data, specific qualities are attributed to particular medicinal models. Tibetan medicine is characterized as safe, natural and gentle, and is believed to be effective for chronic diseases. Western allopathic medicine is said to be the best for emergency situations and for reducing pain. Both weak and strong points were associated with each model. At this stage of the analysis, I examined variables influencing the idiom of disease and views on treatment methods. Then, I made a hypothesis that assumed both of these categories were very much affected by the respondents' level of acculturation and educational background.

7.2.7 Three Levels of Acculturation

One of the final hypotheses tested aimed at explaining the influence of acculturation level on help-seeking behavior. This variable proved useful as a means of understanding the differences in decision-making between models of treatment. It also shed light on the exceptions to the age-based patterns; for example, why some teenagers chose the traditional Tibetan system of medicine even though many young individuals preferred Western medicine. Acculturation has been considered here as a dimensional continuity, which included three main dimensional sub-categories: 1. Involvement with the culture of origin, 2. Involvement with the host culture, and 3. Involvement with Western culture. This division was based on my observations of factors affecting Tibetan culture, ethnic identity, and values.

Involvement with the Culture of Origin

This sub-category describes aspects of the Tibetans' lives that relate to tradition. These include using the mother tongue for communication, eating traditional foods, maintaining affiliation with monasteries, and developing relationships with members of the same community—especially those who share traditional customs, values, and beliefs. Respondents reported that most elderly Tibetans exhibit cultural resistance: in other words, they have a tendency to maintain their traditions and separate themselves from the host culture.

Most of the older Tibetans are active Buddhist devotees who engage in religious practices. These include taking part in pilgrimages, attending public Dharma teachings and audiences, and maintaining affiliations with local monasteries and lamas. Many of them perform religious rituals (*sang*),[13] read sacred texts, practice meditation, chant prayers, repeat mantras, perform prostrations in holy places, circumbulate *stupas*[14] or temples regularly, turn prayer wheels, make offering of butter lamps and prayer flags, give money to monks and lamas, and sponsor religious events—such as gatherings for group recitation of mantras.

Stroem (cited in Von Somm 1988) noted that lay youth brought up in India "have a less experiential, less embodied, and often ambivalent relationship to tradition" (p. 343). Receiving education in a traditional Tibetan school can also be seen as a reflection of the involvement with a culture of origin. Tibetans of all ages, but especially the older generation, wear traditional clothes and stick to traditional Tibetan dietary habits: drink quantities of Tibetan butter tea, and eat *tsampa*, *mo mo*, chowmain, and *thugpa.* In addition, many used the Tibetan language for everyday communication, although a few local dialects could be distinguished.

Involvement with the Host Culture

This sub-category refers to factors that enhance acculturation in the host country. These include establishing relationships with citizens of the host country, learning the prevalent language, employment among citizens the host culture, and adopting Indian cuisine and other aspects of their culture. The younger Tibetans were inclined towards some cultural incorporation or integration, adopting facets of Indian culture while maintaining numerous Tibetan traditional customs. The challenge of creating a new identity can produce inner conflicts as well as cross-cultural disagreements. This assimilation strategy is not only rare, but it is rejected by the chief spiritual authority—the Dalai Lama—who encourages Tibetans to maintain their ethnic identity while adapting to the new situation as best they can.

Exposure to Western Culture

Involvement with Western culture, as distinct from Indian culture, has been set aside as a separate category. The Tibetan settlements in India were in continuous contact with tourists from Europe and America, who were a source of Western influence and contacts. Additionally, many Tibetans (especially the young generation) had access to Western television, movies, and other media. They also tapped into the Internet, which became a source of both friends and sponsors in Western nations.

With respect to cultural influences, three patterns emerged:

1. Older Tibetans who exhibited the highest level of involvement with the culture of origin based their understanding of disease on cultural beliefs, and often sought traditional treatment solutions.
2. Young Tibetans in exile who lived with representatives of the older generation (such as their grandparents) were influenced by their beliefs and used their advice when seeking help.
3. Young Tibetans who presented a higher level of involvement with the host culture as well as exposure to Western culture were more critical of traditional beliefs and behaviors. When choosing medical treatment, the emphasis they placed on quick relief led them to prefer Western allopathic medicine.

Pattern 1: Older Tibetans who exhibited the highest level of involvement with the culture of origin based their understanding of disease on cultural beliefs, and often sought traditional treatment solutions.

Not surprisingly, the older generation were much more involved with tradition. They were often very zealous Buddhist practitioners who regularly engaged in various types of spiritual practices. When they experienced health problems, they often understood them in terms of humoural imbalance, an accumulation of negative karma, or the influence of supernatural forces. For this reason, they tended to use the traditional Tibetan system of medicine and its related paramedical solutions, such as home remedies or healing sessions with shamans.

> Sherab, male, age 17: "When we have conjunctivitis many of us think that using your own urine to clean the eyes will cure it. I came to know about it in my school—TCV—but I didn't believe in it. It really depends on whether the person has been deeply rooted in Tibetan culture or not. If yes, then the belief in

> traditional ways of healing are really strong. Even to the extent that we believe that some of the diseases are caused by provoked by spirits and demons. Many a times we call monks home to pray and drive away or pacify the spirits and demons which are thought to be the root of the problem. Tibetans who have recently arrived in exile might have a greater leaning towards the traditional way of healing."

Pattern 2: Young Tibetans in exile who lived with representatives of the older generation (such as their grandparents) were influenced by their beliefs and used their advice when seeking help.

Many respondents reported that the older generation were the mainstay of Tibetan tradition. Their cultural values, beliefs, and coping strategies were often transmitted to the young, in the processes of conscious and unconscious religious and cultural socialization. While some behavioral patterns were openly taught in the home and at school, others were observed and imitated:

> Chemey, female, age 28: "What is very useful, I think, important to have older people—grandmother and father in the house. It really helped us to spread the culture and religion towards me. I can do it for my children. It goes slowly to the younger generation also. Suppose my family, my parents are going on doing these things. It really influenced me and now I carry out all that, you know. I think it will help the younger generation. It is influencing. The older generation are doing all these things. It really influence slowly. In public also when we discuss these things, these issues come also: 'Also this and this helped me.' And then it influences him to do all these thing . . . him in believing that."

Many respondents reported that it was customary to consult the elderly people when someone experienced health problems or other difficulties. In many cases, they encouraged young people to use the traditional Tibetan system of medicine, as well as paramedical solutions:

> Tsewang, male, age 30: "In Tibet, we would normally seek advice from the elder people—parents, uncles. We would tell them about our problems and ask what to do. Here, I do not have relatives. In some cases I went straight to a practitioner."

Pattern 3: Young Tibetans who presented a higher level of involvement with the host culture as well as exposure to Western culture were more critical of traditional beliefs and behaviors. When choosing medical treatment, the emphasis they placed on quick relief led them to prefer Western allopathic medicine.

Respondents claimed that a large number of young people were influenced by Western culture. This in turn affected their identity, life values, and expectations. Many of them wished to raise their economic standard, and possibly move to a Western country to achieve this end. When young people experienced health problems, they would often neglect them if the symptoms were bearable, and although they shared common views on treatment methods, they were likely to suppress them by means of modern allopathic medicines.

Level of acculturation was an important factor in explaining individual differences in help-seeking behavior. In particular, a high degree of involvement with the host culture was conducive to greater hygienic and sexual awareness. Acculturation level was, in turn, influenced by another variable: the educational background of the respondents.

7.2.8 Educational Background

A number of the health professionals I interviewed confirmed that education was an important factor affecting help-seeking behavior. They compared the older generation—who were often illiterate—with the young Tibetans—most of whom had been to school. Allopathic doctors and Tibetan *amchees* often visited schools and gave talks on hygiene, prophylaxis, disease symptoms, and treatment solutions. According to the respondents, basic knowledge of diseases helped the Tibetans recognize symptoms and seek help at the appropriate facility. Severity of symptoms was the crucial factor in making these decisions:

> Dorjee, male, age 31: "I think, especially here in Dharamsala, there are lot of educated people. They have access to both clinics—the Tibetan medicine and the Western medicine. And since they are more educated, they will normally tend to decide [based] on their own [knowledge], which one to choose for them at a particular time. Here in Dharamsala we would not say, patient would first go to the Tibetan doctor and then consult a Western medicine or the other way round. They will decide according to the problem they have. That might be greatly influenced by the education also, and the knowledge they have. So, since they are more knowledgeable they have higher understanding and education, they will know which is better for them. We say also to them, to the public, normally: it's for the patient to decide which medicine they would choose to have. . . . So, when these people or staff, or community knows about the effectiveness and potential of these different kinds of system they will choose with the right system, for the right disease."

Lack of education was also associated with the strategy of ignoring the symptoms of disease. This was particularly ascribed to the older generation.

> Jigme, male, age 40: "Old age people, they are a little bit uneducated. For example, if they suffer from stomach-ache, like that . . . they think slowly and slowly it will heal automatically without any medicine. They neglect and it grows more severe. Then, they go to the doctor's place."

> Tenpa, male, age 40: "Why neglect? Actually, we can say because of . . . busy, and also . . . you know . . . we can bear the hard things. So, they think, if this is just a small problem. Actually, also most people, the older generation, they don't have much . . . knowledge, I mean, education for this thing. So, they just neglect it. When they are getting old, or become chronic, then they of course want take medicine and of course come to Tibetan medicine. So they take medicine for long time."

It was also reported that uneducated patients had more faith in the doctors and were more inclined to follow their advice. They expected the doctor to give them a clear diagnosis and explain the nature of the disease:

> Jigme, male, age 40: "For doctors, among low intellectual people, uneducated . . . they are much easier to deal with. They listen what the doctor say. Those with the intellectual, they . . . don't like to do as the doctor say. . . . The doctor say: 'Do this kind behavior, do this kind of diet.' Sometimes they listen, sometimes not listening. So, those who uneducated, especially in the rural areas, when they go for the medical . . . for doctors . . . these uneducated people are easier to deal with, to prescribe medicine."

> Tenpa, male, age 40: "It depends upon the education level and understanding. Some people, they might say: 'I don't know why I have this problem.' So, he would come to a doctor, unknowingly, what kind of problem might have caused this problem [symptom]. He does not have a clue that. He is not connecting it either to the stress, either to the diet, or either to the life style or behavior. They say, they don't know why they have this problem and want us to tell them."

Those without educational background were reported more likely to share certain superstitions related to health. An example of such beliefs was presented by Norbu Chophel (1983): "Whether a sick person recuperates or not is not strictly due to the medicines or the medical treatment given him. It is a common belief among the Tibetans that the recuperation of a sick person depends, to a large extent, on the doctor's way of treating the patient, his moral treatment (attitude) and the way he guides the patient, and also the patient's faith in the doctor. Tibetans often say, 'the doctor does not suit me,' when he is not getting well with that particular doctor's treatment or 'the doctor suits me very well,' when he often gets well with this doctor's treatment" (p. 12).

Some respondents reported that public talks given by the doctors and nurses resulted in increased health, hygiene, and sexual awareness in the Tibetan community. This also decreased the rate of certain diseases:

> Dolkar, female, age 50: "Some years back skin diseases were frequent. That is connected with shortage of water and hygienic condition, you know. They used

to get lot of skin disease, like sores, impetigo, skin infection. Now, through constant health education, and facilities it's much better."

7.3 GROUNDED THEORY OF ILLNESS BEHAVIOR

The response of Tibetans to health problems may be described by means of an algorithm. The grounded theory presents a challenging complexity, because individual illness behaviors and help-seeking pathways are diverse and depend on a number of factors, all of which influence one another. The key element of the grounded theory appear below:

Severity symptoms is one of the key variables affecting help-seeking behavior. When the symptoms are mild, they are likely to be ignored, whereas with severe conditions Tibetans tend to seek professional help.

The choice of the treatment model strongly depends on both the severity and the duration of the disease: if symptoms are severe or life-threatening, Tibetans usually turn to the Western allopathic system; whereas in case of chronic diseases they are likely to choose the traditional Tibetan system of medicine.

Important intervening variables that affect this decision-making process are: economic effects, availability of treatment, idiom of disease, views on treatment methods, and the level of acculturation.

Those whose level of income is lower seek less expensive methods of treatment; Tibetan medicine offers treatment at a comparatively lower cost.

Students are more likely to refer to their school dispensaries, where they are offered treatment free of charge (with either Western or Tibetan medicine).

If recovery has not been attained after some time, even considering the long duration of treatment with Tibetan medicine, Tibetans are likely to use specific religious coping strategies: for example, to seek a lama's advice and perform religious activities.

Alternately, in fewer cases, they may visit non-professionals who engage in shamanistic practices.

The higher the patient's involvement with the culture of origin, the higher the probability of their using religious coping strategies.

High involvement with the culture of origin is conducive to using the traditional Tibetan system of medicine; whereas a high level of acculturation will correlate with using Western allopathic medicine more frequently.

High acculturation level is inversely proportional to age: representatives of the older generation will present the greatest level of involvement with the culture of origin, whereas the young generation are more acculturated (involved in the host culture and exposed to Western culture). Individuals with more educational experience will more often rely on their common sense and knowledge gained at school.

NOTES

1. Source: http://www.kunphen.org

2. Modifiers are words, phrases, or clauses that make the meaning of a word more specific by affecting its meaning; that is, they modify the word.

3. Tib. *jam dpal dbyangs*

4. Tib. *sgrol ma*

5. Sanskrit *dharmapala,* Tib. *chos skyong*;

6. Tib. *nag po chen po*

7. Tib. *srung ma*

8. Tib. *zhing skyong*

9. *Tsampa* (Tib. *rtsam pa*) is roasted flour, usually made of barley or sometimes wheat. Tibetans often mix it with their traditional salty butter tea (Tib. *bod cha*).

10. She refers to medical conditions associated with the imbalance of humours. See: "The Three Humours (nepas)" in Chapter Five.

11. Tib. *mog mog*

12. A school set up by the Tibetan government to meet the needs of Tibetan refugees (up to the age of thirty) who have not had or had little formal education in Tibet.

13. A *sang* (Tib. *bsang*) is a fire ritual in which smoke is produced and offered up to deities. Special substances are burned in the fire, including *tsampa,* incense, and juniper branches. The most common *sang* is done in honor of higher beings, in order to bring down blessings. It is believed that the ritual cleanses, sanctifies, and brings "good energy" to the people and place involved. There are also other types of *sang,* where the smoke is offered to the sacred principles of Buddhism. In Tibet, *sang* was traditionally performed as part of welcoming a hallowed guest, such as a high lama. (Duff 2003)

14. A *stupa* (Tib. *mchod rten*) is a physical representation of the enlightened mind. Originating in India, the first *stupas* were simple mounds of earth crowned with umbrella-like ornaments. Elaborations on this simple structure gradually became stylized, and eventually, eight specific types of *stupa* were enumerated in the Buddhist traditions of India and Tibet. They are called the eight types of *stupa (*Tib. *mchod rten brgyad*). Despite the formalization of the style in later times, a *stupa* in fact is any spiral-shaped representation of the enlightened mind (Duff 2003).

Chapter Eight

Discussion and Conclusions

8.1 The Idiom of Disease in the Tibetan Community
8.2 Perception and Assessment of Treatment Methods
8.3 Common Help-Seeking Pathways
8.4 Variables Affecting Illness and Help-Seeking Behavior
8.5 Religion and Illness Behavior
8.6 Conclusions

In Chapter Seven, I sequentially analyzed the qualitative material to produce a grounded theory of illness behavior among members of the Tibetan diaspora. Grounded theory is a descriptive narrative "grounded" in data: in this case, data about the core category of illness behavior. The concept of illness behavior refers to various phenomena associated with health difficulties. These include perception and interpretation of symptoms or discomfort and their causes; the suspected outcome; perception and assessment of potential treatments; and ways of communicating one's suffering. It also involves help-seeking pathways—a theoretical concept that refers to the process of decision-making: whether to seek help and if so, where to look for advice, support, and treatment.

As a result of this analysis, a number of patterns and intervening variables emerged, and I examined the relationships between them. The overriding purpose of the analysis was to answer the following questions:

1. How do contemporary Tibetans construct the idiom of disease? How do they perceive and interpret their health problems?
2. How do Tibetans perceive and assess potential treatment methods?
3. What are the common help-seeking pathways?

4. What factors affect illness behavior and help-seeking pathways, and how?
5. What is the relationship between religion and illness behavior among Tibetans?

In this section, I would like to discuss my research findings, making reference to the theoretical framework explained in Chapters One, Two, and Three. The discussion will be organized according to these five research problems.

8.1 THE IDIOM OF DISEASE IN THE TIBETAN COMMUNITY

The analysis of qualitative data supported the general notion that culture is a meaning-making device for interpretation of health problems. It determines the way in which patients and everyone else who plays a role in the clinical setting understand the symptoms, and what value is ascribed to these symptoms (Kleinmann 1980). The idiom of disease constructed by Tibetans can be associated with both folk (local) categories and explanatory models. The former refers to ways in which people in different societies recognize and label mental illness (Tseng 2001). However, this notion could be used for health problems in general. In this study, the subjects were approached from a wide perspective and no special distinction was made between physical and mental problems, disease and illness. Explanatory models (EMs), on the other hand, are notions about a particular episode of sickness and its treatment, employed by all those involved in the clinical process (Kleinmann 1980).

Data revealed that the idiom of disease in the Tibetan community was mediated by traditional beliefs present in the Tibetan system of medicine and the teachings of Dharma. According to both Dharma and Tibetan traditional medicine, ultimate health is only possible when *liberation* has been achieved. As long as individuals have ego-clinging, they are bound to suffer from the three mind poisons (anger, desire, and ignorance), which results in the imbalance of the three humours or *nepas*—Wind, Bile, and Phlegm. The imbalance of these three humours is believed to be one of the major causes of disease.

In most cases, Tibetans would interpret their dysfunctions in terms of Wind, Bile, or Phlegm imbalance. Many would also associate the onset of disease with the accumulation of negative karma, and sometimes with supernatural, malignant forces. Whereas all experiences can be understood in terms of the effects of positive or negative karma, some disorders are classified specifically as "karmic diseases," and cannot be cured by medicine. Special spiritual methods must be used to treat such conditions. This confirms the findings of Pathak (2003), whose respondents recognized supernatural intrusion, ghost possession, or imbalance of body constituents as potential causes of their ailments.

The explanatory models held by the patient may differ from those of the clinician (Kleinmann 1980). In a Tibetan context this was exemplified by Jacobson (2002), and also confirmed by the field data in the present study. For instance, whereas some patients would describe their symptoms as a *rLung* (wind) disorder, others may classify the very same symptoms in terms of anxiety disorder or depression—from the standpoint of the Western psychiatric diagnostic system.

Some people may also acknowledge that they are suffering from depression, yet use Tibetan herbs to balance their *rLung* at the same time. This may support the findings of Joel et al (2003) that an individual can hold diverse and contradictory beliefs simultaneously. Field data also revealed that some Tibetans would not even hold a notion of depression or other mental disorders in their minds, and may thus ignore such symptoms. Because of this cultural condition, health education was conducted in Tibetan settlements in order to promote awareness of and sensitivity to such problems.

In some cases, disorders were also understood in terms of biological causes or the effect of psychological disturbances and stress. A number of variables that affect Tibetans' explanatory models have been revealed. For example, the more educated individuals may be dismissive of interpreting certain symptoms in terms of spirit possession. On the other hand, traditional cultural beliefs were found to be common among most Tibetans, irrespective of age and education level. It is possible that some of them would hold conflicting beliefs about health, and, for example, seek help from allopathic doctors or nurses, while allowing for the possibility that their condition is due to the curse of serpent deities.

To summarize the above, various idioms of disease were identified in the field study. These idioms can be referred to the models of Murdock and Foster (cited in Garro 2000) as discussed in Chapter Two, "Health and Illness Behaviors." Both models describe different causations of ailments and seem complementary to each other. Murdock describes two types of causation in his model: natural and supernatural. The first one (natural) is congruent with modern science and includes infection, stress, organic deterioration, or accident. Such understanding of the causes of disease was reported by a number of Tibetan respondents. Supernatural causation includes mystical causation, as through karma; magical causation, as through sorcery or the evil eye, and animistic causation, as with the curse of the *nagas* (serpent deities; the respondents made frequent reference to these).

Foster's classification (cited in Garro 2000) describes naturalistic versus personalistic systems. Naturalistic refers to imbalance of the natural forces or conditions, for example, the three humours, or the five elements (Earth, Water, Fire, Wind, and Space). Personalistic, on the other hand, refers to the purposeful intervention of an agent, such as a sorcerer, angry ghost, evil spirit, or deity. Patients' explanatory models were either compatible with modern medical science, with the traditional Tibetan system of medicine, or both. The fact that some Tibetans have confidence in both systems simultaneously has created situations of conflict in their medical decision-making. As a result, the Tibetan authorities have carried out an intensive program of patient education, to help Tibetans use both systems complementarily, not alternatively.

8.2 PERCEPTION AND ASSESSMENT OF TREATMENT METHODS

How patients perceive and assess treatment methods is another component of the explanatory models described by Kleinmann (1980). In the course of my field work, I identified a number of treatment solutions that were available in Tibetan settlements. These were the traditional Tibetan system of medicine, paramedical solutions (including home treatments, shamanistic practices, spiritual methods, and counseling), and Western allopathic medicine. The Tibetan and Western medical models were the ones mentioned most frequently by the respondents.

The traditional Tibetan system of medicine was characterized as safe, natural, gentle, and as removing the underlying causes of a disease rather than its symptoms. At the same time, numerous respondents reported that it worked slowly and required diligence to administer. It was believed to be more effective in case of chronic diseases and symptoms that were less severe. Western allopathic medicine was praised for its effectiveness, and its ability to help acute, life-threatening conditions and reduce their symptoms. On the other hand, it was associated with side effects and symptomatic rather than causal treatment.

These findings are consistent with Pathak (2004), who wrote that Tibetans older than age 50 assessed the traditional Tibetan system of medicine as effective for all kinds of ailments, although they preferred to use this method for chronic conditions. They believed that it would provide a permanent cure, even though the treatments take more time. Patients in Pathak's study also reported that Tibetan medicine was less expensive. They admitted, however, that it needed further improvement (e.g., making administration of the herbal pills easier or modifying their taste. In my research, some respondents also complained that Tibetan herbal pills had an unpleasant (bitter or sour) taste, and that the treatment regimens required too much effort (for example, taking pills with hot water at particular times of the day, before or after meals, or at night).

The perception of treatment methods was mediated to a large extent by education and health campaigns run by the Tibetan Department of Health. Numerous talks on prophylaxis and hygiene were conducted at schools, and also provided to the general public. Doctors representing both medicinal systems often spoke about prevention and treatment of different disorders. Moreover, it was observed that Tibetans often shared among themselves their knowledge and views on health-related topics. Subsequently, they often described both treatment modalities using very similar phrases; see Section 7.2.6, "Views on Treatment Methods," in Chapter Seven.

8.3 COMMON HELP-SEEKING PATHWAYS

The concept of help-seeking pathways refers to whether and how patients seek help when they experience health problems. In his study, Pathak (2004) presents quantitative data related to Tibetans' use of healthcare services. His findings reveal that 80.2 percent of the older generation of Tibetans preferred Tibetan traditional medicine for chronic ailments, and 15 percent of this age group reported consulting healers. In the same study, he found that 80 percent of patients younger than age 50 visited Delek Hospital, or other allopathic clinics and private practitioners, for all kinds of ailments. Young individuals also visited Men-Tsee-Khang, for treatment with traditional Tibetan medicine.

Respondents mentioned several possible patterns of help-seeking behavior: ignoring symptoms, referring to family and friends for advice or support, consulting health professionals or spiritual teachers (lamas), and visiting faith healers. Some of these solutions could be used simultaneously or sequentially. For example, a person might ignore the symptoms until they grew more severe, and then consult a medical doctor. Like some other Asian minority groups (Chung and Lin 1994), Tibetans reported using dual healthcare systems: for example, they would take Western allopathic medicines alongside Tibetan herbal pills. They might also treat themselves according to Western medical science, but consult lamas about spiritual methods that would help during the recovery process.

There were also individuals who refrained from any kind of medical treatment, and instead, concentrated on spiritual practices alone. This could be due to their own explanatory models for illness, or for economic reasons. Many

Tibetans reported that they would seek help and advice from family and friends in a difficult situation. This strategy is also common in other collectivistic societies. For example, Yeh et al (2003) note that Asians are more likely to seek help from intimates than a stranger (such as a counselor). My field data also confirmed the observations of Crescenzi et al (2002) that Tibetans often express emotional distress through somatic symptoms.

Like some other Asian populations (Speller 2005), Tibetans may see psychological problems as a sign of weakness. Faced with this type of problem, they may seek medical help instead of psychological counseling—which is not present in traditional Asian cultures outside the counseling role of spiritual teachers. Individual differences in help-seeking pathways resulted from a number of intervening variables.

8.4 VARIABLES AFFECTING ILLNESS AND HELP-SEEKING BEHAVIOR

As they affected help-seeking pathways, the variables that emerged in my study resembled those presented by Cummings, Becker, and Maile (cited in Pillay 1996): age of the patient, severity of symptoms, duration of treatment, economic conditions, availability of treatment, the idiom of disease, the patient's views on treatment methods, and their acculturation level and educational background.

Age

The first factor to be identified and analyzed was the age of the study subjects. Research data revealed that the older generation of Tibetan migrants were more likely to maintain traditional customs and values, and refer to their traditional cultural beliefs, so as to make meaning of their new experiences (Tseng 2001; Vang and Flores 1999; Kwak and Berry 2001; Misra 2003; Penny-Dimri 2003). Older Tibetan migrants were also reported as being more likely to use the traditional Tibetan system of medicine, as was also observed by Pathak (2004). This can be explained in terms of acculturation, and is also consistent with the observation of Chung (2001), who found an association between higher use of indigenous healing methods and lower education and literacy.

Transmission of the traditional cultural beliefs and values to the young generation was observed in the sample as well. Young Tibetans were exposed to cultural and religious socialization from an early age—for example, in their homes, and in the Tibetan schools. Like other minority groups (Tseng 2001;

Gil, Vega, and Dimas 1994; Vang and Flores 1999; Kwak and Berry 2001; Anderson and Kagawa-Singer 1996; Ausubel 1960; Speller 2005; Von Somm 1998), the more they were exposed to Western culture, the faster they would acculturate, and the more likely they were to use Western allopathic medicine.

This was observed in other Asian migrant groups by Chung and Lin (1994), who noted that exposure to Western culture, and the availability of Western medicine, were important variables in the shift from indigenous medicine to higher use of mainstream services. In the present study, a higher level of acculturation (which involves contact with Indian as well as with Western culture) was associated with greater use of Western medicine. Its quick alleviation of symptoms made it the treatment mode of choice for the more acculturated Tibetans, who were concerned about missing time from work or school.

Severity of Symptoms

Another important factor affecting illness behavior was the severity of symptoms. I observed that while patients were likely to ignore milder symptoms, they tended to seek professional help when the symptoms were severe. In addition to this, I found that they made their choice of the appropriate treatment modality based on the affliction and the severity of its symptoms. For milder illnesses, Tibetans were likely to use home methods, whereas for more serious ones, they would consult a biomedical doctor, *amchee,* or a lama (depending on their explanatory models). This is consistent with the patterns observed in other Asian minority groups by Uehara (2001).

There may be several reasons why the Tibetans relocated to India tend to neglect mild symptoms. First of all, they may be concentrating their attention on their economic pursuits, and efforts to adapt themselves to new and demanding life circumstances. Suffering associated with symptoms may be perceived as less important than potential economic hardship—especially in light of the fact that treatment will cost money.

Secondly, ignoring symptoms (and suffering in general) may be understood as a defense mechanism—denying worrying thoughts may help Tibetans cope with difficulties and sustain the brave face that is so highly valued in Asian populations (see Speller 2005). To achieve such an appearance of stoicism, some also rationalize that disease is empty in nature—that is, its existence is merely an illusion—and so they believe they can overcome it by using the power of the mind and performing certain rituals. With this in mind, they may feel that they have gained control over the situation (see Pargament, Koenig, and Perez 2000; Hood et al. 1996). However, if they have not mastered meditation techniques well enough and the conditions grow more severe or become life threatening, these individuals are likely to experience anxiety and react to the situation by seeking medical help, or further advice from spiritual advisors.

Tibetans attributed different qualities to the available medicinal models in relation to their effectiveness in particular cases. To choose the right method of treatment, they would consider the severity and duration of disease: if symptoms were severe or life-threatening Tibetans usually turned to the Western allopathic system; whereas in case of chronic diseases they were likely to choose the traditional Tibetan system of medicine. Most of those interviewed for this study—both caregivers and patients—reported this algorithm. When Western medicine became available to the Tibetans, it had to be incorporated into their system of meaning. Tibetans had to learn what they could expect from each system of medicine, respectively. Not only their level of formal education, but their shared experiences within each system, played an important role in this process.

Explanatory Models

Patients' perception of symptoms (both mental and physical) and their response to them is culturally determined. Whether the causes of disease are understood in terms of infection, biochemical imbalance, stress, imbalance of the three humours, or the influence of supernatural forces, depends on the "mind software" (Hofstede 1991) that helps people make meaning of a given situation. People will act according to their learned patterns of behavior; and it is worth noting that some of these patterns are culturally accepted and others are not.

For example, it is not culturally appropriate in a Tibetan community to express depressive symptoms, sit and cry, or show self-pity and despondency due to hardships and setbacks. This would be associated with being weak. On the other hand, it is acceptable to experience headaches, tiredness, or stomach problems, and then seek professional help in response to such problems. While monks are not expected to exhibit anger or sexual drive, somatization and seeking solitude fall within the range of normal behaviors for them.

These observations are in line with what Speller (2005) reported among other Asian emigrant groups. In Tibetan communities, it is improper to reveal emotional conflicts in public, or to exhibit disruptive behaviors. This was also observed by Jacobson (2002). Tibetans are likely to be ashamed of psychiatric disorders—even though cases of psychosis, epilepsy, mania, anxiety, and depression are recorded at the clinics. On the other hand, many young girls and sometimes boys were reported as being victims of spirit possession. Behavior attributed to possession included becoming excessively angry, throwing stones at people and calling them names, or losing consciousness. For the Tibetans, spirit possession appears to be more culturally accepted than having psychiatric problems. This may be understood in terms of the pathoplastic function of culture. Another example of it relates chronic skin problems, that are generally attributed to the curse of the *nagas* (not necessarily poor hygiene or water pollution). Tibetans often perform spiritual actions to appease these beings.

The explanatory models held by the Tibetans affect their help-seeking pathways. These determine whether Tibetan patients will seek support from their family and friends, from Western medical doctors and *amchees,* or from lamas and faith healers. A good example was presented by one of the respondents who developed symptoms of a swollen penis. He explained that normally Tibetans might believe that such a condition was caused by the *nagas*, who punished him for urinating onto the trees, or into rivers and ponds—places he believed were inhabited by these deities. His other explanation was that the organ was swollen due to infection caused by intercourse with a prostitute. This understanding may stem from health education and disease prevention campaigns. In general, if a condition is understood in terms of demonic or spirit influence, the individual is unlikely to seek medical help from a doctor trained in allopathy. He or she would rather consult a lama or an *amchee.* Even if the patient had his broken limb x-rayed and put into a plaster cast at the hospital, he or she might still make use of Tibetan herbal medicine, to augment Western medical treatment.

Economic Effects and Availability Factor

Two other variables affecting help-seeking pathways are the economic effects factor, and the availability of various forms of treatment. My field data analysis affirmed the tendency of migrant populations to seek out cost-effective treatment solutions. Tibetans who had limited budgets were likely to seek out low-cost healthcare solutions, as well as those most easily available to them; for example, students were more likely to use school dispensaries or consult school nurses and doctors.

Acculturation

Finally, we come to the issue of cultural transformation, which emerged as an important variable affecting help-seeking behavior. What I observed among Tibetans in the present study is characteristic of various ethnic minorities in the course of the acculturation process (see Tseng 2001). Most Tibetans living in India identify themselves as refugees. Many have obtained Indian documents that allow them to work in the host country, travel abroad and then back to India. Many experience high levels of stress, as they attempt to find an occupation, adjust to different climatic conditions, foods, and customs, and otherwise strive to adapt themselves to their new environment. Subsequently, some develop physical and psychological symptoms associated with that change (see Tseng 2001; Vang and Flores 1999; Torres and Rollock 2004). Examples of how acculturative stress affects physical and mental well-being were presented in Chapter One, "Tibetan Culture, Religion, and Acculturation."

Even though most Tibetans reveal a tendency to keep close to their countrymen and resist assimilation, some degree of integration has been inevitable. In order to survive and communicate well in the host country, Tibetans have had to learn its language, symbols, customs, and laws. Nevertheless, many refugees still resist coming into closer contact with Indians—interracial marriages or cases of Tibetans working for Indians are barely reported. In a community of people who were deprived of their land and possessions, such an acculturation strategy may be understood as a struggle to maintain their cultural heritage, traditional values, and ethnic identity. It may also be seen as an expression of prejudice against members of the host culture. Although Tibetans are encouraged to exhibit kindness to all (which has become a cultural norm), on a deeper level some may feel threatened by the Indian way of life, and behave so as to preserve and protect their own culture.

The analysis of field data revealed the following pattern: While the older generation of Tibetans favor treatment based on the traditional Tibetan system of medicine and home remedies, the young generation prefer Western allopathic medicine, mostly to obtain quick relief. The older generation reveal a greater tendency to use spiritual strategies to enhance the recovery process or cope with the situation more efficiently. This strategy is also reported by the young generation, but its frequency decreases in parallel with the age of the subjects. The older generation reveal a greater tendency to use shamanistic methods and "tantric power" to deal with difficult situations; these strategies occur much less frequently among the young generation.

Such findings may be explained in terms of acculturation. It is apparent that older people who are naturally more involved with the culture of origin are more likely to use its traditional patterns of behavior or coping styles (also noted by Chung 2001). Some young individuals are also highly involved with the culture of origin, often because they live close to their grandparents, or observe traditional customs practiced at home. For this reason, they may copy the older generation's traditional patterns of behavior. Similarly, Yeh et al (2003) note that those who interact with family and other members of their own ethnic group are more likely to endorse traditional cultural norms.

Older Tibetans who resist acculturation may reject (or even fear) methods promoted in a modern society. Some also perceive the changes happening in the community as a sign of degradation or degeneration and express worry that the traditional values and cultural heritage will be lost. Subsequently, they praise old methods and show distrust towards modern medicine. Despite that, examples may be found of elderly Tibetans who maintain a very pragmatic attitude: they claim that Western medicine can help them deal with acute problems or even save lives, and use Tibetan medicine to complement modern biomedicine. Tibetans who remained more involved with the culture of origin reported more frequent use of spiritual coping strategies. On the other hand, when faced with a crisis, even young and highly acculturated individuals would sometimes use this approach to make meaning of their situation, and find comfort and reassurance.

8.5 RELIGION AND ILLNESS BEHAVIOR

Numerous authors have identified religion as an important salutary agent (Sosis and Alcorta 2003; Ferraro and Albrecht-Jensen 1991; Koenig 2001, 2002, 2004; Koenig et al. 2004; Kendler et al. 2003; Oman and Thoresen 2002). This is also well exemplified by the Tibetan diaspora. Most Tibetans, irrespective of age, identify themselves as Tibetan Buddhists. Together with other ethnic markers, religion helps them maintain a sense of identity and belonging, despite being deprived of their homeland.

His Holiness the Dalai Lama is a crucial figure for most Tibetans. Even those who disagree with his policies still show respect for their leader. Religion also equips Tibetans with a variety of skillful means for coping with suffering. It is a source of practical methods, symbolic language such as mantras, liturgical objects, and rituals that can be used for healing practices. This symbolic aspect, was also described by McGuire (1987). The concept of karma, seemingly familiar to all Tibetans, is conducive to self-directing religious coping styles (Pargement 1997). Relying on Dharma, Tibetan Buddhists feel responsible for everything they experience, as part of their karma, which comes about as a result of their previous actions. Subsequently, they are stimulated to involve themselves in virtuous actions, which they believe will produce favorable results in the future.

While the Tibetans pray to Buddha for his blessings, they believe that improvement of their situation might not manifest itself until their next lifetime. In doing so, they did not bind Buddha with particular expectations as to how his blessings might be expressed. For example, they would not pray for a sick person to be cured if it was better for that person to die and have a better life upon his or her rebirth. Tibetan Buddhists are also discouraged from asking for specific solutions or gains for themselves. Instead, they are advised to pray for the benefit of all: "May all sentient beings be happy and free from suffering." This protects them from ever feeling ignored, abandoned or punished by the Higher Power.[1]

When Tibetans get involved in some new undertaking, such as study, a journey, or a new business, they often pray that all the benefits produced by this action may be a source of happiness for all. Asking Buddha for trivial things, such as curing one's body or making good business, is compared to asking a king to get off his throne and sweep the floor (Lhalungpa 1979). In spite of this, many Tibetans reported asking Buddha for success in their exams, protection from the authorities, and so on. If they failed to achieve what they had expected, instead of saying: "I am not good enough and Buddha punished me," they were more inclined to think: "Despite Buddha's perfect benevolence I was unable to enjoy his blessing due to my karma." Many Tibetans use specific contemplative instructions, to overcome difficult emotions, or to find more inner strength and hope. Consulting lamas and following their advice is a popular way of coping.

The findings of the present study are consistent with what is described in the literature on religious coping. Tibetan Buddhism is a system that offers meaning, a sense of control, comfort, and intimacy, through fostering social solidarity. It also encourages life transformation. Referring to Dharma practice helps Tibetans overcome situations of crisis, find explanations for negative experiences, and develop a sense of peace and security. It can protect Tibetans from acculturative stress. It also helps them deal with the issue of death and dying, so much elaborated on in Buddhist teachings. These aspects of religion are discussed by various authors, including Pargament, Koenig, and Perez (2000), Sosis and Alcorta (2003), Vanderpool (1980), Hood et al. (1996), Koenig et al. (2004), Kamaya (1997), and Osborne and Vandenberg (2003)

8.6 CONCLUSIONS

During the course of this study, I gathered a great deal of interesting information and insights. It has broadened my own understanding of the phenomena associated with culture and health. It also provided fascinating live examples of the issues outlined in my theoretical framework. I discovered these examples in a very specific context: a community being affected by gross cultural changes, one that will soon cease to exist in its traditional form. Because the research context was new to me, I used a grounded theory methodology.

This allowed for an inductive approach, through which I could examine a vast number of phenomena. From these, I was able to develop my core category, along with the variables affecting it. Relationships between illness behavior and factors affecting it were analyzed in detail. One of the weaknesses of this research is that data was mostly gathered from authority figures. In the future, it would be still more challenging to do a follow-up study of a larger sample of Tibetans, in which quantitative data could be triangulated with qualitative data.

NOTE

1. Examples of the negative religious coping were discussed in Chapter Three, Section 3.8: "Pathogenic and Pathoplastic Functions of Religion."

Appendix: Frequently Reported Complaints

The most frequent health complaints reported among the Tibetan diaspora, as cited by the Tibetan Department of Health, were classified as follows: respiratory infections, diarrhea, dysentery, skin and infectious diseases, trauma, and infection. This information can be supported and supplemented with statements given by the respondents:

> Yeshi, female, 50: "Most often they suffer from food problems, indigestion, headaches. There are some cases of asthma and arthritis because they use air-conditioning quite frequently. It is not good for them, I tell them."

> Dolkar, female, 50: "In the society, you will find that most Tibetan people seem to have hypertension—maybe due to the diet, you know . . . because we butter tea . . . high intake of butter and oily things. It could be due to heart or whatever. Then arthritic diseases among the older people. For the children, it's mostly seasonal diarrhea or upper respiratory infections, you know. Because of the altitude and all that. And some years back it used to be . . . skin . . . but now through constant health education, the facilities. . . . That is connected with shortage of water and hygienic condition, you know. They used to get lot of skin disease, like sores, impetigo, skin infection. Now, it's much better. There are also seasonal diseases: allergies, seasonal diarrhea. You heard about this . . . chicken pox. If one person gets this, those who never had it before, they will get the attack. So, you have, like sometimes due to the weather, if you have water polluted and then you have the epidemic of gastric problems—like vomiting and diarrhea together. Among the older people you will find like . . . joint . . . like arthritis, you know—rheumatics or osteoarthritis. It's very common. You will see that most of them are taking Tibetan medicine, you know. And for [rLung]."

The concept of *rLung*—which refers to the element Wind or "life-wind"-—is said to govern mental problems, such as anxiety and depression. A few

Tibetan health professionals reported that psychological problems were frequent among Tibetans, although patients did not often complain about them. Instead, they were more likely to somatize these complaints, as was observed by Crescenzi et al. (2002): "The high levels of anxiety and depression in the Tibetan community is consistent with our clinical experience. Patients typically seek help by presenting headaches, stomach pain, body-aches, fits, medically unexplained paralysis, feelings of unhappiness, palpitations, insomnia, discomfort with anger, and difficulties concentrating and learning" (p. 374).

A counsellor from Delek Hospital reported that symptoms of depression were the most frequently observed mental health problem, but that they were barely expressed during the initial interview.

> Dolma, female, 39: "The problem of our Tibetan community is, they are still not aware of mental disease and most of them come with a somatized complain: 'I have a headache, I have a back pain.' They never say that: 'I am unhappy' or 'I am depressed' or 'I am anxious.'"

Tibetan doctors also reported referring Western patients to Men-Tsee-Khang or private clinics:

> Tenpa, male, 40: "Here in Dharamsala, we have a lot of [Tibetan] patients with arthritis, sometimes also with hypertension, and see . . . here . . . lots of Westerners are also coming here. They also have some minor problems, like cold, diarrhea, dysentery. So, it depends upon place to place. Whereas in the plains we have lot of Indian patients. So they have common problems with diabetes."

Appendix: Medical Institutions

The Tibetan medical institutions in India are managed by the Department of Health (DoH) of the Tibetan Government-in-Exile. DoH runs forty-four health clinics, nine primary healthcare centers, one mobile clinic, and seven hospitals in the Tibetan communities in India and Nepal (CTA).[1] DoH aims at promoting an integrated approach in treatment, where the allopathic Primary Health Care (PHC) is combined with the traditional system of Tibetan medicine. These two systems of medicine run in parallel to each other and there is a referral process between them. Allopathic treatment is offered by the following institutions:

Northern India
Tibetan Delek Hospital, Dharamsala
Tibetan Health Center, Dekyiling
Primary Healthcare: Paonta Sahib, Bir, Dalhousie, Chauntra, Delhi, Tashi Jong
Health Clinics: Sataun, Puruwala
Southern India
Tsojhe Khangsar Hospital, Bylakuppe
Doeguling Tibetan Resettlement Hospital, Mundgod
Dhondenling Van Thiel Hospital, Kollegal
Phende Hospital, Hunsur
Central India
Menlha Hospital, Orissa
Primary Healthcare: Bandhara, Mainpat

Treatment with the traditional Tibetan system of medicine is available at the Tibetan Medical and Astro Institute (TMAI), also known as Men-tsee-khang.[2] TMAI was founded in 1961 as a small dispensary of traditional

Tibetan medicine, to cope with the health problems of Tibetan refugees who were continuously arriving in Dharamsala. Today it is a huge complex that includes a dispensary, an inpatient unit, and a surgical ward. TMAI also carries out extensive research. The Institute produces about 200 different types of pills, and other forms of medicine, including salves, herb teas, and incense. These are distributed to their branch clinics in India and Nepal. TMAI runs 48 branch clinics worldwide:

North Indian States

Gangchen Kyishong, McLeod Ganj, Ladakh Choglamsar, Cultural Center Ladakh, Poanta Sahib, Danglob, Maj-nu-ka-tilla (Delhi), Nizammudin (New Delhi), Dalhousie, Shimla, Dekyiling, Bir, Manali, Jispa, Rajpur and Meerut.

Northeastern Indian States

Darjeeling, Bomdila, Tawang, Salugara, Shillong, Miao, Jaigaon, Rawangla, Tezu, Gangtok, Kolkata, Kalimpong and Itanagar.

Eastern/Western/Central Indian States

Orrisa Phuntsokling, Bhubaneshwar, Mumbai, Bhandara and Mainpat.

South India (Karnataka)

Bylakupee, Sera, Hunsur, Kollegal, Bangalore, Mundgod Third Camp and Mundgod Sixth Camp.

The other branch clinics operate in Nepal (Solokhumbu, Tashi Palkyi, Jampaling, Chabahil and Chatrapatti), USA (Spring Green, Wisconsin) and Netherlands (Amsterdam).

TMAI also houses an Astrological Department, which provides training in the art of Tibetan astrology. It offers other special services, such as individual horoscope interpretations, and the manufacture of amulets (for general and individual needs), and publishes an annual lunar calendar based on the Tibetan system of astrological calculations.

Apart from providing basic healthcare for both Tibetans and Indians in refugee settlements and indigenous villages, the Department of Health also conducts healthcare programs and education campaigns. Health promotion in the Tibetan community is focused on the expansion of health awareness regarding disease prevention, hygiene, healthier lifestyles, and a cleaner environment. The Department of Health reports: "In the two decades of its existence, the DoH has been able to establish Health Centers in almost every

Tibetan refugee settlement in India and Nepal. At least one Community Health Worker (CHW) attends to the preventive and curative health care needs through the centers as well as providing health promotion in the community."

Gradually, the services they provide have expanded from immunization and TB control to antenatal care, family planning, HIV/AIDS education, among other programs. In 1993 the Department of Health initiated a program that addressed the needs of torture victims. In 1996, this became known as the Tibetan Torture Survivor Program (Sadutsang 2002).

Appendix: Health, Hygienic, and Sexual Awareness

Some respondents touched upon the issue of health, hygiene, and sexual awareness in relation to the idiom of illness. Several statements referred to both young and old individuals being ignorant of these issues. The degree of health, hygiene, and sexual awareness was related to educational background and life experiences. Thanks to educational campaigns, more and more Tibetans (especially the young) have acquired knowledge about birth control and prevention of sexually transmitted diseases. Doctors or nurses frequently give talks on hygiene, substance dependence, contagious diseases, and sex education. Pathak (2004) observes: "Literacy mission, occupational mobility, and the mass media promote health awareness among the Tibetan youth. Data also reveal that younger generation is conscious about immunisation of their children. They consult doctors for major and minor ailments" (p. 87). One of the Tibetan *amchees* reported:

> Norbu, male, age 40: "In Tibetan settlement, doctor used to give a lecture to the old people and educated people also. They gather in hall and he would talk on the Tibetan medicine. Sometimes we would go for a particular topic. And suppose . . . rheumatic, suppose hepatitis B, now there is many hepatitis in Tibetan also. So for that they are giving a talk, each and every different topic . . . . So now this, and there is no anymore [uneducated] Tibetan. . . . In 1960, 70's, 80's—that time, most of the people, Tibetan people are quite uneducated."

Sexual matters were likely to be avoided, even by professionals who provided education. Some reported sex to be one of the taboo topics:

> Dolma, female, age 39: "We had [talks on sex] some time ago in TCV but the headmaster said it was wrong, because children only get more interested in sex. 'You encourage them to do this,' he said."

A number of respondents claimed that Tibetans (especially the older generation) avoided talking about intimate relationships, tended to hide their nudity (even in front of their partners), and exhibited attitudes marked by shame. Only one of the respondents maintained that he felt at ease talking about any issue (including intimate matters), while most interviewees blushed, giggled, became nervous, or simply avoided answering questions related to sex.

> Dolma, female, age 39: "Tibetans are ashamed to talk about sex. They get angry, when you mention. They say they do not have such needs."

The Tibetans' level of openness about these subjects could be related to their degree of exposure to Western culture, as observed by a health professional from TCV Hospital. She maintained that it was more natural for the younger people to talk about sex. They also felt less restrained in their actions:

> Dolkar, female, age 50: "We don't talk about sex so openly, you know. You feel very shy and you never express anything of that sort in front of your teacher, your elders, or your parents. Now the Western influence is so great in Dharamsala. Now, it's 21st century . . . so different and everybody seems to change. The world . . . it's easier to learn the bad habits. Nobody has to teach you, you just learn by yourself so fast. And the good habits, no matter how much you impose, it takes lot of time to catch them, isn't it? Like that . . . the 20th and 21st century . . . sex has become so open and everybody seems to talk, seems to be so free and there is no shyness, you know. So, in a way, I feel that is not too good. Maybe I am a little old-fashioned."

A few statements referred to the lack of knowledge about functioning of the human body and its processes, pregnancy, and sexual development.

> Dolma, female, 39: "One girl got her . . . blood . . . first menstruation. Other children saw it and then ask: 'Where is that blood come from?' She was very ashamed and said it is from here [points at her side, above hips]. She was so ashamed. . . . Some girls are afraid if they can get pregnant through kiss. There is no sexual education at school. . . . A boy came to me one. . . .a street boy. He asked if he can get some [talks in a very low voice] arse condoms. I ask him: 'What you need this for?' He say that the other boys using him and someone told him that he will get pregnant. He asked me if that was true. I tell him: 'Of course not! You are a boy. You can't get pregnant. Only girls can get pregnant!' I asked him about the other boys and told him, they should not do that. I said that if they still do that, he should send them to me. . . . They never talk about homosexuality. Most might think it is because of evil spirits. Possessed. I saw a friend and

she showed me a picture. She said, that girl who rented her flat was a lesbian [talks in a low voice, blushes]. I was shocked and I asked: 'How do you know this?' She said: 'Why are you so surprised?'"

Hygiene was one of the topics that triggered cross-cultural conflicts among the Tibetans. Indeed, a few respondents admitted that some Tibetans neglected hygiene. It thus become one of the key issues addressed by the health education program organized by the Department of Health.

> Sherab, M 17: "Hygiene—they [older Tibetans] were not that clean. But it is a stereotypical description. They would not wash . . . after going to the toilet and stuff, which is the same with the youngsters as well . . . yeah . . . I mean they didn't wash their hands and stuff. My friends from school as well . . . and the teachers and nurses use to give a lot of health and hygiene talks. They used to check whether we had clean clothes and nails, hair without lice and stuff."

Another respondent recalled visiting a nunnery in the early 1990s. She claimed that the nuns lacked proper health and hygienic education. During menstruation, instead of sanitary towels the nuns used old socks, which they later washed and re-used. For many nuns, bleeding presented a serious problem—not only in terms of physical discomfort, but also emotionally: they were very much ashamed of this side of their femininity. The same nuns often consumed old food, affected by mold, because the refrigerator was often switched off at dusk to save electricity.

Health education varies in different places. In some Tibetan schools, fundamental principles of the traditional Tibetan system of medicine were introduced, together with lectures on hygiene. In others, education focused on disease prevention. This could perhaps be explained in terms of the availability of appropriate healthcare professionals. A school principal from southern India reported that an American doctor and some Tibetan physicians visited his institution and gave talks on hygiene. They spoke about washing hands before and after eating, and drinking clean water—but there were no talks whatsoever on Tibetan medicine.

Appendix: RCOPE

RCOPE Subscales and Definitions of Religious Coping Methods by Pargament, Koenig, & Perez 2000, p. 522-524

Religious Methods of Coping to Find Meaning

1. Benevolent Religious Reappraisal—redefining the stressor through religion as benevolent and potentially beneficial.
2. Punishing God Reappraisal—redefining the stressor as a punishment from God for the individual's sins
3. Demonic Reappraisal—redefining the stressor as an act of the Devil
4. Reappraisal of God's Powers—redefining God's power to influence the stressful situation

Religious Methods of Coping to Gain Control

1. Collaborative Religious Coping—seeking control through a partnership with God in problem solving.
2. Active Religious Surrender—an active giving up of control to God in coping
3. Passive Religious Deferral—passive waiting for God to control the situation
4. Pleading for Direct Intercession—seeking control indirectly by pleading to God for a miracle or dive intercession.
5. Self-Directing Religious Coping—seeking control directly through individual initiative rather than help from God.

Religious Methods of Coping to Gain Comfort and Closeness to God

1. Seeking Spiritual Support—searching for comfort and reassurance through God's love and care.
2. Religious Focus—engaging in religious activities to shift focus from the stressor.
3. Religious Purification—searching for spiritual cleansing through religious actions.
4. Spiritual Connection—experiencing a sense of connectedness with forces that transcend the individual.
5. Spiritual Discontent—expressing confusion and dissatisfaction with God's relationship to the individual in the stressful situation.
6. Marking Religious Boundaries—clearly demarcating acceptable from unacceptable religious behaviour and remaining within religious boundaries.

Religious Methods of Coping to Gain Intimacy with Others and Closeness to God

1. Seeking Support from Clergy or Members—searching for comfort and reassurance through the love and care of congregation members and clergy.
2. Religious Helping—attempting to provide spiritual support and comfort to others.
3. Interpersonal Religious Discontent—expressing confusion and dissatisfaction with the relationship of clergy or members to the individual in the stressful situation.

Religious Methods of Coping to Achieve a Life Transformation

1. Seeking Religious Direction—looking to religion for assistance in finding a new direction for living when the old one may no longer be viable.
2. Religious Conversion—looking to religion for a radical changes in life.
3. Religious Forgiving—looking to religion for help in shifting from anger, hurt, and fear associated with an offence to peace.

NOTES

1. CTA: Department of Health [On-line] Available at: http://www.tibet.net/health
2. Tib. *sman rtsis khang*

Bibliography

Abbott, M.W., Wong, S., Williams, M., Au, M., Young, W. (1999). Chinese migrants' mental health and adjustment to life in New Zealand. *Australian and New Zealand Journal of Psychiatry*, 33, 13–21.

Addington, J., Mastrigt, S. van, Hurchinson, J., Addington, D. (2002). Pathways to care: help-seeking behaviour in first episode psychosis. *Acta Psychiatirca Scandinavica*, 106, 358–364.

Ai, A.L., Bolling, S.F., Peterson, C. (2000). The Use of Prayer by Coronary Artery Bypass Patients. *The International Journal For the Psychology of Religion*, 10(4), 205–220.

Allen, M., Naka, K., Ishizu, H. (2004). Attacked by the gods or by mental illness? Hybridizing mental and spiritual health in Okinawa. *Mental Health, Religion and Culture*, Vol. 7, No. 2, 83–107.

Antonovsky, A. (1990). "Salutogenesis. Studying Health vs. Studying Disease." Lecture at the Congress for Clinical Psychology and Psychotherapy, Berlin, 19 February 1990, Available online: http://www.ensp.unl.pt/saboga/soc/pulic/soc_AAconference_berlim_91.pdf

Ashwin-Hirst, M. (2001). *Dissertation guidelines for students and staff*. London Southbank University, Available online: http://www.lsbu.ac.uk/sbbsmktg/dissertation/ba_dissertationguide.doc

Aull, F. (2005). Telling and Listening: Constraints and Opportunities. *Narrative*, Vol. 13, No. 3, 281–293.

American Psychiatric Association (2000). *Diagnostic and Statistical Manual of Mental Disorders DSM-IV-TR*. Washington, DC: American Psychiatric Association.

Anand, D. (2000). (Re)imagining nationalism: identity and representation in the Tibetan diaspora of South Asia. *Contemporary South Asia*, Issue 9(3), 271–287.

Anand, D. (2003). A Contemporary Story of 'Diaspora': The Tibetan Version. *Diaspora*, 12:2, Available online: http://staff.bath.ac.uk/ecsda/DAnand-Diaspora Article.pdf

Anderson, N., Kagawa-Singer, M. (1996). Policy recommendations for the ethnic-minority adolescent health issues: A paradigm shift. In: M. Kagawa-Singer, P. Katz, D. Taylor, J. Vanderyn (Eds.), *Health issues for minority adolescent.* (217–242) Lincoln, NE: University of Nebraska Press.

Apte, R.Z., Edwards, A.R. (2001). *Tibet: Enduring Spirit, Exploited Land.* New Mexico: Heartsfire Books.

Ausubel, D.P. (1960). Acculturative Stress in Modern Maori Adolescence. *Child Development*, 31, 617–631.

Babchuk, W.A. (1996). *Glaser or Strauss? Grounded theory and adult education.* Presented at the Midwest Research-to-Practice Conference in Adult, Continuing, and Community Education, University of Nebraska, October 17–19, Available online: http://www.iupui.edu/~adulted/mwr2p/prior/gradpr96.htm

Baer, R.D., Weller, S.C., Garcia, J.G.D.A., Glazer, M., Trotter, R., Pachter, L., Klein, R.E. (2003). A Cross-Cultural Approach to the Study of the Folk Illness Nervios. *Culture, Medicine and Psychiatry*, 27, 315–337.

Barbaro, B., de. (2002). Opetanie: Kategoria Teologiczna czy Psychiatryczna? *Nomos*, 39/40, 67–78.

Bartholomew, R.E. (1999). Penis Panics. The Psychology of Penis-Shrinking Mass Hysterias. *Skeptic*, Vol. 7, No. 4, 45–49.

Batson, C.D., Schoenrade, P., Ventis, W.L. (1993). *Religion and the individual.* New York: Oxford University Press.

Bazaron, E. (1991). *Medycyna Tybetanska.* Bialystok: Wydawnictwo Rewers.

Beiser, M., Simich, L., Pandalangat, N. (2003). Community in Distress: Mental Health Needs and Help-Seeking in the Tamil Community in Toronto. *International Migration*, Vol. 41, No. 5, 233–245.

Bemak, F., Chung, R.C., Bornemann, T.H. (1996). Counseling and psychotherapy with refugees. In: P.B. Pedersen, J.G. Draguns, W.J. Lonner, J.E. Trimble (Eds.), *Counseling across cultures*, 4th edition, (243–265) Thousand Oaks, CA: Sage Publications.

Berry, J.W. (2001). A Psychology of Immigration. *Journal of Social Issues*, Vol. 57, No. 3, 615–631.

Berzin, A. (2004). *The Heart Sutra. The Heart of Far-Reaching Discriminating Awareness, the Vanquishing Lady Surpassing All.* Translation from the Tibetan. Available online: http://www.berzinarchives.com/sutra/sutra_level_2/heart_sutra.htm

Bhugra, D. (2004). Migration and mental health. *Acta Psychiatrica Scandinavica*, 109, 243–258.

Bhui, K. (1999). Common mental disorders among people with origins in or immigrant from India and Pakistan. *International Review of Psychiatry*, 11, 136–144.

Bokar Rinpoche, Khenpo Donyo. (1994). *Profound Wisdom of the Heart Sutra and Other Teachings.* California: Clear Point Press.

Bokar Rinpoche. (1996). *Opening The Door to Certainty.* California: Clear Point Press.

Bosworth, H.B., Park, K., McQuoid, D.R., Hays, J.C., Steffens, D.C. (2003). The impact of religious practice and religious coping on geriatric depression. *International Journal of Geriatric Psychiatry*, 18, 905–914.

Bourhis, R., Moise, L.C., Perreault, S., Senecal, S. (1997). Towards an Interactive Acculturation Model: A Social Psychological Approach. *International Journal of Psychology*, Vol. 32, No. 6, 369–386.

Brennan, B. (1998). *Hands of Light: A Guide to Healing Through the Human Energy Field*, New York: Bantam.

Buchung, K.T. (2005). Tibetan Culture in the 21st Century. *The Times of Tibet*. Available online: http://www.timesoftibet.com/articles/433/1/Tibetan-Culture-in-the-21st-Century

Caaps, L. (1999). Fright Illness in Hmong Children *Pediatric Nursing*, Vol. 25, Issue 4, 378–384.

Castro, R., Eroza, E. (1998). Research notes on social order and subjectivity: Individuals' experience of susto and fallen fontanelle in a rural community in Central Mexico. *Culture, Medicine and Psychiatry*, 22, 203–230.

Cawthron, L. (2003). Supporting Tibetans in Tezu. *Tibet Foundation Newsletter*, No. 39, 16–17.

Cetrez, Ö. (2005). *Meaning-Making Variations in Acculturation and Ritualization.* Uppsala: Uppsala Universitet.

Chanchani, S., Theivanathampillai, P. (2002). *Typologies of Culture*. University of Otago, Available online: www.commerce.otago.ac.nz/research/working_paper.html

Chung, R.C. (2001). Psychosocial Adjustment of Cambodian Refugee Women: Implications for Mental Health Counseling. *Journal of Mental Health Counseling*, Vol. 23, No. 2, 115–126.

Chung, R.C., Lin, K. (1994). Help-Seeking Behavior Among Southeast Asian Refugees. *Journal of Community Psychology*. Vol. 22, 109–120.

Chowdhury, A.N., Bera, N.K. (1994). Koro following cannabis smoking: two case reports. *Addiction*, 89, 1017–1020.

Clifford, T. (1994). *Tibetan Buddhist Medicine and Psychiatry. The Diamond Healing*. New Delhi: Shri Jainendra Press.

Cohen, A.B., Koenig, H.G. (2003) Religion, Religiosity and Spirituality in the Biopsychosocial Model of Health and Aging. *Aging International*, Vol. 28, No. 3. 215–241.

Crescenzi, A., Ketzer, E., Ommeren, M.V., Phunstok, K., Komproe, I., Jong, J.T.V.M., de. (2002). Effect of Political Imprisonment and Trauma History on Recent Tibetan Refugees in India. *Journal of Traumatic Stress*, Vol. 15, No. 5, 369–375.

Culver, J.L., Arena, P.L., Wimberly, S.R., Antoni, M.H., Carver, C.S. (2002). Coping Among African-American, Hispanic, and Non-Hispanic White Women Recently Treated for Early Stage Breast Cancer. *Psychology and Health*, Vol. 19, No. 2, 157–166.

Dagthon, J.G. (1995). The Importance of Astro. Science in Medicine. In: *Tibetan Astronomy and Astrology* (29–37). Dharamsala: Men-Tsee-Khang.

Dalai Lama. (1997). *The Four Noble Truths*. India: HarperCollins Publishers.

Davis-Floyd, R., St. John, G. (1998). *From Doctor to Healer: The Transformative Journey*. New Jersey: Rutgers University Press.

Dechen Khando, Sither, T.M. (2004). Shattering the Shangri-La Stereotype: Tibetans re-branded. *Tibetan Review*. Available online: http://www.tibet.ca/en/wtnarchive/2004/12/4_8.html

Department of Information and International Relationships. (2002). *Tibet. The Facts*. Dharamsala.

Department of Health, The. (2002–2003). *Healthcare of Tibetans In-Exile*. Dharamsala: Department of Health.

Dewaraja, R., Sasaki, Y. (1991). Semen-Loss Syndrome: A Comparison between Sri Lanka and Japan. *American Journal of Psychotherapy*, Vol. XLV, No. 1, 14–20.

Dick, B. (2005). *Grounded theory: a thumbnail sketch*. Available online: http://www.scu.edu.au/schools/gcm/ar/arp/grounded.html

Diki Tsering. (2002). *Dalai Lama, my son: a mother's story*. New York: Penguin Group.

Dilgo Khyentse Rinpoche. (2002). *The Hundred Verses of Advice of Padampa Sahgye*. Nepal: Shechen Publications.

Dolkar Khangkar. (1998). *The Buddhist Way of Healing*. New Delhi: Lustre Press Roli Books.

Dona, G., Berry, J.W. (1994). Acculturation Attitudes and Acculturative Stress of Central American Refugees. *International Journal of Psychology*, Vol. 29, No. 1, 57–70.

Dorje Reptan Neshar. (2003). Tibetan medicine—An introduction. The Experience Festival 2003. Available online: http://www.experiencefestival.com/a/Tibetan_Medicine/id/1867

Dorjee, T., Giles, H. (2005). Cultural Identity in Tibetan Diasporas. *Journal of Multilingual and Multicultural Development*, Vol. 26, No. 2, 138–157.

Duff, T. (2003). *The Illuminator Tibetan-English Encyclopaedic Dictionary. Electronic Version*. Padma Karpo Translation Committee.

Dummer, T. (1988). *Tibetan Medicine and Other Holistic Health-Care Systems*. New Delhi: Paljor Publication.

Ellison, C.G. (1993). Religious Involvement and Self-Perception among Black Americans. *Social Forces,* Vol. 71, No. 4, 1027–1055.

Escobar, J.I. (2004). Transcultural Aspects of Dissociative and Somatoform Disorders. *Psychiatric Times*, April Special Edition, 10–12.

Ferraro, K.F., Albrecht-Jensen, C.M. (1991). Does Religion Influence Adult Health? *Journal for the Scientific Study of Religion,* Vol. 30, No. 2, 193–202.

Ferraro, K.F., Koch, J.R. (1994). Religion and Health Among Black and White Adults: Examining Social Support and Consolation. *Journal for the Scientific Study of Religion,* Vol. 33. No. 4, 362–375.

Ferraro, K.F., Kelley-Moore, J.A. (2001). Religious seeking among affiliates and non-affiliates: do mental and physical health problems spur religious coping? *Review of Religious Research*, Vol. 42, No. 3, 229–251.

Fielding, N. (1994). Getting Into Computer-Aided Qualitative Data Analysis. *Data Archive Bulletin*, Available online: http://caqdas.soc.surrey.ac.uk/fieldinggettinginto.pdf

Finerman, R. (1998). Zaburzenia specyficzne kulturowo. In: S. Puzynski, J. Wciorka (Eds.), *Klasyfikacja zaburzen psychicznych i zaburzen zachowania w ICD-10. Badawcze kryteria diagnostyczne*. (154–162) Krakow-Warszawa: Uniwersyteckie Wydawnictwo Medyczne "Vesalius." Instytut Psychiatrii i Neurologii.

Fishbain, D.A., Barsky, S., Goldberg, M. (1989). "Koro" (Genital Retraction Syndrome): Psychotherapeutic Interventions. *American Journal of Psychotherapy*, Vol. XLIII, No. 1, 87–91.

Flannelly, K.J., Weaver, A.J., Larson, D.B., Koenig, H.G. (2002). A Review of Mortality Research on Clergy and Other Religious Professionals. *Journal of Religion and Health*, Vol. 41, No. 1, 57–68.

Gampopa. (1995). *The Precious Garland of the Sublime Path*. Boudhanah: Rangjung Yeshe Publications.

Garro, L. (2000). Cultural meaning, explanations of illness, and the development of comparative frameworks. *Ethnology*, Vol. 39, No. 4, 305–334.

Gil, A.G., Vega, W.A., Dimas, J.M. (1994). Acculturative Stress and Personal Adjustment Among Hispanic Adolescent Boys. *Journal of Community Psychology*, Vol. 22, January, 43–54.

Glaser, B. (2004). Remodeling Grounded Theory. *The Grounded Theory Review: An International Journal*. Vol. 4, No. 1, 1–24.

Glaser, B. (2004). Naturalist Inquiry and Grounded Theory. *Forum: Qualitative Social Research*. Vol. 5, No. 1, Art. 7, Available online: http://www.qualitative-research.net/fqs/

Gomez, S.L., Kelsey, J.L., Glaser, S.K., Lee, M.M., Sidney, S. (2004). Immigration and Acculturation in Relation to Health and Health-Related Risk Factors Among Specific Asian Subgroups in a Health Maintenance Organization. *American Journal of Public Health*, Vol. 94, No. 11, 1977–1984.

Greenberg, D., Stravynski, A., Bilu, Y. (2004). Social phobia in ultra-orthodox Jewish males: culture-bound syndrome or virtue? *Mental Health, Religion and Culture*, Vol. 7, No. 4, 289–305.

Grigsby, R.K., Thyer, B.A., Waller, R.J., Johnston, G.A. (1999). Chalk Eating in Middle Georgia: A Culture-Bound Syndrome of Pica? *Southern Medical Journal*, Vol. 92, No. 2, 190–192.

Grzymala-Moszczynska, H. (2004). *Religia a kultura.* Krakow: Wydawnictwo Uniwersytetu Jagiellon´skiego.

Guarnaccia, P.J., Rogler, L.H. (1999). Research on Culture-Bound Syndromes: New Directions. *The American Journal of Psychiatry*, Vol. 156, No. 9, 1322–1327.

Haar, G., ter. (1987). Religion and Healing: the Case of Milingo. *Social Compass*, XXXIV/4, 475–493.

Haig, B.D. (2008). *Grounded Theory as Scientific Method*. University of Canterbury, Available online: http://www.ed.uiuc.edu/EPS/PES-Yearbook/95_docs/haig.html

Harrison, M.O., Koenig, H.G., Hays, J.C., Eme-Akwari, A.G., Pargament, K. (2001). The epidemiology of religious coping: a review of recent literature. *International Review of Psychiatry*, 13, 86–93.

Hawley, R.M., Owen, J.H. (1988). Koro: its presentation in an elderly male. *International Journal of Geriatric Psychiatry*, Vol. 3, 69–72.

Hirini, P., Flett, R., Long, N., Millar, M. (2005). Frequency of Traumatic Events, Physical and Psychological Health among Maori. *New Zealand Journal of Psychology*, Vol. 34, No. 1, 20–27.

Hofstede, G. (1991). *Cultures and organizations: software of the mind*. New York: McGraw-Hill International.

Hood, R., Spilka, B., Hunsberger, B., Gorsuch, R. (1996). *The Psychology of Religion*. New York: The Guilford Press.

Howard, J., Ramsell, J. (1990). *The Original Writings of Edward Bach*. Norfolk: C.W. Daniel Company Ltd.

Hovey, J.D. (2000). Psychosocial Predictors of Acculturative Stress in Mexican Immigrants. *The Journal of Psychology*, Vol. 134, No. 5, 490–502.

Hummer, R.A., Ellison, C.G., Rogers, R.G., Moulton, B.E., Romero, R.R. (2004). Religious Involvement and Adult Mortality in the United States: Review and Perspective. *Southern Medical Journal*, Vol. 97, No. 12, 1223–1230.

Hyman, I., Dussault, G. (2000). Negative Consequences of Acculturation on Health Behaviour, Social Support and Stress among Pregnant Southeast Asian Immigrant Women in Montreal: An Exploratory Study. *Canadian Journal of Public Health*, Vol. 91, No. 5, 357–360.

Jacobson, E. (2002). Panic attack in a context of comorbid anxiety and depression in a Tibetan refugee. Clinical History. *Culture, Medicine and Psychiatry*, 26, 259–279.

Jamgon Kongtrul Rinpoche. (2003). *The Torch of Certainty*. Shambhala.

Jegede, A.S. (2005). The Notion of "Were" in Yoruba Conception of Mental Illness. *Nordic Journal of African Studies*, Vol. 14, No. 1, 117–126.

Jhampa Kalsang. (1995). Traditional Community Role of the Astro-Practitioner. In: *Tibetan Astronomy and Astrology* (19–28). Dharamsala: Men-Tsee-Khang.

Joel, D., Sathyaseelan, M., Jayakaran, R., Vijayakumar, C., Muthurathnam, S., Jacob, K.S. (2003). Explanatory models of psychosis among community health workers in South India. *Acta Psychiarica Scandinavica*, 108, 66–69.

Jones, J.W. (2004). Religion, Health, and the Psychology of Religion: How the Research on Religion and Health Helps Us Understand Religion. Journal of Religion and Health, Vol. 43, No. 4, 317–328.

Kagitcibasi, C., Berry, J.W. (1989), Cross-cultural Psychology: Current Research and Trends. *Annual Review of Psychology*, 40, 493–531.

Kalu Rinpoche. (1995a). *Profound Buddhism. From Hinayana to Vajrayana*. California: ClearPoint Press.

Kalu Rinpoche. (1995b). *Secret Buddhism. Vajrayana Practices*. California: ClearPoint Press.

Kalu Rinpoche. (1997). *Luminous Mind. The way of the Buddha*. Boston: Wisdom Publications.

Kamya, H.A. (1997). African Immigrants in the United States: The Challenge for Research and Practice. *Social Work*, Vol. 42, No. 2, 154–165.

Katsavdakis, K.A. (2001), Book reviews. Personality disorders and culture: Clinical and conceptual interactions. *Bulletin of the Menniner Clinic*, Vol. 65, No. 1, 120–122.

Kendler, K.S., Liu, X., Gardner, C., McCullough, M.E., Larson, D., Prescott, C.A. (2003). Dimensions of Religiosity and Their Relationship to Lifetime Psychiatric and Substance Use Disorders. *American Journal of Psychiatry*, 160/3, 496–503.

Kennedy, B. (1991). Classification of Koro. *The American Journal of Psychiatry*, Vol. 148, No. 9, 1278–1279.

Khenpo Ngawang Pelzang. (2004). *A Guide to the Words of My Perfect Teacher*. Boston: Shambhala Publications Inc.

Khndro Rinpoche. (2003). *This Precious Life. Tibetan Buddhist Teachings on the Path to Enlightenment*. Boston: Shambhala Publications Inc.

Kim, L.I., Kim, G.I. (1998). Searching for and defining a Korean American identity in a multicultural society. In: Y.I. Song, A. Moon (Eds.), *Korean American women: From tradition to modern feminism* (115–125) Westport, CT: Praeger Publishers.

Kim Yeshi. (2008). *The Tibetan Buddhist view of the Environment*. Available online: http://www.tibet.com/Eco/eco8.html

Kleinman, A. (1981). *Patients and Healers in the Context of Culture.* London: University of California Press.

Kleinman, A., Eisenberg, L., Good, B. (1978). Culture, Illness, and Care. Clinical Lessons from Anthropologic and Cross-Cultural Research. *Annals of Internal Medicine*, 88, 251–258.

Knipscheer, J.W., Jong, E.E.M. de, Lamptey, E. (2000). Ghanaian migrants in the Netherlands: General health, acculturative stress and utilization of mental health care. *Journal of Community Psychology*, Vol. 28, No. 4, 459–476.

Koenig, H.G., Larson, D.B. (1999). Use of Hospital Services, Religious Attendance, and Religious Affiliation. *Southern Medical Journal*, Vol. 91, No. 10, 925–932.

Koenig, H.G., Larson, D.B. (2001). Religion and mental health: evidence for an association. *International Review of Psychiatry*, 13, 67–78.

Koenig, H.G. (2002). Religion, Congestive Heart Failure, and Chronic Pulmonary Disease. *Journal of Religion and Health*, Vol. 41, No. 3, 263–278.

Koenig, H.G. (2004). Religion, Spirituality, and Medicine: Research Findings and Implications for Clinical Practice, *Southern Medical Journal*, Vol. 97, No. 12, 1194–1200.

Koenig, H.G., George, L.K., Titus, P. (2004). Religion, Spirituality, and Health in Medically Ill Hospitalized Older Patients. *Journal of the American Geriatrics Society*, 53, 554–562.

Kolas, A. (2004). *Ethnic Tourism In Shangrila. Representations of Place and Tibetan Identity*. Thesis submitted in partial fulfillment of the requirements for the Dr. Polit. Degree, Department of Social Anthropology, University of Oslo.

Korzenny, F., Abravanel, R. (1998). Acculturation: conceptualization and measurement. Quirk's Marketing Research Review, No. 0324, Available online: www.quirks.com

Kosic, A. (2002). Acculturation Attitudes, Need for Cognitive Closure, and Adaptation of Immigrants. *The Journal of Social Psychology*, Vol. 142, No. 2, 269–278.

Kosic, A. (2004). Acculturation strategies, coping process and acculturative stress. *Scandinavian Journal of Psychology*, 45, 269–278.

Kozielecki, J. (1997). *Transgresja i kultura*. Krakow: Wydawnictwo Akademickie 'Zak'.

Kraszewski, P. (2003). Typologia migracji. In: J. Bursztyn, J. Serwanski (Eds.), *Migracja - Europa - Polska* (11–16). Poznan: Zaklad Badan Narodowosciowych PAN.

Kubler-Ross, E. (1997). *On Death and Dying*. New York: Scribner Book Company.

Kwak, K., Berry, J.W. (2001). Generational differences in acculturation among Asian families in Canada: A comparison of Vietnamese, Korean, and East-Indian groups. *International Journal of Psychology*, Vol. 36, No. 3, 152–162.

Laarivaara, P., Kiuttu, J., Taanila, A. (2001). The patient-centered interview: the key to biopsychosocial diagnosis and treatment. *Scandinavian Journal of Primary Health Care,* 19:1, 8–13.

Lama Karma Samten. (2002). Suicide and Depression. Transcript of a lecture given at Auckland University School of Performing Arts on 20 March 2002. *Darmachakra*, Marpa Activities, March/June, 27–29.

Lama Mipham. (1973a). The Wheel of Analytic Meditation. In: *Calm and Clear* (29–55). California: Dharma Publishing.

Lama Mipham. (1973b). Instructions on Vision in the Middle Way. In: *Calm and Clear*. California: Dharma Publishing.

Lester, R. (2004). Commentary: Eating Disorders and the Problem of "Culture" in Acculturation. *Culture, Medicine and Psychiatry*, 28, 607–615.

Lester, R. (2007). Critical Therapeutics: Cultural Politics and Clinical Reality in Two Eating Disorder Treatment Centers. *Medical Anthropology Quarterly*, Vol. 21, No. 4 369-387

Lhalungpa, L.P. (1979). *The Life of Milarepa*. New Delhi: Book Faith India.

Lhawang, Namgyal Qusar, Namgyal Tenzin. (1995). The Knowledge of Skin Care in Tibetan Medicine: as explained in the Upadesa Tantra. *sMan-rTsis*, Vol. 1, No. 1, 47–61.

Lin, E.H.B., Carter, W.B., Kleinman, A.M. (1985). An Exploration of Somatization among Asian Refugees and Immigrants in Primary Care. *American Journal Of Public Health*, Vol. 75, No. 9, 1080–1084.

Littlewood, R. (2004). Commentary: Globalization, Culture, Body Image and Eating Disorders. *Culture, Medicine and Psychiatry*, 28, 597–602.

Lobsang Dolma Khangkar. (1986). *Lectures on Tibetan Medicine*. New Delhi: Library of Tibetan Works and Archives.

Lopsang Rapgay. (1996). *The Tibetan Book of Healing*. Varanassi: Pilgrims Publishing.

Lobsang Rapgay. (1981). *rLung (Vata) Diseases: Diagnostic and Cure*. Dharamsala.

Lobsang Tsultrim Tsona, Tenzin Dakpa. (1981). *Fundamentals of Tibetan Medicine*. Dharamsala: Men-Tsee-Khang.

Lobsang Wangyal. (1995). Practice and Principle of Diagnosis in Tibetan Medicine. *sMan-rTsis*, Vol. 1, No. 1, 32–46.

Lotsawa Kawa Paltseg. (1992). *A Manual of Key Buddhist Terms. Categorization of Buddhist Terminology with Commentary*. New Delhi: Library of Tibetan Works and Archives.

Lorenz, K.A., Hays, R.D., Shapiro, M.F., Cleary, P.D., Wenger, N.S. (2005). Religiousness and Spirituality Among HIV-Infected Americans. *Journal of Palliative Medicine*, Vol. 8, No. 4, 774–781.

Manjula, M., Prasadarao, P.S.D.V., Kumaraiah, V., Mishra, H., Raguram, R. (2003). Sexual Dysfunction in Single Males: A Perspective from India. *Journal of Clinical Psychology*, Vol. 59, No. 6, 701–713.

Maynard, E.A., Gorsuch, R.L., Bjorck, J.P. (2001). Religious Coping Style, Concept of God, and Personal Religious Variables in Threat, Loss, and Challenge Situations. *Journal for the Scientific Study of Religion*, Vol. 40, No. 1, 65–74.

McGuire, M.B. (1987). Ritual, Symbolism and Healing. *Social Compass*, XXXIV/4, 365–379.

McQueen, A., Greg, J., Bray, J.H. (2003). Acculturation, Substance Use, and Deviant Behavior: Examining Separation and Family Conflict as Mediators. *Child Development*, Vol. 74, No. 6, 1737–1750.

Men-Tsee-Khang. (2001). Tibetan medicine: A holistic approach. *Men-tsee-khang News*, Vol. 9, No. 2, 1.

Mercer, S.W., Ager, A., Ruwanpura, E. (2005). Psychosocial distress of Tibetans in exile: integrating Western interventions with traditional beliefs and practice. *Social Science and Medicine*, Vol. 60, No. 1, 179–189.

Miles, M.B., Huberman, A.M. (1994). *Qualitative Data Analysis*. Sage Publications.

Miller, D.J. (1999). Nomads of the Tibetan Plateau. Rangelands in Western China. *Rangelands,* Vol. 21, No. 1, 17–19.

Misra, A. (2003). A Nation in Exile: Tibetan Diaspora and the Dynamics of Long Distance Nationalism. *Asian Ethnicity,* Vol. 4, No.2, 189–206.

Miranda, A.O., Fraser, L.D. (2002). Culture-bound Syndromes: Initial Perspectives from Individual Psychology. *The Journal of Individual Psychology*, Vol. 58, No. 4, 422–433.

Mol, H. (1979). The Identity Model of Religion: How It Compares with Nine Other Theories of Religion and How It Might Apply to Japan. *Japanese Journal of Religious Studies,* Vol. 6, No. 1–2, 11–38.

Myers, M. D. (1997). *Qualitative Research in Information Systems*. MISQ Discovery, archival version. Available online: www.qual.auckland.ac.nz

Myss, C. (1996). *Anatomy of the Spirit*. New York: Random House.

Mysyk, A. (1998). Susto: An Illness of the Poor. *Dialectical Anthropology*, 23, 187–202.

Nairn, R.V., Merluzzi, T.V. (2003). The role of religious coping in adjustment to cancer. *Psycho-Oncology*, 12, 428–441.

National Child Traumatic Stress Network (2003). *Review of Child and Adolescent Refugee Mental Health. White Paper from the National Child Traumatic Stress Network Refugee Trauma Task Force*. Boston, Massachusetts: National Child Traumatic Stress Network.

Neto, F. (2002). Social Adaptation Difficulties of Adolescents with Immigrant Backgrounds. *Social Behavior and Personality*, Vol. 30, No. 4, 335–346.

Ng, B.Y. (1998). Wei han zheng (frigophobia): a culture-related psychiatric syndrome. *Australian and New Zealand Journal of Psychiatry*, 32, 582–585.

Noh, S., Kaspar, V. (2003). Perceived Discrimination and Depression: Moderating Effects of Coping, Acculturation, and Ethnic Support. *American Journal of Public Health*, Vol. 93, No. 2, 232–238.

Norbu Chophel. (1983). *Folk Culture of Tibet*. New Delhi: The Library of Tibetan Works and Archives.

Nuland, S. (1994). *How We Die.* New York: Alfred A. Knopf.

Office of Tibet, The. (2001). *A Guide to Little Lhasa in India*. Available online: http://www.tibet.com/dasaguide.html

Oh, Y., Koeske, G.F., Sales, E. (2002). Acculturation, Stress, and Depressive Symptoms Among Korean Immigrants in the United States. *The Journal of Social Psychology*, Vol. 142, No. 4, 511–526.

Oman, D., Thoresen, C.E. (2002). "Does Religion Cause Health?": Differing Interpretations and Diverse Meanings. *Journal of Health Psychology,* Vol. 7(4), 365–380.

Oppedal, B., Røysamb, E., Lackland, S, D. (2004). The effect of acculturation and social support on change in mental health among young immigrants. *International Journal of Behavioral Development,* Vol. 28, No. 6, 481–494.

Osborne, T.L., Vandenberg, B. (2003). Situational and Denominational Differences in Religious Coping. *The International Journal for the Psychology of Religion*, 13(2), 111–122.

Pargament, K.I. (1997). *The psychology of religion and coming: theory, research, practice.* New York: The Guilford Press.

Pargament, K.I., Smith, B.W., Koenig, H.G., Perez, L. (1998). Patterns of Positive and Negative Religious Coping with Major Life Stressors, Journal for the Scientific Study of Religion, Vol. 37, No. 4, 710–724.

Pargament, K.I., Koenig, H.G., Perez, L.M. (2000). The Many Methods of Religious Coping: Development and Initial Validation of the RCOPE. *Journal of Clinical Psychology*, Vol. 56(4), 519–543.

Pargament, K., Tarakeshwar, N., Ellison, C.G., Wulff, K.M. (2001). Religious Coping Among the Religious: The Relationships Between Religious Coping and Well-Being in a National Sample of Presbyterian Clergy, Elders, and Members. *Journal for the Scientific Study of Religion*, Vol. 40, No. 3, 497–513.

Pargament, K.I., Zinnbauer, B.J., Scott, A.B., Zerowin, J., Stanik, P. (2003). Red Flags and Religious Coping: Identifying Some Religious Warning Signs Among People in Crisis. *Journal of Clinical Psychology*, Vol. 59, No. 12, 1335–1348.

Pargament, K., Emery, E.E. (2004). The many faces of religious coping in late life: conceptualization, and link to well-being. *Aging International*, Vol. 29, No. 1, 3–27.

Pasang Yonten. (1989). A History of the Tibetan Medical System. *Tibetan Medicine*, No. 12, 32–51.

Pathak, N. (2003). The Response of Immigrant Tibetans towards Cultural Iatrogenesis in Contemporary Health Care System in India, *The Tibet Journal*, Vol. XXVIII, No. 3, 43–52.

Pathak, N. (2004). Revitalisation Movement Gripping the Exile Tibetan Diaspora: A Model of Non-violent Struggle for Peace. *The Tibet Journal*, Vol. 29, Issue 1, 85–90.

Patrul Rinpoche. (1998). *The Words of My Perfect Teacher*. Boston: Shambhala.

Pema Chodron. (2001). *Tonglen. The Path of Transformation*. Halifax: Vajradhatu Publications.

Pema Dorjee. (2002). Importance of Saving the Himalayas. A Tibetan medical practitioner's perspective. *Men-Tsee-Khang News*, Vol. IX, No. 3, Available online: http://www.men-tsee-khang.org/newsletter

Pema Dorjee. (2008). *An explanation of Tibetan Medicine from my own experience*. Available online: www.men-tsee-khang.org/publication/article.htm

Pema Dorji. (1989). Introductory Notes on Tibetan Medicine. *Tibetan Medicine*, No. 12, 52–62.

Penny-Dimri, S. (1994). Conflict amongst the Tibetans and Indians of North India: communal violence and welfare dollars. *The Australian Journal of Anthropology*, Vol. 5, No. 3, 280–304.

Phinney, J.S., Horenczyk, G., Liebkind, K., Vedder, P. (2001). Ethnic Identity, Immigration, and Well-Being: An Interactional Perspective. *Journal of Social Issues*, Vol. 57, No. 3, 493–510.

Pietkiewicz, I. (2002). Disease—remedy per se? Reflections on the informative-adaptive-transgressive role of disease. *XII European Symposium of Somatotherapy, V European Symposium of Psychosomatic Education.*

Pietkiewicz, I. (2004). The phenomena of suffering from the perspective of the Tibetan Buddhist philosophy. *Sztuka Leczenia*, Vol. 10, No. 3–4, 35–41.

Pillay, B.J. (1996). A model of help-seeking behaviour for urban blacks. *South African Journal of Psychology*, Vol. 26, No. 1, 4–9.

Pires, G.D., Stanton, P.J. (2000). Ethnicity and Acculturation in a Culturally Diverse Country: Identifying Ethnic Markets., *Journal of Multilingual and Multicultural Development,* Vol. 21, No.1, 42–57.

Powers, J. (1999). *Wprowadzenie do Buddyzmu Tybetanskiego*. Krakow: Wydawnictwo "A."

Ray, O. (2004). How the Mind Hurts and Heals the Body. *American Psychologist,* Vol. 59, No. 1, 29–40.

Ramos, B.M. (2005). Acculturation and Depression among Puerto Ricans in the Mainland. *Social Work Research*, Vol. 29, No. 2, 95–105.

Ritchie, I.D. (2004). African Religion and Culture. Internet: www3.sympatico.ca/ian.ritchie/ATSC.Chapter4.htm

Ritchie, J., Lewis, J. (2003). *Qualitative Research Practice*. London: Sage Publications.

Rogers, S.A., Poey, E.L., Reger, G.M., Tepper, L., Coleman, E.M. (2002). Religious coping among those with persistent mental illness. *The International Journal for the Psychology of Religion*, 12(3), 161–175.

Rudmin, F. W. (2003). Catalogue of acculturation constructs: Descriptions of 126 taxonomies, 1918–2003. In: W. J. Lonner, D. L. Dinnel, S. A. Hayes, D. N. Sattler (Eds.), *Online Readings in Psychology and Culture* (Unit 8, Chapter 8), (http://www.wwu.edu/~culture), Center for Cross-Cultural Research, Western Washington University, Bellingham, Washington.

Rudmin, F.W. (2005). *Debate in Science: The Case of Acculturation.* Tromso: University of Tromso.

Ryan, M., Dhadon Jamling. (1995). Study of Tibetan Medicine on Arthritis—A Research Report. *sMan-rTsis*, Vol. 1, No. 2, 11–20.

Sadutsang, T. (2002). *Psychosocial Development Aid in Traumatized Communities*. Paper from the seminar "New Challenges in the Treatment of Traumatized Refugees," hosted by OASIS, Denmark. Available online: http://www.oasis-rehab.dk/Sider/Bibliotek/Artikler/Tsadutshang.pdf

Santina, P.D. (1997). *The Tree of Enlightenment*. Chico Dharma Study Foundation.

Shantideva. (1979). *A Guide to the Bodhisattva's Way of Life*. Dharamsala: Library of Tibetan Works and Archives.

Shome, S., Bhutia, M.S., Gautam, R.K. (1993). Culture-Bound Trichotillomania. *The American Journal of Psychiatry*, Vol. 150, No. 4, 674.

Schwimmer, B. (2008). "Method and Theory in Cultural Anthropology." Description of a course in cultural anthropology. Department of Anthropology, University of Mantioba. Available online: http://www.umanitoba.ca/faculties/arts/anthropology/courses/122/module1/dimensions.html

Sieradzan, J., Jaworski, W., Dziwisz, M. (1987). *Buddyzm*. Krakow: Krakowskie Wydawnictwo Prasowe RSW.

Singh, S. (2004). Tears from the land of snow: health and human rights in Tibet. *Phayul*. Available online: http://www.studentsforafreetibet.org/article.php?id=479

Smart, J.F., Smart, D.W. (1995). Acculturative Stress of Hispanics: Loss and Challenge. *Journal of Counseling and Development*, March/April, 390–396.

Snodgrass, L.L., Yamamoto, J., Frederick, C., Ton-That, N., Foy, D.W., Chan, L., Wu, J., Hahn, P.H., Shinh, D.Y., Nguyen, L.H., Jonge, J. de, Fairbanks, L. (1993). Vietnamese Refugees with PTSD Symptomatology: Intervention Via a Coping Skills Model. *Journal of Traumatic Stress*, Vol. 6, No. 4, 569–575.

Somm, C., von. (1998). Tibetan Culture in the Diaspora. *Journal of Buddhist Ethics*, Vol. 5, 339–346.

Songwathana, P., Manderson, L. (1998). Perceptions of HIV/AIDS and caring for people with terminal AIDS in southern Thailand. *AIDS Care*, Vol. 10, Issue 2, 155–166.

Soothill, K., Morris, S.M., Harman, J.C., Thomas, C., Francis, B., McIllmurray, M.B. (2002). Cancer and faith. Having faith—does it make a difference among patients and their informal carers? *Scandinavian Journal of Caring Sciences*, 16, 256–263.

Sosis, R., Alcorta, C. (2003). Signaling, Solidarity, and the Sacred: The Evolution of Religious Behaviour. *Evolutionary Anthropology*, Vol. 12, 264–274.

Speller, H. (2005). Asian Americans and Mental Health. *Elements*, Vol. 1, Spring, 69–78.

Spiritual Cinema Circle, The, (2005). *The Yogis of Tibet*. California: The Spiritual Cinema Circle.

Strahl, H. (2003). Cultural interpretations of an emerging health problem: blood pressure in Dar es Salaam, Tanzania. *Anthropology and Medicine*, Vol. 10, No. 3, 309–324.

Strauss, A., Corbin, J. (1990). *Basics of Qualitative Research. Grounded Theory Procedures and Techniques*. Sage Publications.

Suzuki, K., Takei, N., Kawai, M., Minabe, Y., Mori, N. (2003). Is Taijin Kyofusho a culture-bound syndrome? *The American Journal of Psychiatry*, Vol. 160, No. 7, 1358.

Szawarski, Z. (1996) Dwa rodzaje wiedzy medycznej. *Sztuka Leczenia,* vol. 2, no. 3, 27–35.

Takeuchi, D.T., Adair, R.K. (1992). The Exposure and Vulnerability of Ethnic Minorities to Life Events. *Research in Community and Mental Health*, Vol. 7, 111–124.

Tarthang Tulku Rinpoche. (1973a). Commentary on The Wheel of Analytic Meditation by Lama Mipham. In: *Calm and Clear*. California: Dharma Publishing.

Tarthang Tulku Rinpoche. (1973b). Commentary to Instructions on Vision in the Middle Way by Lama Miphan. In: *Calm and Clear*. California: Dharma Publishing.

Josayma, T.T., K. Dhondup. (1990). *Dolma and Dolkar: Mother and Daughter of Tibetan Medicine.* New Delhi: Yarlung Publications.

Taylor, R.J., Chatters, L.M., Jayakody, R., Levin, J.S. (1996) Black and White Differences in Religious Participation: A Multisample Comparison. *Journal for the Scientific Study of Religion*, Vo. 35, No. 4, 403–410.

Taylor, R.J., Ellison, C.G., Chatters, L.M., Levin, J.S., Lincoln, K.D. (2000). Mental Health Services in Faith Communities: The Role of Clergy in Black Churches, Social Work, Vol. 45, No. 1, 73–87.

Tenzin Choedrak. (1995). A Lecture on AIDS and Tibetan Medicine. *sMan-rTsis Journal*, Vol. 1, No. 1, 26–31.

Tenzin Namdul. (2000). Diet and Lifestyle in Harmony with the Season., *sMan-rTsis Journal*, Vol. 2, No. 2, 72–78.

Terheggen, M.A., Stroebe, M.S., Kleber, R.J. (2001). Western Conceptualizations and Eastern Experience. A Cross-Cultural Study of Traumatic Stress Reactions Among Tibetan Refugees in India. *Journal of Traumatic Stress*, Vol. 14, No. 2, 391–403.

Thrangu Rinpoche, K. (1981). *The Three Vehicles of Buddhist Practice*. Prepublication Edition, Namo Buddha Seminar.

Thrangu Rinpoche. (2001). *Ten Teachings from the 100,000 Songs of Milarepa*. New Delhi: Sri Satguru Publications.

Thrangu Rinpoche. (2002). *The Seven Points of Mind Training*. New Delhi: Sri Satguru Publications.

Tibetan Centre for Human Rights and Democracy (2000a). *Religious Repression in Tibet*. Dharamsala: TCHRD.

Tibetan Centre for Human Rights and Democracy. (2000b). *Torture in Tibet*. Dharamsala: TCHRD.

Tobten Tsering. (2004). Identity Interrupted: The story of exile Tibetan Youth. *The Times of Tibet*, 27.12.2004, Available online: http://www.timesoftibet.com/articles/140/1

Tobten Tsering. (2005). We are no monks: a film review. *The Times of Tibet*, 20.04.2005, Available online: http://www.timesoftibet.com/articles/435/1/-We-are-no-Monks%3A-A-film-review

Tompenaars, F., Hampden-Turner, C. (1997). *Riding the waves of culture.* London: Nicholas Brealey Publishing.

Torres, L., Rollock, D. (2004). Acculturative Distress among Hispanics: The Role of Acculturation, Coping, and Intercultural Competence. *Journal of Multicultural Counseling and Development*, Vol. 32, July, 155–167.

Tseng, W. (2001). *Handbook of Cultural Psychiatry*. London: Academic Press.

Tsering Dhundup. (2001). Tibetan Personal Names and Their Meanings. *Tibet Foundation Newsletter*, No. 31, 4–5.

Tsering Dhondup. (2003). *How to study Tibetan Medicine. A commentary on the Root Tantra*. Diss. Kangra: Dolmaling Institute.

Tsering, F. (2003). *Tibetan Medicine. A Unique and Comprehensive Amalgamation of Science, Art and Philosophy*. New Delhi.

Tsering Gellek. (2001). *The Role of Buddhist Institutions in the Tibetan Diaspora*. Medford: Feinstein International Famine Center, Working Paper No. 4.

Uehara, E.S. (2001). Understanding the dynamics of illness and help-seeking: event-structure analysis and a Cambodian-American narrative of "Spirit Invasion." *Social Science and Medicine*, 52, 519–536.

United Nations High Commissioner for Refugees (UNHCR). (1996). *Convention and Protocol Relating to the Status of Refugees*. Geneva: United Nations High Commissioner For Refugees.

United Nations High Commissioner for Refugees (UNHCR). (2006). *2005 Global Refugee Trends. Statistical Overview of Populations of Refugees, Asylum-Seekers, Internally Displaced Persons, Stateless Persons, and Other Persons of Concern to UNHCR*. Geneva: Field Information and Coordination Support Section Division of Operational Services UNHCR. Available online: www.unhcr.org/statistics.

Vanderpool, H.Y. (1980) Religion and Medicine: A Theoretical Overview. *Journal of Religion and Health*, Vol. 19, No. 1, 7–17.

Van Ness, P.H., Kasl, S.V., Jones, B.A. (2002). Are Religious Women More Likely to Have Breast Cancer Screening? *Journal of Religion and Health*, Vol. 41, No. 4, 333–346.

Vang, T., Flores, J. (1999). The Hmong Americans: Identity, Conflict, and Opportunity. *Multicultural Perspectives*, Vol. 1, No. 4, 9–14.

Verkuyten, M. (1998). Perceived Discrimination and Self-Esteem Among Ethnic Minority Adolescents. *The Journal of Social Psychology*, Vol. 138, No. 4, 479–493.

Verma, R.K., Sharma, S., Singh, R., Rangaiyan, G., Pelto, P. (2003). Beliefs concerning sexual health problems and treatment seeking among men in an Indian slum community. *Culture, Health and Sexuality*, Vol. 5, No. 3, 265–276.

Vertovec, S. (1999). Three meanings of "diaspora." exemplified among South Asian religions. *Diaspora,* 7(2), Available online: http://www.transcomm.ox.ac.uk/working%20papers/diaspora.pdf

Vertovec, S. (2000). Religion and Diaspora. *Paper presented at the conference on "New Landscapes of Religion in the West,"* University of Oxford, September 2000, Available online: http://www.transcomm.ox.ac.uk/working%20papers/Vertovec01.PDF

Vinokurov, A., Trickett, E.J., Birman, D. (2002). Acculturative Hassles and Immigrant Adolescents: A Life-Domain Assessment for Soviet Jewish Refugees. *The Journal of Social Psychology*, Vol. 142, No. 4, 425–445.

Vollebergh, W.A.M., Huiberts, A.M. (1997). Stress and Ethnic Identity in Ethnic Minority Youth in the Netherlands. *Social Behavior and Personality*, Vol. 25, No. 3, 249–258.

Weine, S., Muzurovic, N., Kulauzovic, Y., Besic, S., Lezic, A., Mujagic, A., Muzurovic, J., Spahovic, D., Feetham, S., Ware, N., Knafl, K., Pavkovic, I. (2004). Family Consequences of Refugee Trauma. *Family Process*, Vol. 43, No. 2, 147–160.

White, A.M., Grilo, C.M. (2005). Ethnic Differences in the Prediction of Eating and Body Image Disturbances among Female Adolescent Psychiatric Inpatients. *International Journal of Eating Disorders*, 38, 78–84.

Wilson, B.R. (1988), The Functions of Religion: A Reappraisal. *Religion,* Vol. 18, 199–216.

Williams, D.R., Willims-Morris, R. (2000). Racism and Mental Health: the African American Experience. *Ethnicity and Health*, Vol. 5, No. 3⁄4, 243–268.

World Health Organization. (1994). *Qualitative Research for Health Programmes*. Geneva: WHO.

Wrona-Polanska, H. (2000). Czlowiek wobec powaznej choroby somatycznej—proba syntezy. *Sztuka Leczenia*, Vol. VI, No. 3, 77–84.

Yamamoto, J.I. (2005). *Tibetan Buddhists: Exiled from Their Homeland, Extolled in the West*. Christian Research Institute, Available online: http://www.equip.org/free/DB565-4.pdf

Yangarber-Hicks, N. (2004). Religious coping styles and recovery from serious mental illness. *Journal of Psychology and Theology*, Vol. 32, No. 4, 305–317.

Ye, J. (2005). Acculturative Stress and Use of the Internet among East Asian International Students in the United States. *CyberPsychology and Behavior*, Vol. 8, No. 2, 154–161.

Yeh, C.J., Arora, A.K., Inose, M., Okubo, Y., Li, R.H., Greene, P. (2003), The cultural adjustment and mental health of Japanese immigrant youth. *Adoloscence*, Vol. 38, No. 151, 481-500

Yeo, S.S., Meiser, B., Barlow-Stewart, K., Goldstein, D., Tucker, K., Eisenbruch, M. (2005). Understanding community beliefs of Chinese-Australians about cancer: initial insights using an ethnographic approach. *Psycho-Oncology*, 14, 174–186.

Yeshi Dhonden. (1977). *The Ambrosia Heart Tantra*. Dharamsala: Library of Tibetan Works and Archives.

Yick, A.G. (2000). Predictors of Physical Spousal/Intimate Violence in Chinese American Families. *Journal of Family Violence*, Vol. 15, No. 3, 249–262.

Ying, Y.W., Akutsu, P.D. (1997). Psychological Adjustment of Southeast Asian Refugees: The Contribution of Sense of Coherence. *Journal of Community Psychology*, Vol. 25, No. 2, 125–139.

Ziegahn, L. (2001). *Considering Culture in the Selection of Teaching Approaches for Adults*. Ohio State University, Available online: www.cete.org/acve/docs/dig231.pdf

Index

abhisheka (or abisheka), 34, 141
abortion, 95–96
absolute truth. *See* truth in Buddhism
accessory therapy in Tibetan System of Medicine, 155–56
acculturation, xi, 5, 16–33, 201, 232–36; styles/patterns/attitudes, 20–22; stages, 22, 24–25, 198; affecting factors, 22–33
acculturative stress, 53, 58, 249, 251
acupuncture, 43, 92–93, 155, 161, 186, 194
acute condition. *See* course of sickness
AIDS, 42, 57, 82, 107, 144, 188, 208–9, 257
alcohol, 47, 55, 56–57, 60, 65, 81, 101–2, 153–54, 202
allopathic medicines. *See* Western/allopathic medicines
ambiguity tolerance, 6, 59, 105
amchee/amchi (Tibetan Medicine practitioner), v, 91, 93, 151, 164, 186, 191, 193–94, 210–12, 215, 221, 229, 230, 232, 236, 246, 248, 259
amok, 68
anaemia, 107
anal intercourse, 260
anthropometry, 47, 52, 93
antibiotics, 205
anxiety. *See* depression & anxiety
aphrodisiacs, 146
ascribed identity, 50
assimilation. *See* acculturation styles
asthma, 143, 210, 215, 253
astrology, 82, 154, 159–61, 186, 206, 256
Atisia, 120, 133
aura. *See* energy field
automatized adaptive behavior, 105
Avalokiteshvara (Chenrezi). *See* bodhisattva of love and compassion
Ayurveda. S*ee* ethnomedicine

bacteria, 38, 44, 215. *See also* germs
bile (mkhris pa). *See* humours in the Tibetan System Medicine
bioethics, 95, 147
biomedicine, 36–40, 42–43, 87, 89, 187–88, 211–12, 215–16, 232, 236, 246–47, 250. See *also* Western allopathic medicines
biopsychosocial model of medicine. *See* humanistic medicine
birth control, 72, 96, 259
black magic, 70, 81–82, 242
blessed/holy pills. *See* lama medicine
blood, 157–58, 192, 205, 216; beliefs related to, 69, 82, 96; in Tibetan

System of Medicine, 91, 145–47, 151–52, 155, 161; letting, 146, 155; menstruation, 260; pressure, 56, 62, 98, 101, 210, 253–54; transfusions, 90
blushing phobia in Japan, 74. See *also* culture-bound syndromes
bodhicitta (enlightened attitude), 135, 203
bodhisattva, 108, 127, 140, 199, 201, 202; of love and compassion (*see* Chenrezi)
body odor phobia in Japan, 74. See *also* culture-bound syndromes
Bön tradition, 118–19, 145, 187
Buddha, 34,117–18, 121, 124, 127–28, 132–34, 140, 146, 151, 155, 161–62, 200, 202–3, 250–51
buddhahood, 123, 127–28, 133, 135, 141, 200, 202–3
butter lamp, 4–5, 136, 187, 200, 209, 233
butter tea, 34, 143, 152, 157, 222, 233, 239

calm-abiding meditation (shine), 133–34, 156–57
Cambodians, 18, 25–26, 85, 87–88
cancer, 42, 81–82, 103–4, 106–8, 111, 114, 143, 210, 223
chakra, 43, 43, 93
chang, 4, 34, 145
chaplains in hospitals, 94
Chenrezi, 120–21, 200; mantra of, 92
ch'i energy, 43, 92–93
childbirth, 23, 56–57, 72, 75, 157, 159
Chinatown, 23
Chinese Americans, 23, 48
Chinese Medicine. *See* ethnomedicine
Chinese repression, xi, 14, 121–22, 185–86, 228; torture, 18, 121, 228. See *also* Torture Survivor Program
Chinese-Vietnamese, 25, 87
chiropractic therapy, 43
cholera, 32
chronic ailments. *See* course of sickness
chuba. *See* clothing
circumambulating holy places, 4–5, 92, 137, 182, 187, 201–2, 233
civic identity, 49. See *also* identity
clothing, 4–5, 20, 22, 31, 33, 51, 67, 122, 137, 154, 186, 225, 233
coherence, sense of, 25–26, 34, 105
collaborative coping style. *See* religious coping styles
complementary & alternative medicine, 41, 46, 185–87, 206
concept of God, 101, 112, 199, 202–3
condoms, 260
conflicting explanatory models. *See* explanatory models
counseling: psychological c., 80, 185, 188, 190, 207, 243, 245; spiritual c., 95, 110, 196–98, 204, 245
counter-transference, 38, 92
course of sickness: acute condition, 38, 69, 74, 79, 90, 117, 192, 210–11, 213, 215, 227, 230, 232, 243, 250; chronic ailments, 79, 81, 89, 101, 107, 109, 152, 177, 191, 210–12, 214, 217, 220, 230–32, 237–38, 243–44, 247–48; severity of symptoms, 69, 75, 79, 80, 85–86, 88–90, 96, 101, 107–8, 111–13, 143, 157–58, 167, 177, 180, 188, 190–91, 209–13, 215–16, 230, 232, 236, 238, 243–47
culture: as meaning-making device, 2, 3, 46, 50, 54, 56, 72, 77–84, 241–43, 247; cultural differences, 22–24, 33, 63–65, 87; cultural values, 2–6, 8, 19–20, 24–27, 31, 47, 64, 138, 235, 246; defining, 1–2; dimensions of, 6–7; levels of, 2–5; prejudice against, 23; shock/stress/fatigue (*see* acculturative stress)
culture and health: pathogenic function, 46, 54–67; pathoplastic aspect, 46, 67–77; salutary function, 46–54
culture bound (or culture specific) syndromes, 67–77, 79

culture-broker role, 59
cyclic existence (samsara), 119, 124–26, 128, 133, 135

Dalai Lama, 4, 14–16, 19, 30–31, 120–23, 126, 138, 144, 157, 165–66, 186, 202, 204, 216, 234, 250
death, 10, 18, 69, 71, 81–83, 90, 102, 107–9, 114, 143, 190, 213; in medical paradigms and healthcare, 37, 39–40, 42–43, 96; in Tibetan belief system, 117, 119, 124–28, 130–32, 148–49, 157–60, 199, 206, 214, 223, 251
deferring coping style. *See* religious coping styles
delusions of guilt, punishment, damnation, 96
demonology in Tibetan tradition, 157–58, 160
depression & anxiety, 16–17, 43, 53, 55, 59, 68–72, 75–76, 83, 96, 99, 101; associated with acculturation, 59–62, 64–65; in Tibetan population, 18, 87, 90–91, 203, 207, 224, 228, 247, 253–54; in Tibetan System of Medicine, 151, 221, 228, 242
Dewachen (the Pure Land of Buddha Amitabha), 198
Dharma (Buddhist teachings), 8, 12, 33, 51, 85, 116–40, 146–47, 199, 204, 233, 241, 250–51. See *also* protectors; Wheel of Dharma
Dharma protectors. *See* protectors
diagnosis, 37–40, 42, 45, 84, 104, 142, 196, 231, 237. See *also* disease diagnosis and treatment in Tibetan System of Medicine
Diamond Way/Path/Vehicle. *See* vajrayana
diet, 18, 33, 39, 43–44, 47, 54–56, 81, 92–93, 149–50, 152–54, 160, 186, 213–14, 221–22, 233, 237, 253
discrimination, 20, 32–33, 49, 59–61, 63, 67, 112; perceived d., 53, 58–59, 62, 66; personal versus group d., 62
disease, 32, 38, 41, 44–45, 56–57, 101, 106–7, 143, 210; diagnosis and treatment in Tibetan System of Medicine, 147, 151–56, 160–61, 186, 212, 216, 221, 224; holistic approach to, 44–46; in biomedicine, 37, 84; in Buddhist teaching, 124–25, 156, 159; in Tibetan System of Medicine, 146–62, 185; karmic diseases, 91, 149, 217, 222–23, 241; reaction to (*see* illness behavior); versus illness (*see* illness versus disease); informative, adaptive and transgressive function of, 45. See *also* idiom of health and disease/illness
dispensary, 188, 191, 218–19, 238, 248, 255–56
divination, 54, 187, 195–97, 200, 217, 225
doctor-patient communication, 38, 40–41, 46, 152
dorje, 187. See *also* ritual objects
Dorje Sempa (Vajrasattva), 135; Hundred-syllable mantra of, 135
driggu, 187. See *also* ritual objects
Drugpa Kunley, 8
drugs, 55–57, 65, 79, 81, 101–2, 104
dukha. *See* suffering in Buddhist teaching

earth. *See* elements
East-Indians, 24–25
eating disorders, 17, 55–56, 101; binge eating, 55–56; obesity, 56, 93
education, 7, 11, 15–16, 22, 23, 30– 31, 44, 57, 58, 62, 70, 81, 84–85, 88, 93, 109, 111–12, 123, 139, 144, 159, 185, 188, 190, 208–9, 213, 217, 221, 230, 232–33, 236–39, 242, 245, 248, 253, 256–57, 259–61; health education, 44, 57, 144, 188, 208, 217, 221, 236–38, 242, 248, 253, 256–57, 259, 261; medical training,

38, 45, 95, 122, 144, 187–88, 228, 248
elements, 43, 78, 145, 147–48, 159–60, 243, 253–54
emchi. *See* amchee
emic, vi, xiv, 116
enculturation, 2, 11, 24, 26, 49–50, 199, 235, 249
enemas, 155
energy field and channels, 43, 45, 93
epilepsy, 83, 89, 115, 143, 210, 247
ethnic group, 50
ethnic identity. *See* identity
ethnic markers (labels), xi, 4, 29, 49, 51, 138, 204, 250
ethnicity, 48–50, 55, 110, 112
ethnomedicine, 39, 43, 80; Chinese Medicine, 43; Indian ayurveda, 43, 93, 146, 187, 206; Tibetan folk treatment methods, 145, 186, 191–92. See *also* Tibetan System of Medicine
ethnopharmacology. *See* Tibetan herbal medicines
etic. *See* emic
etiology of illness/disease: natural causes theory, 78; supernatural causation, 71, 78–79, 81–82, 88, 217, 221, 223, 227, 234, 241–42, 247. See *also* explanatory models; folk categories
euthanasia, 95–96
evil eye, 217, 242
evil spirits. *See* spirits
explanatory models (EMs), 40, 72, 77–85, 90–92, 161, 221, 228–32, 241–44, 246–48; conflicting EMs, 80–81, 83, 228, 242
expressing emotions, 7–8, 24, 33, 64, 76, 81, 207–9, 247; through somatic symptoms (*see* somatization)
eye-to-eye contact phobia in Japan, 74. See *also* culture-bound syndromes

fallen fontanelle, 72. See *also* culture-bound syndromes
feng-shui. *See* geomancy
fire. *See* elements
flower remedies, 43, 45
folk categories, 68, 77–85, 241
frigophobia (fear of cold temperatures) in Singapore, 74

gau, 5
Gelukpa. *See* sects in Tibetan Buddhism
generation gap, 5, 24–25,
genitalia loss, 68–71, 73.
geomancy (feng-shui), 82
germs, 44, 79, 82. See *also* bacteria
ghost, 68, 77–78, 88, 124, 157–58, 223–24, 226, 242, 243. See *also* possession
globalization, 12
golden hammer, 153, 155, 194
Guru Rinpoche, 119, 226

handicraft, 16, 28–29, 32, 165, 218
healers: holistic h., 39, 43–44, 39, 46; indigenous h., 73–74, 85, 88–89, 96–97, 187, 205, 217, 227, 244, 248. See *also* shamanism
health education. *See* education
health insurance, 88, 218–19; companies, 39, 46
healthy migrant effect, 47
help-seeking behavior. *See* illness behavior
help-seeking pathways, 74, 87–92, 103–4, 160, 193, 195–96, 205–6, 208–18, 220, 244–45
hepatitis, 148, 210, 215, 259
herbs, 41, 154, 186, 191–94, 219, 231, 242. See *also* Tibetan herbal medicines
hikikomori, 74
hinayana, 118. See *also* Wheel of Dharma
Hispanics, 19, 56, 58, 66, 86, 111
Hmong, 24–25, 47, 72, 80, 83, 87
holistc approach in healthcare, 36–37, 40, 43- 47, 78–79, 93, 95

homeopathy, 43, 45, 219
homosexuality, 96, 114, 260–61
hospitals. *See* medical institutions
humanistic approach in healthcare, 37, 40–43, 46, 95, 215–16
humours in Tibetan System Medicine, 90–91, 148–52, 154, 212, 221–22, 228–29, 242, 253
hydrotherapy, 155, 161, 186
hypertension. *See* blood pressure

identity, 4–5, 26–28, 33, 48–48, 108; ethnic identity, 49–50; types, 48–49
idiom of health and disease/illness, 40, 44, 77–79, 80–83, 85, 88, 91, 94–96, 148–50, 153–54, 157–58, 160, 167, 195, 198, 203, 217, 221–22, 228–29, 241–44, 259; conceptions of mental health, 99–100; folk beliefs, 37, 81–82. See *also* folk categories; explanatory models
ignorance concept in Tibetan Buddhism and Medicine, 124, 126, 129, 130, 135, 150, 241
illness, 18, 32, 42, 46, 68, 71–73, 77, 86, 89–90, 100–101, 104, 154, 156, 158, 190, 212; illness versus disease, 41–42, 77, 84; illness narrative, 40; mental illness, 76, 79–80, 84, 99, 110–11, 158, 228–29, 241. *See also* idiom of health and disease/illness
illness behavior, 1, 74, 84–86, 88–92, 104, 107–9, 112, 180, 188–91, 193–94, 238, 240, 245–51. See *also* help-seeking pathways
immunization, 144, 257, 259
impermanence, 106, 109, 125–26, 130, 134
indigenous beliefs about illness. *See* folk categories
indiginous systems of medicine. *See* ethnomedicine
insurance. *See* health insurance
integration. *See* acculturation styles
Internet services, xi, xiv, 31, 53–54, 180, 234
interpretative control. *See* religious coping effects
intuition in healthcare, 43, 45

jaundice, 148, 210, 212–13. See *also* hepatitis

Kagyupa. *See* sects in Tibetan Buddhism
Kalachakra, 159
Kanjur, 117, 140
karma, 8, 26, 81–82, 91, 117–18, 125, 128–29, 132, 134–35, 147, 149, 153, 160, 187, 192, 198–200, 203, 214, 217, 221–24, 241–42, 250–51
Karmapa, 9, 120
karmic diseases, 149
kathak, 4–5, 33, 51–52
kinship, 19, 53, 64
kora. *See* circumambulating holy places
Koreans, 24–25, 47, 64–65
koro. *See* genitalia loss; culture-bound syndromes

lama medicine (blessed or holy pills), 92, 149, 181, 187, 192–93, 212
language, 2, 4, 9, 19–26, 29, 37, 41, 49, 53, 57–60, 63, 66, 88, 167, 169, 173, 175, 179, 187, 207, 228, 233, 249–50
Laotians, 25, 57, 87
Lesbian. *See* homosexuality
Little Lhasa, xi, 23
local categories. *See* folk categories

Mahakala, 199, 239. See *also* protectors
mahayana, 118, 120, 127. See *also* Wheel of Dharma
mala (rosary), 5, 31, 137, 196, 203
malaria, 32, 143
mania, 115, 247
Mañjushri, 196

mantra, 4, 31, 92, 97, 109, 135, 137, 187, 196–97, 201–3, 209, 226–27, 233, 251
mantra pills. *See* lama medicine
mantrayana. *See* vajrayana
Maori community, 63–64
marginalization. *See* acculturation styles
marriage, 19, 29, 32–33, 61, 159, 249
mass media, 5, 19, 20, 31, 54, 56, 74, 82, 234, 259
massage, 41, 43, 149, 156, 161, 164, 186–87, 206–7, 218
masturbation, 69, 71
medical institutions, 16, 28, 32, 39, 43, 46, 89, 90, 92–93, 96, 103, 141, 144, 145, 156, 166, 179, 185–88, 191, 193–96, 207, 212, 215, 218–21, 228–29, 231, 236, 244, 247–48. See *also* private sector in healthcare
medical jargon, 39
medical training. *See* education
Medicine Buddha (Sangye Menla), 146, 150, 155
meditation, 9, 44, 96, 101, 111, 130–31, 133–35, 136, 141, 156, 161, 201, 203, 209, 213–14, 233
men drub. *See* lama medicine
menstruation, 148, 260, 261
mental health, 17, 46, 50, 54–55, 59, 66, 68–69, 76, 78–79, 80, 83–84, 86–87, 89, 90, 94, 98–103, 110, 113–14, 124, 134, 142–43, 150, 152, 156, 158, 166–67, 188, 207, 217, 228, 241–42, 247, 249, 253–54; and religion, 98–104; problems in migrant population (*see* acculturative stress; depression & anxiety associated with acculturation; migration risk factors)
Men-Tsee-Khang. *See* Tibetan Medical and Astro Institute
meridian, 43, 92–93
merits, accumulation of, 118, 135–36, 199
methodology: data analysis, 177–80; grounded theory, 169–70, 238–39; theoretical sensitivity, 169–70; qualitative data, 170–77; qualitative research methodology, 167–69
Mexicans, 20, 48, 56, 59, 72
migration: typologies of, 12; phases of enforced migration, 16–17; risk factors, 16–18, 54–55; 62–63; results of (*see* acculturation)
Milarepa, 4, 159
mo. *See* divination
mo mo (Tibetan dumplings), 4, 33–34, 157, 218, 233
monasteries. *See* religious institutions
monks. *See* ordained individuals
moxibustion (applying moxa), 91, 93, 146, 153, 155, 161, 186, 194
mudra, 4, 187
multiculturalism. *See* acculturation styles
Muslims, 32, 75, 82, 145

nadis. *See* energy field and channels
naga. *See* serpent deities
nepas. *See* humours
nervios. 68, 72
ngakpa, 205. *See also* yogi
nirvana, 119, 128, 133. See *also* buddhahood
nunneries. *See* religious institutions
nuns. *See* ordained individuals
nurse, 39, 96, 164, 188, 195, 207, 218, 220–21, 230, 237, 242, 248, 259, 261
Nyigmapa. *See* sects in Tibetan Buddhism

obsessive religious thoughts, 96
operation. *See* surgery
ordained individuals, 5, 7, 14, 30, 33–34, 54, 73, 88, 92, 119–23, 139, 160, 186–87, 200–202, 209, 218–20, 225, 227, 233, 235, 247, 261

Padmasambhava. *See* Guru Rinpoche
pain killer, 193, 207, 211, 213, 231
Panchen Lama, 9, 122
paramitas (perfections), 133
patronage system, 29, 92, 119–20, 136, 139, 200, 222, 227, 233. See *also* sponsorships
penis, 69–71, 229, 248
pharmaceuticals, 144, 188, 192, 211–12, 215, 218–21, 228, 230–31, 237, 244. See *also* Tibetan herbal medicines; Western/allopathic medicines
pharmacology, 39, 41, 44–45, 146
pharmacy, 188, 193. See *also* dispensary
phlegm (bad kan). *See* humours in the Tibetan System Medicine
phurba, 187. *See also* ritual objects
pica, 73
pilgrimage, 27, 92, 137, 187, 200, 233
poison, 82, 149, 220; mental poisons, 125, 129, 150, 241; food poisoning, 210, 212, 229
Portuguese, 23–24
possession by spirits, 74, 76, 81, 83, 87, 95–96, 115, 119, 205, 223–27, 242, 247–48, 260
post traumatic stress disorder (PTSD), 18, 207
poverty, 17, 26, 30, 32, 70, 81, 88, 111–12, 142, 160, 200, 204, 218
prana, 43, 92
pranic healing, 187
prayer flags, 5, 28, 137–38, 187, 200, 233
prayer wheel, 31, 201, 203, 233
praying, 74–75, 82, 96–98, 101, 104, 109–11, 122, 137, 155, 159, 160, 187, 200–205, 209, 217, 229, 233
precious pills (rinchen rilbu), 154–55
predictive control. *See* religious coping effects
pregnancy, 32, 56–57, 61, 75, 81, 260
prejudice, 23, 28, 32–33, 49, 60–61, 66–67, 115, 249
pre-migratory expectations, 20, 22
prevention of disease, 144, 153, 244, 256, 259, 261
private sector in healthcare, 43, 46, 89, 185–87, 196, 211–12, 220, 244, 254. See *also* medical institutions
prostitution, 82, 248
prostrations, 122, 187
protector deities (or Dharma protectors), 119, 160, 199–200, 202, 227
protectors of Dharma, 199
psychiatry, 18, 42, 55, 57, 60, 68, 78, 83, 86, 95–96, 98–99, 101, 149, 167, 217, 228, 242, 247–48
psychoneuroimmunology (PNI), 97, 102
psychosis, 80, 81, 86, 115, 247
psychosomatics, 17, 45, 59, 97
psychotherapy, 44, 99
puja, 192, 197, 200, 203–4, 217, 222
pulse reading or testing, 146, 152, 186, 224. See *also* disease diagnosis and treatment in Tibetan System of Medicine
punishing God/deity reappraisal, 71, 95–96, 113, 223, 248, 251, 263
Pure Land of Amitabha (Opame). *See* Dewachen
purification (religious. of negative karma), 34, 134–35, 199–200, 203, 212, 222, 264
pyretic treatment, 155

racism, 60–62, 111
radio. *See* mass media
realms of existence, 119, 124–25, 133
rebirth, 117, 119, 124–25, 128, 131, 140, 198, 214, 223, 251
re-education campaign, xi, 122
reflexology, 43, 187
Refuge, taking or going for, 133–35, 202–3
refugees, 12–18, 25–27, 52, 58, 132, 137
Reiki, 43, 187, 206

reincarnation. *See* rebirth
relative truth. *See* truth in Buddhism
relaxation response, 98
religion: and meaning, 10–12, 26, 52, 54, 95, 97, 101, 105–7, 109, 115, 117, 134, 138, 198, 203, 222, 241–42, 245, 251, 263; as coping strategy (*see* religious coping); defining, 9–11; extrinsic (means), intrinsic (end), and quest dimensions, 98–100; latent functions of, 10, 120–21
religion and medicine: and general health, 1, 36–38, 90, 94–115, 241, 250–51; and health behavior, 101–3, 106, 109; ethics in medicine (*see* bioethics); faith or spiritual healing, 73, 89, 96–97, 102, 156, 187, 205, 248; pathogenic and pathoplastic function of religion, 113–15. See *also* mental health and religion
religious activities. *See* circumambulating holy places; mantra; meditation; pilgrimage; prayer flags; praying; prostration; sang (smoke offering) ritual; stupa
religious coping, 10–11, 26, 94–95, 98–99, 102–13, 117, 132–34, 138, 187, 195–202, 203–4, 209, 222–23, 227–28, 235, 250–51, 263–64; effects of, 105; predictors of, 110–13; RCOPE, 107, 202, 263–64; styles, 106–7, 113–14
religious institutions, 8, 14, 27, 53, 103, 119–23, 136–40, 166, 186–87, 200, 202–3, 218, 233
religious language, 97. See *also* mantras
religious offerings, 4, 82, 88, 136–38, 187, 196, 199–200, 202, 206, 209, 223, 227, 233. See *also* butter lamps; merits; prayer flags
religious symbols, 4–5, 10, 96–97, 133, 136, 149, 187, 203, 206, 239, 249, 251
renouncing, 135, 203
rinpoche, 9, 34, 197, 200, 202–3, 206, 225, 227
ritual objects, 97, 187, 205

Sakyapa. *See* sects in Tibetan Buddhism
samsara. *See* cyclic existence
sang (smoke offering) ritual, 137–38, 200, 233, 239
Sangha, 103, 133, 136
sects in Tibetan Buddhism, 120, 192
self-directing coping style. *See* religious coping styles
semen, 68–69, 76–77
separation. *See* acculturation styles
serpent deities (nagas), 9, 88, 158, 199, 217, 223, 229, 242, 248
severity of symptoms. *See* course of sickness
sexual activity and herbal medicines, 146, 155
sexuality: as taboo, 32, 208, 260–61; homosexuality, 96, 114, 260–61; in Asian populations, 32, 67–71, 260; of ordained individuals, 247; risky sexual behaviors, 102; sexual abuse, 18, 129; sexual awareness, 57, 69, 236–37, 259–61
sexually transmitted diseases, 57, 82, 229
shamanism, 83, 96, 115, 118, 145, 185, 187, 190, 205–6, 235, 239, 243, 249
shiatsu massage, 187
shine. *See* calm-abiding meditation
shrinking penis syndrome (koro). *See* genitalia loss
significants, 104–6
sinbyong in Korea, 115
skin diseases, 44, 143, 152, 210, 224–25, 237–38, 248, 253
smoking, 44, 47, 55–57, 81, 102–3, 202
social phobia (azmat zibur) in Jewish culture, 74–75
somatization, 77, 75–76, 87, 90–91, 207, 245, 247, 254

sorcery. *See* witchcraft; magic
soul, 37–38, 41, 43, 68, 71, 78, 83, 117
Southeast Asians, 25, 47, 56
space. *See* elements
spirits, 78, 81–82, 88, 96–97, 119, 146, 149, 152, 157–58, 160, 199, 205, 217, 222–26, 243, 260
sponsorships, 29–32, 234. See *also* patronage system
steroids, 44
stigmatization: associated with mental problems, 76, 89, 247; of minority groups, 61
stupa, 138, 200, 233, 239
suffering in Buddhist teaching, 124–32
suicidal: behavior, 60, 65, 86, 101; ideation, 17, 88
superior vision meditation, 156
supernatural: beings, 9–10, 71, 83; causation (*see* etiology of illness/disease). See *also* spirits, idiom of
surgery, 48, 109, 153, 155–56, 188, 196, 218
survivor's guilt, 18
susto, 68, 71–72, 76. See *also* culture bound syndromes
sutra, 34, 127, 140, 146

taijin kyofusho in Japan, 74. See *also* culture bound syndromes
tantra, 120, 140–41, 146, 159, 162; Medical Tantra, 146–47, 154, 158, 161; tantric power, 97, 187, 190, 205–6, 249; tantric practices, 34, 118
tantrayana. *See* vajrayana
technocratic model of medicine. *See* biomedicine
television. *See* mass media
Tenjur, 117, 140
Thanka (Tibetan painting), 8, 156, 218, 133
Three Jewels, 133, 136, 149, 203. See *also* Buddha; Dharma; Sangha
thugpa, 4, 34, 233
Tibetan Centre for Human Rights and Democracy (TCHRD), 17, 117, 122–23, 140
Tibetan herbal medicines, 72, 89, 153–54, 186, 191–95, 211–17, 219–22, 230–32, 237, 242–44, 250, 256. See *also* lama medicine
Tibetan Medical and Astro Institute, 144, 156, 166, 186, 194–95, 212, 216, 219, 244, 254–56
Tibetan System of Medicine, 46, 89, 144, 145, 147–62, 185–86, 216, 220–21, 236–38, 244, 255–57; history of, 145–47. See *also* disease diagnosis and treatment in Tibetan System of Medicine; Tibetan herbal medicines
tigle (energy drops), 76–77
Ting Moong (dummy personality), 18
TMAI. *See* Tibetan Medical and Astro Institute
tobacco chewing, 57
tong len (giving and taking meditation), 134, 156, 198
torture, 16, 18, 121, 143, 228, 257. See *also* Chinese repression
Torture Survivor Program, 144–45, 188, 257
trance, 45, 115, 205
trauma, 16–18, 26, 55, 68, 72, 87, 90, 112, 132, 146, 165–66, 207, 228, 253
trichotillomania, 73
truth in Buddhism, 127, 123–32
tsampa, 4, 34, 138, 206, 233, 239
tuberculosis, 32, 140, 143–44, 188, 210, 215, 229
tulku, 120, 140

United Nations High Commissioner for Refugees (UNHCR), 13–16

vajrayana, 118, 156, 158, 162, 187. See *also* Wheel of Dharma

Vayrasattva. *See* Dorje Sempa
vegetarianism, 33, 96, 142–43
vicarious control. *See* religious coping effects
Vietnamese, 24–25, 47, 56, 70, 87
virus, 38, 107
vows, 34, 203, 215

water. *See* elements
Western/allopathic medicines, 89, 188, 192–93, 195, 211–16, 218, 228, 230–31, 236–37, 244
Western medicine. *See* biomedicine
wheel of cyclic existence. *See* cyclic existence
Wheel of Dharma, 123, 146, 161–62
wind (rLung). *See* elements; humours in the Tibetan System Medicine
witchcraft, 78–79, 83, 242. See *also* black magic

x-ray, 195, 219, 248

yoga, 93, 159
yogi, 4, 8, 137, 156, 159, 187, 205, 217, 227